trim
healthy
mama
cookbook

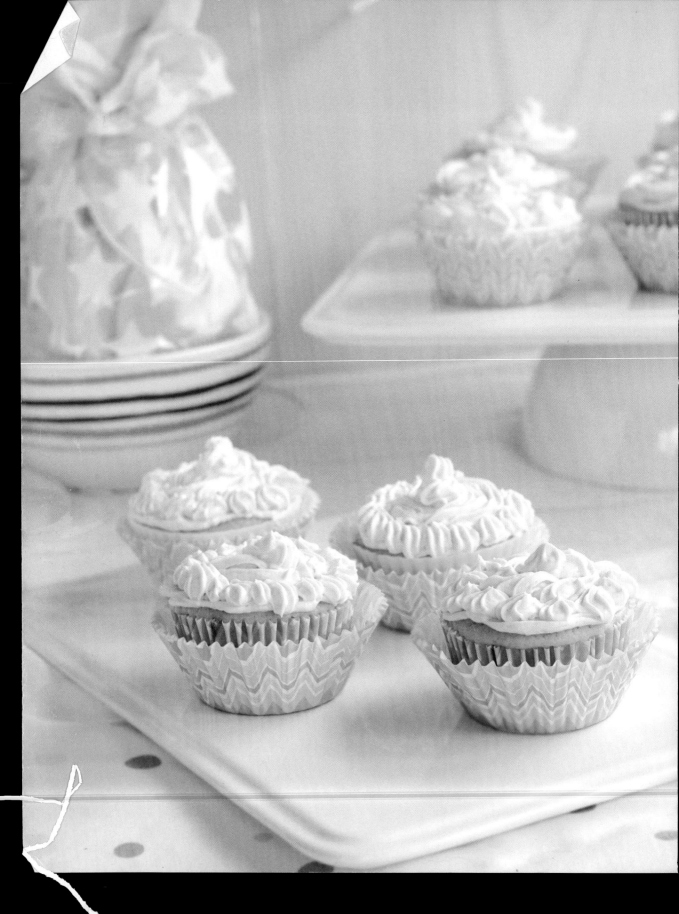

trim
healthy
mama
cookbook

EAT UP AND SLIM DOWN WITH
MORE THAN 350 HEALTHY RECIPES

Pearl Barrett and Serene Allison

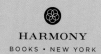

HARMONY
BOOKS · NEW YORK

Published in the United States by Harmony Books, an imprint of the
Crown Publishing Group, a division of Penguin Random House LLC, New York.
www.crownpublishing.com

Harmony Books is a registered trademark, and the Circle colophon
is a trademark of Penguin Random House LLC.

Library of Congress Cataloging-in-Publication Data
Barrett, Pearl.
Trim healthy mama cookbook / Pearl Barrett and Serene Allison.
pages   cm
1. Reducing diets—Recipes. I. Allison, Serene. II. Title.
RM222.2.B3847   2015
641.5'635—dc23   2015022057

ISBN 978-1-101-90266-0
eBook ISBN 978-1-101-90267-7

Printed in the United States of America

Photographs by Rohnda Monroy (Rohnda's blog can be found at rohndasue.com)
Cover photographs by David Bean/Visual Reserve

10 9 8 7 6 5 4 3 2 1

First Edition

To all our Trim Healthy Mama Sisters around the globe . . . this one is for you! You spread the word and turned this thing into a movement. How could we not give you what you were asking for? Here's your big ol' book full of recipes with the pictures you asked us for. Enjoy. We hope it helps keeps you and your family well-fed, happy, and satisfied for years to come.

A special shout-out to Rohnda Monroy, who took all the recipe photographs for this book and went above and beyond what we asked for. She never considered herself a professional photographer, just a Mama at home who loved taking pictures of her Trim Healthy Mama food, but we sensed something special in her pictures. She not only made all the recipes, then took the beautiful pictures of them, but also gave us lots of feedback on whether she and her family loved the recipe or whether it still needed some work. Rohnda is an incredible cook, so getting a thumbs-up from her was a big deal for us.

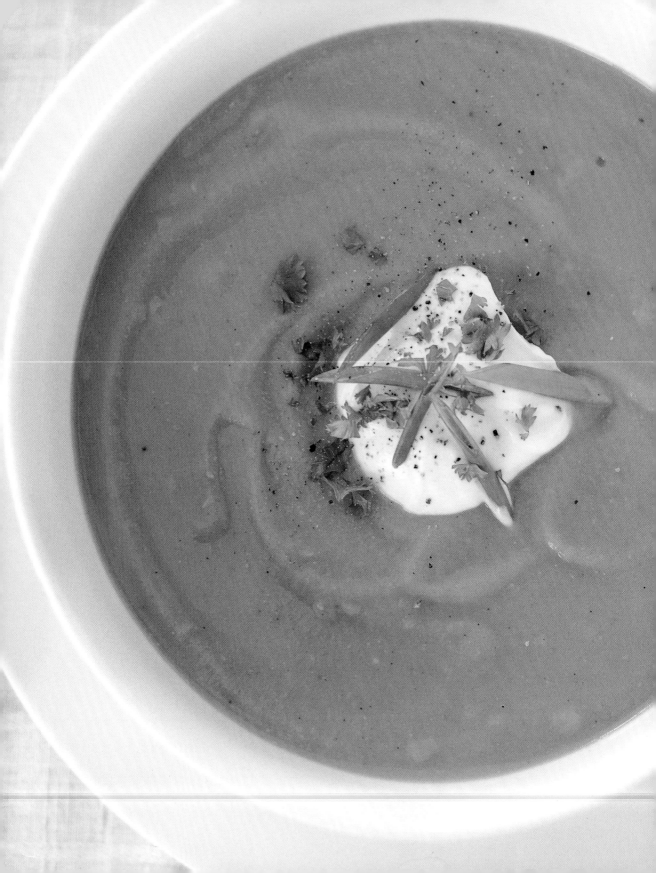

contents

SWEET TREATS

BEVERAGES

ALL THINGS SMOOTH AND CRUNCHY

introduction
LET'S EAT!

Get ready to feast on foods that are both delicious and trimming! It's time to mesh these two food worlds that seldom meet. Mouthwatering and waist whittling—can the two ever really go together?

Yes, beyond your wildest dreams!

You won't find Spartan diet foods in these pages. Food Freedom is our mantra, so now it's time to get practical and stick our forks into the succulent pie!

If you want cake for breakfast, then by golly, you shall have it! Why not, when Trim Healthy Mama sweet treats are brimming with health benefits and packed with protein, and won't spike your blood sugar. Rather dig into a hearty sausage and egg breakfast? If that is what Mama wants, that is what Mama gets!

You want quick and easy? We hear ya, so do we. Most of our breakfasts and lunches take only 5 to 10 minutes to make (some are quicker than that). Dinners don't have to be laborious, either: enjoy our no-fuss, save-your-sanity crockpot meals or quicky-quick one-pot skillet dishes. Or, pull a steaming, traditional meatloaf or tasty lasagna out of the oven and watch your family's eyes light up. If you are a foodie and want a bit of a culinary adventure, we've got some recipes here for you, too. One of us has a purist, foodie brain, while the other is mostly concerned with shortcuts to get 'er done. You get the best of both worlds.

SERVING SIZES AND PORTIONS

The Food Freedom mantra of Trim Healthy Mama (THM) means we don't dictate your every bite or tell you exactly when you should feel full. You will not see any suggested serving sizes indicating you must eat only one sliver of cake or only one baked chicken leg. You're going to be the boss of you. If we tell you exactly how much of each recipe you may or may not eat, that's our decision, not yours—our eating plan, not yours. We want you to learn that you—not us—are the key to your lifelong success. We are *all* so unique. A hungry nursing mama running around after multiple children all day and a postmenopausal computer technician sitting at her desk all day are going to want and need different serving sizes.

But, of course, you want to know how much a recipe makes so you don't go wasting ingredients. Most of the recipes in this book are divided into three groups:

Single Serve – A generous one-person meal, dessert, side, snack, or drink.

Family Serve – Enough food to feed a large family (of 6–8 people). If your family is smaller (or you are single), you will simply halve or quarter the ingredients—or better yet, make the full meal and then freeze the leftovers for other "no-think" meals.

Multiple Serve – This category is used for recipes like sauces, crackers, cookies, and the like. You won't see us saying "Eat only one cookie" or "Use only 1 tablespoon of dressing or gravy." You'll use your discretion and common sense.

You're going to learn how to tune in to your own hunger and full signals. That won't happen perfectly at first; it takes time. You might find some of your favorite recipes in the book and eat too much of them in the beginning weeks or months. Or, perhaps it will take some time to ditch a "dieting" mindset and you will eat too little. Give yourself some grace. The signals of hunger and of feeling full will become clearer to you the longer you are on plan, and as your blood sugar and insulin levels balance.

You'll notice we sometimes suggest 3 to 6 ounces of chicken, beef, or salmon to top a salad or to put in your single size soup. That is only a suggestion; some of us may need (or want) only 4 ounces of meat on our salad, while others might want or need 8 or 9 ounces—or more. If your guy is on plan with you, you sure don't want to limit him to tiny portions! We have made some suggestions here, simply because they are generally the amounts we personally eat, but you can overrule them. This is not a numbers game, where you have to feel constantly restricted by ounce amounts or calorie counts. (The exception to this is if you are actually setting out to have a Fuel Pull meal, which is described in the Appendix—that is the only time we put a limit on protein portions.)

KNOW THE PLAN

A big welcome back to all our Mama peeps! Our Trim Healthy Mama "lifers" by now can probably explain the Trim Healthy Mama principles better than we can. It's so fun to be here with you again. You've been on our minds and in our hearts as we created each recipe. Your insistence that we do a separate recipe book is why this big ol' chunky book is sitting on your lap now.

If you're new to the Trim Healthy Mama plan, a huge Hi! to you. Welcome to the THM sisterhood; you're going to rock this! The recipes in this book will only be truly understood and work in your trimming favor if you understand the concepts behind Trim Healthy Mama. While the food lists for each meal type are summarized in lists at the back of this book ("The Meal Recap") for your convenience, this lifestyle cannot be lived from a bunch of lists—ugh! You need to understand the "whys" and the spirit behind this plan. It sure won't happen by committing to memory a list of do's and don'ts.

The companion book *Trim Healthy Mama Plan* will get you started on the right track. It's not a hard read; we have a lot of fun in those pages as we walk you through the basics. If your

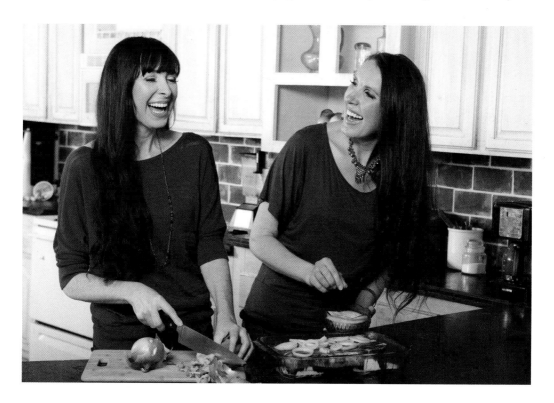

budget is tight, borrow it from the library or a friend (if she'll part with it). It will help you understand the principles, and then hold your hand as you begin practicing the lifestyle (with lots of mess-ups along the way, of course—don't expect perfection from yourself). As much as we said we don't want to dictate your portion sizes and that you must make your own decisions, there are some basic principles that are crucial for this way of eating to work in your favor. We don't get all bogged down with numbers, but we do heed safe blood sugar–fuel boundaries. These are not diet prison bars; they are safe picket fences that keep you in trim and healthy pastureland.

True understanding of the plan will be your path to victory. As we mentioned, you won't count calories, but you won't abuse them, either—and that beautiful balance will only come from juggling your food fuels in what we call "freestyling." The **S** (Satisfying), **E** (Energizing), and **FP** (Fuel Pull) recipes in this book will begin to make sense as you practice this freestyling by eating both fats and carbs (always anchored by protein), but not always in the same meals. You'll change your meals every day and every week according to your needs, wants, and unique "life happens" challenges. Pregnant and nursing Mamas and those at goal weight will sometimes merge **S** and **E** fuels into what we call "Crossovers." (You can read about those in more detail in the *Trim Healthy Mama Plan,* or look at the quick reference Appendix at the back of this book.)

DESSERT FOR BREAKFAST

You'll notice that the recipes in this book have not been categorized into breakfast, lunch, and dinner, with dessert tacked on at the end. We don't even have a desserts chapter, so don't go looking for it. Is it because we left out desserts? No way! You almost made us spit out our Good Girl Moonshine (page 397) with that question! It's because desserts can be eaten for breakfast, lunch, or dinner, if desired. Of course, you'll eat a lot of greens, fruits, certain grains, and nourishing proteins, too. Balance is the key to this lifestyle, but freedom is the delight of it!

TOOLS FOR YOUR KITCHEN

You don't need to go to a whole bunch of expense to set up your Trim Healthy kitchen. You probably have all the gadgets you need already, like baking dishes, cookie sheets, a griddle, a large soup pot, a big and a little skillet, and, of course, the basics like knives and so on. Don't think you have to go to an expensive specialty store and purchase only the best. Most of our knives can barely slice cheese, but we make them work. There are some gadgets sitting on your counter now that you will probably be able to just pack away. We keep it simple.

Do make room for the big three: a blender, a food processor, and a crockpot. Each deserves a little chat. Leave these out on your counter. If you have to put your blender away after every time you use it, and then drag it out again, that will become way too much work—and you may want to go take a nap instead of making yourself a treat.

BLENDER – Truth is, for years we used cheapo blenders that took a lot of cajoling, so if you don't have the bucks for a high-end blender, don't for a moment think you can't blend your way to Trim. Most of our trademark drinks (yes, even the Fat-Stripping Frappas, page 418) were invented with a cheapo $20 blender. That's not saying we didn't have to do some dangerous tricks, like stabbing a wooden spoon into the blender while it was running to help break up the ice, but we also wore our son's motor cross goggles for protection while doing it! We sure don't recommend you do the same such tricks, though. A sweet Trim Healthy Mama gifted us each a Blend Tech right after we released our first self-published book three years ago. We've been enjoying blending with those machines ever since, no goggles or wooden spoons needed. Still, you don't have to fork out hundreds of dollars for a high-end blender like a Blend Tech or a Vitamix (although we love 'em). There are middle-of-the-road blenders (like the Ninja) that make many a Mama perfectly happy.

A blender is a Trim Healthy Mama's best friend, so do put your dream blender on your Christmas and birthday list and accidentally let the list fall out of your purse next to your wealthy aunt (or, if you don't have a wealthy aunt, perhaps ten or fifteen poor relatives could get the job done).

NOTE

We do use hot (not boiling) liquids in some of our blended recipes, so please follow your manufacturer's directions for safety with hot liquids. We periodically vent for safety and/or hold our hands tightly over the lid to help it stay sealed. It is best not to use those tiny one-serving blenders when using hot liquids, as there is not enough room for the steam to rise and the container may burst. Stick blenders can come in handy for hot drinks.

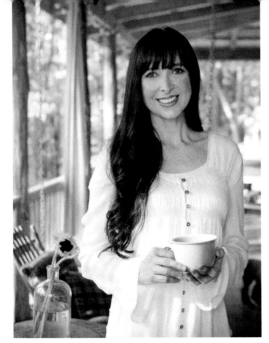
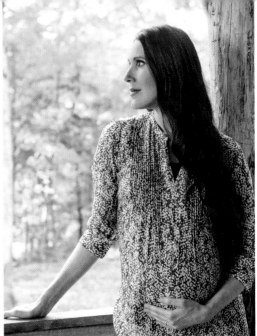

FOOD PROCESSOR – We have had no better luck with high-end processors than with cheapo ones. In fact, we are always on the lookout for a good five-buck garage-sale food processor score. Don't spend an arm and a leg for yours; any old one should do the job.

CROCKPOT – Again, oldies are sometimes goodies here, and garage sales can be a huge help for finding a crockpot or two. Even if you find one the color of seventies green shag carpet, don't pass it by; it will still make awesome lentil soup. Actually, some of the new fancy-schmancy crocks cook at too high a temperature. You want a cooker with a removable ceramic insert that heats all the way around, not just on the bottom. If you do have a big family, that would be one reason to shed some dollars for the largest cooker you can find; you could take a swim in Serene's giant crockpot.

We hate calling the above three "must haves," but if you don't have one of them, you might find yourself a tad frustrated. And trust us: investing in these "helpers" will save you time, money, and stress later!

We do have two more items to mention that are not as crucial but are useful little gadgets and are also easy on your budget.

TROODLE – This fun tool (or toy) gives you noodles with just a simple zucchini and a couple of minutes. We call it the Troodle because your noodles will be trimming instead of fattening. What a happy thought! You can find it on our website, www.trimhealthy mama.com. There are other spiral cutters available from online sources, if you think we're being shamelessly salesy about our own products, or you can find it at the occasional store if you're lucky.

COFFEE GRINDER – You'll be good to go with a separate grinder instead of using one you might have for actually grinding coffee (although not all of us grind our own coffee, Serene! There is such a thing as a shiny packet of Dunkin' Donuts pre-ground coffee!). Trust us; if you are using one coffee grinder for dual purposes, bad things can happen. Sleepy Mamas who wake up to discover they have oats or some Super Sweet Blend jammed around their coffee blades and need to spend ten minutes doing a deep clean before any coffee ever touches their lips might want to throw such coffee grinder out the window. Do yourself a favor and get a second one. You may sometimes have to grind small amounts of oats or sweeteners, and those amounts won't be large enough to spin properly in a blender. Thrift stores are the best places to get awesome coffee grinders for just a couple of bucks, but they are reasonably inexpensive in stores like Walmart and Target.

STOCK YOUR KITCHEN

We cannot give you a set grocery list because your food preferences will be vastly different from the next woman (or guy). Even our own cupboards and fridges don't look all matchy-matchy. Serene is the purist, while Pearl is 63.9 percent Drive Thru Sue (self-diagnosed). Even though we are united on the core principles of the plan, we live them out differently.

Purists (like Serene) seldom veer from using only pure foods, with nary a tiny toxin to be seen. Drive Thru Sue's (like Pearl) use some slightly imperfect store-bought items now and then to make this thing doable—like a low-carb wrap. (Gasp!) Or, some fat-free Reddi-wip. (Gulp!) Those items that we officially term "personal choice" (but Serene calls "Frankenfoods") are not mainstays. They simply make it easier so we don't set ourselves up for failure by having to prepare everything from scratch and then give up because of all the time it takes. The all-or-nothing approach will only make you miserable—and derail your efforts. We don't want you to get caught up in that mindset. Life happens, and you don't have to be perfect. But if being absolutely perfect with all your food choices makes you happy, then more power to ya!

There are some staple ingredients all of us will share, like berries, fruits, leafy greens, nonstarchy veggies, eggs, dairy, and meat (although if you have food intolerances, we've got plenty of wonderful substitutes for you). Fresh leafy greens will always be in your grocery cart, but frozen veggies are biggies on the Trim Healthy Mama plan, too. Don't look down on them as less superior to fresh veggies—they are inexpensive, picked at the height of freshness, and often easier and quicker to cook because they require less prep. Canned veggies and beans can also be your BFF. Many stores are now carrying BPA (bisphenol A)-free cans, and we encourage you to choose them over regular when possible. BPA is a synthetic estrogen and a known hormone disrupter that hampers the body's natural hormone balance, which is responsible for metabolism and reproduction.

NO SPECIAL INGREDIENTS?

You can do Trim Healthy Mama with basic ingredients from any grocery store. If you want to stick to only everyday foods, look for "NSI" on our recipes. This means you won't need any special ingredients to whip it up. But even if you do see a recipe with a specialty ingredient or two, don't gloss over it, deciding you'll never make it. Most of the time you can substitute other "easy to find" ingredients for the more special ones called for, simply by reading our tips in the "Special Mention Foods" list that follows.

You certainly don't have to buy our products to see success on the plan. We use these ingredients in some recipes because we have sourced the most pure and effective versions and have discovered they give the best results in our recipes. But there are many ways to skin a cat (what a weird saying!). If you find similar products you can access easier, use them with our blessing (or should we say, partial blessing). Full blessing goes to our products (kidding . . . kinda). In all seriousness, diet plans that make their own brand of ingredients mandatory are repulsive to us, and that's not what is going on here. We want you to have successful recipe outcomes, but we also want what is easiest and most doable for you—and what can work within your budget, no matter how tight. Our greatest desire is for you to feel that you can do this, that it is not something too hard to keep up for life. For some, that means enjoying playing with a whole bunch of fun special ingredients; for others, it means sticking to everyday foods and ignoring the special stuff. So, yep, you're going to see some ingredients listed that you may have never heard of before. Don't throw your hands up defeated—there are ways around them.

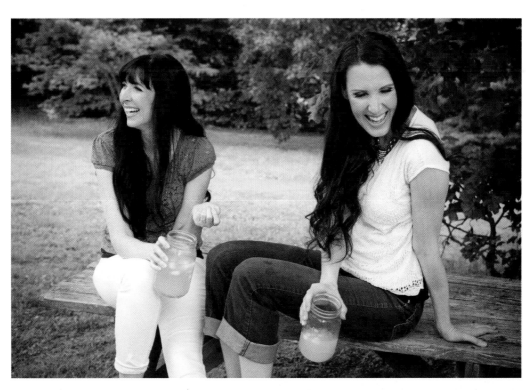

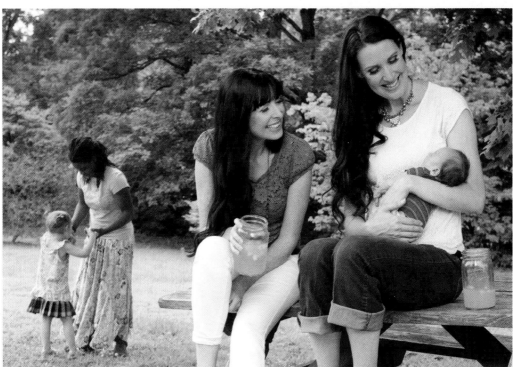

SPECIAL MENTION FOODS

OKRA – Every good little Trim Healthy Mama will have a few bags of frozen okra in her freezer. Now, before you say "yuck" or "gross" or "what have I gotten myself into?" we're not going to make you sit down to a bowl of okra, for goodness sakes! Okra has powerful blood sugar–regulating, gut-healing, and slimming powers. You have our word: you will not be slimed out or grossified by any of our recipes that contain okra. Try our Cry-No-More Brownies (page 314) if you don't believe us. Buy frozen whole okra and frozen diced okra, as they have different uses in the recipes. Thankfully, frozen okra is an extremely affordable veggie. Note: We recommend that you keep your okra use a secret from picky children. We have adamant okra haters in our families, who remain blissfully unaware they are frequently eating it. In fact, they beg for seconds—or thirds—and we just smile and say, "Sure, honey!"

RADISHES – Since radishes lose all their bitter bite once they are cooked, they are fabulous potato replacements. In fact, they look like little red potatoes while cooking. Radishes are in the category of the lowest calorie but highest nutrient-dense veggies, right up there with our beloved okra. They can soothe the digestion, come to the rescue for constipation, help fight cancer, cleanse the liver, aid the gall bladder, fight infections, regulate the metabolism, assist with weight loss—and the list goes on from here. You'll buy them fresh. And another fist pump is in order, because they are blessedly cheap. You can buy the little 4-ounce bags of matchstick-cut radishes for hash brown replacements with eggs for breakfast, or the 1-pound bags of whole radishes to throw into pot roasts or soups, or roast as a side item for dinner with butter or coconut oil. You can also grow a bunch of radishes in your garden—if you are the gardening type.

CAULIFLOWER – What a versatile vegetable this is. Frozen cauliflower florets are often cheaper and easier than a head of fresh, but go with your own preference. We keep a stash of frozen bags in our freezer to make mashed-potato and rice replacements (there are recipes for those on pages 219 and 225). You'll also want to try Fooled Ya Pizza (page 214). Talk about a yummy way to get healthy veggies into your family while they happily eat piece after piece. Cauliflower is divine when roasted with seasonings and butter, or steamed and topped with goodies like butter, Mineral Salt, and grated cheese. Here's a cool piece of news: a large frozen foods brand has just come out with pre-crumbled cauliflower. You can now find bags of these cauliflower crumbles in the frozen vegetables section of many grocery stores. This heralded "Hooray!" from thousands of Drive Thru Sue–minded Trim Healthy Mamas who now have one less prep step when they make pizza or rice with cauliflower. (Thanks for tuning in to the needs of the THM community, Green Giant—love you for this!)

ZUCCHINI – It makes fabulous noodles! The easy recipe for Troodles (trim noodles) can be found on page 222. It's also the reason for the wonderfully moist texture of the Trimtastic Chocolate Zucchini Cake on page 296. Buy it fresh or grow lots of it in your garden.

SEASONING BLEND – This stuff can save you hours of prep work. It is simply an inexpensive frozen blend of finely diced onion, celery, and green pepper. We call for it in many of the fussless crockpot, soup, and skillet recipes. But don't stress out if you cannot find it in the frozen veggies case of your grocery store. It is not a mandatory ingredient; you can always dice up an onion, but do keep an eye out for it, then buy up big if you see it (Walmart carries it).

BERRIES – Buying frozen berries rather than fresh will save you money. We throw frozen berries into smoothies, shakes, whips, and ice cream. However, in the summer there's nothing better than chowing down on some fresh berries. Watch for sales, or take a fun family trip to a berry field in your area and get picking.

MINERAL SALT – Whenever we call for salt in a recipe, that is what you'll read. High-mineral salt is helpful rather than harmful to your body. You can read about all of its health benefits in the "Specialty Food Stars" chapter of *Trim Healthy Mama Plan*. You'll know if your salt contains a high mineral content by its color: regular table salt is white, which means it has been refined and depleted of its minerals. Salt containing lots of minerals is either gray (from the sea) or pink (from deep within the earth) and is unrefined. Our Trim Healthy brand of salt (available at www.trimhealthymama.com) is a beautiful, rich pink color and has the highest mineral content available. Playing with it in recipes brings us lots of happiness from the sheer prettiness of its color. We even put small amounts of it in desserts! It has a lot of salty strength, so you may find you need less salt than you normally would; it is finely ground so it can work in any recipe. Additionally, you can find other forms of mineral-rich salt at health food stores, from online distributors, or sometimes in the natural food aisles of certain grocery stores. Look for rich color—then you know you have something special. But, hey, if you can't locate Mineral Salt, don't throw in the towel. This is not a deal breaker. You can still do the plan using any old salt from your local grocery store.

COCOA POWDER – You'll see a lot of our recipes call for unsweetened cocoa powder because—well, don't ya dare pull chocolate from a Mama's life, right? It must always be in its unsweetened version, though (don't buy pre-sweetened cocoa). Purists (like Serene) may want to stick to the natural version, rather than Dutch-processed, because the original is higher in antioxidants, but if you like special dark cocoa, that's fine, too.

EXTRACTS – We use a lot of them to bring varied flavors to our treats. Whenever possible, choose "pure" versions of vanilla, orange, peppermint, and almond. Many pure extracts can be found at any grocery store, so buy up. Pure versions of extracts like banana and caramel are a little harder to find at regular grocery stores, but they are available at natural food stores or from online distributors. Purists will, of course, want to stick to pure versions of all extracts, while our Drive Thru Sue's may not care so much if the banana extract is not quite up to snuff. Nobody's going to judge. Do your best and baby-step the rest.

ALUMINUM-FREE BAKING POWDER – You'll notice we call for aluminum-free baking powder in all our recipes. It's not an expensive item, so it's an easy fix. We don't like to condemn a bunch of foods or fantasize that almost any packaged item will kill us, but when you can find the aluminum-free version right next to the regular stuff, why not choose it? It's a no-brainer—you don't want to serve aluminum with your cake. But again, this is not a deal breaker; if you really like your regular baking powder, use the stuff you prefer.

TRIM HEALTHY MAMA BAKING BLEND – We worked for months, with much trial and error, to put together the flours that would make the best all-purpose baking flour: gluten free, superfood rich, not too calorie heavy, kind to blood sugar. My, oh my, do we have some fabulous recipes with it! But you can absolutely do the plan without using our baking blend (we did for years). Thankfully, most grocery stores (including Walmart and Target) carry brands of golden flaxseed meal, coconut flour, and almond flour. Golden flaxseed meal and coconut flour are very affordable; almond flour is not as affordable, but at least it is readily available. We made sure to include wonderful baked recipes using those flours in this book, so you don't have to buy our products online, if that freaks you out or does not fit into your budget.

Oat fiber is another great low-glycemic baking flour and is super-inexpensive. Mix that with a few of the other baking flours, and experiment with your own baking blend as an alternative. Your own flour blend may not be perfectly Fuel Pullish, as our blend is, but **S** treats are completely fine on the plan. Almond flour is welcome, and you can make some lovely baked goods, but be careful about overdoing it—it is very calorie dense. Remember, while we are not afraid of calories, we don't abuse them, either. Blending almond flour with lighter flours like coconut flour will be a great idea if you plan to use it a lot.

ON-PLAN SWEETENERS – We all have different tastes when it comes to how sweet we like things. For this reason, we offer alternative sweetening options, and you'll soon figure out which ones suit you best. If you are in weight-loss mode on Trim Healthy Mama, you will be primarily sweetening with stevia-based sweeteners. Once you get closer to your goal weight, you can bring a little more raw honey (or coconut sugar) back into your life along with stevia. It is true that stevia can taste disgustingly bitter, but once you figure out what type to use, how to use it, and then give your taste buds time to adjust, you'll never want to go back to sugar. Sounds crazy right now, but we predict you'll come to love it!

Pure Stevia Extract: This is the most budget-friendly option of all our natural sweeteners. It is several hundred times sweeter than sugar, so when you sweeten with it, you "doonk." (That's our made-up name for the action of putting a tiny $1/32$ of a teaspoon amount into your treat. Check out our free video on our website or YouTube on how to "doonk.") One little pouch of stevia extract can last you a few months, and it tastes fabulous in tea, in all our All-Day Sipper drinks (pages 396–406) and in berry- or fruit-flavored smoothies or whips. But it's more difficult to bake with stevia extract, so here's where two other sweeteners can come to your aid.

Gentle Sweet: This is a blend of stevia, erythritol, and xylitol (the latter two are sugar alcohols that have negligible impact on your blood sugar and actually have some health benefits). Gentle Sweet tastes most like sugar; it also produces fantastic baking results. If you are new to plan and have not yet developed a taste for stevia, Gentle Sweet can be your lifeboat to navigate those first few weeks of sugar detox and withdrawal. It is still about twice as sweet

> **NOTE**
>
> Gentle Sweet (or any other blend containing xylitol) can be harmful to dogs—even fatal if they consume too much. So keep any treats you make with it away from your doggy friends. (Dogs are also intolerant to chocolate, so be careful with that, too.) If you're worried about it, use the Super Sweet Blend option or straight erythritol.

as sugar, so don't go throwing cupfuls of it in your treats. You'll use teaspoon-size amounts; the most you'll ever use will be ¾ cup in a large batch of brownies or in a cake. Many people like the taste of xylitol alone, and buy bagful after bagful of it, but we see some problems with that. It has calories that can add up through overuse, and because it is not very sweet by itself, you need to use a lot to get anything sweet enough. Yet using too much can cause some gas or even diarrhea for certain people, and we don't want to take the blame for your becoming known as the Tooting Mama. Mixing it as we do with stevia and erythritol makes most of these problems disappear. Gentle Sweet is also ground finely, so you don't have to bother grinding it for recipes such as Skinny Chocolate (page 377) when you want a smooth taste and mouth feel.

Super Sweet Blend: This is your most budget-friendly blend. It is at least four times sweeter than sugar, and since it does not contain xylitol, you don't have to worry about your dog stealing the treats cooling on your counter. Super Sweet Blend shines with a clean, smooth taste, but it won't be as forgiving if you throw too much into a recipe. There are tens of thousands of Mamas who love it in all their baked goods, but they have learned that less

DON'T WANT TO USE OUR SWEETENERS?

That's fine (our fingers had trouble typing that). Many grocery stores now carry stevia-based sweeteners, and you can probably find one locally that suits your needs. You'll need to be savvy about what you purchase, though, as many stevia brands have started to flood the market, and too many of them contain low-grade stevia extracts with added ingredients; those won't do your blood sugar, health, or waistline any favors. You can use any pure stevia or stevia blend with erythritol, xylitol, monk fruit extract, or chicory root, but please avoid the following fillers: sugar, dextrose, fructose, maltodextrin, agave.

We encourage you to seek non-GMO sources and to use brands that do not contain "natural flavors," which is sometimes code for MSG. There is no good reason to put "natural flavors" in stevia, which is already naturally sweet. But the GMO/MSG thing is a personal choice, not a commandment, so don't get hung up on it. If you're the type who doesn't have much of a sweet tooth, and will very rarely make a sweet treat or drink, then enjoying the rare sweetened treat with raw honey or coconut sugar will be your unique approach; so long as that doesn't happen too frequently, it should not hinder your trimming progress. Fresh fruit is on plan and is naturally sweet, so you won't feel deprived.

is more. You'll only use 1 or 2 teaspoons in a smoothie, or ¼ cup at the very most in a large batch of 12 muffins.

You'll notice most of the time, when we list sweeteners in a recipe, we will call for either Super Sweet Blend or Pure Stevia Extract. This is because they'll be the easiest on your budget and will last you the longest. But if you can't seem to make them work for your tastes, just use Gentle Sweet and double the amounts that would be used for Super Sweet Blend. If we do call for Gentle Sweet as the only sweetener, then know that this will give you the best results—that we've tried it both ways. If you are worried about the xylitol in Gentle Sweet because of canine family members, simply add 1½ bags of erythritol to a bag of Super Sweet Blend, and that will give you a blend about the same strength of sweetness as Gentle Sweet. Put this in a container and use it whenever Gentle Sweet is called for, using the same amounts.

COCONUT OIL AND MCT OIL – Just a few years ago it was difficult to find extra-virgin coconut oil in grocery stores, now lucky for you, it is everywhere—even budget stores like Aldi carry it! Brimming with health benefits, it is a staple on our plan. If you detest the taste of coconut oil, though, you can find tasteless versions. They don't carry all the same health benefits, but they still provide middle-chain fatty acids, which are helpful for your weight-loss goals. Louanna is a brand that many coconut-taste-despising Mamas use to sauté their meats and veggies or put into their Skinny Chocolate (page 377). We enjoy using coconut oil spray for baking and sometimes for light sautéing—there are even purist-approved versions of this available without any soy lecithin.

MCT oil is like coconut oil on steroids when it comes to firing up your metabolism and protecting your brain from diseases such as Alzheimer's. It is not found in stores (it is found on our website—shameless plug), but don't fret because it is absolutely not a crucial ingredient for you to have on the plan. Since it is tasteless, we love it in our Trimmaccinos (pages 427–433), poured over our salads, and in other treats when a coconut taste is not desired. If you're the "no special ingredients" type, you can stick to simple cream or half-and-half in your coffee, and we'll still be super proud of you.

JUST GELATIN – You'll see this ingredient called for in many of our recipes. This refers to the traditional unsweetened powdered gelatin that turns a liquid into a gel. Perhaps you only thought of it as something used to make a jiggly red dessert, but we have so many other wonderful uses for it. Gelatin is a fantastic source of fat-busting protein. It moisturizes and protects the mucosal lining of your intestinal tract, and brings healing to an irritated bowel. It is hydrophilic in nature, which means it attracts water. Hydrophilic foods support proper digestion and assimilation of your nutrients. Years ago, doctors were advising gelatin consumption for gut healing, rheumatoid arthritis, allergies, and inflammatory bowel disorders.

Don't buy flavored gelatin (Jell-o or similar products) from your grocery store, however. They are full of dyes and sugar, or artificial sweeteners. Seek out unflavored gelatin, optimally from the bones of grass-fed beef. Grocery store unflavored gelatin (Knox brand) is usually made from pork. It can work in our recipes, but it does not have the same health benefits. If you don't care about those health benefits, one ¼-ounce packet of unflavored Knox gelatin is about 2½ teaspoons. It can still be used to make our Key Lime Pie (page 326) and other recipes. You can find Just Gelatin at www.trimhealthymama.com or find another clean source online.

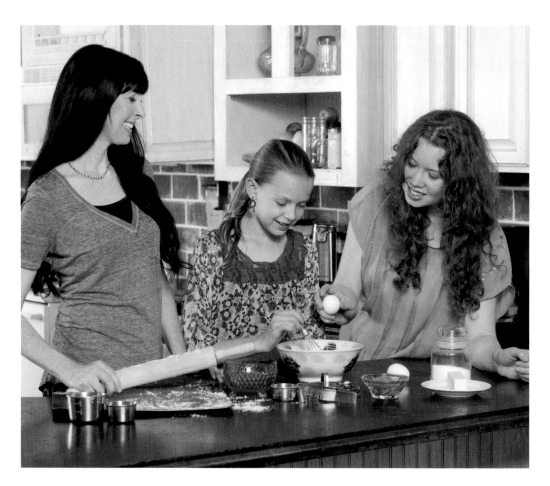

INTEGRAL COLLAGEN — While this is not a mandatory ingredient, it is a superfood of superfoods! It is simply gelatin broken down into smaller chains called peptides (through a natural process with a pineapple enzyme). You can put it in anything because it doesn't gel and it dissolves rather easily when whisked. It is a wonderful protein supplement for anyone with dairy allergies, and it helps stimulate glucagon, which is the fat-releasing hormone in your body. We make yummy recipes with it, even put it in our coffee, but it is also used therapeutically to help joint pain, arthritis, muscle repair, insomnia relief, and liver detoxification. It helps improve hormone balance, skin, teeth, and hair. Rich in glycine, it soothes the nervous system and helps to influence a quieting and anti-stress effect. You won't usually find collagen in stores, but it can be found online at www.trimhealthymama.com or at other online nutritional support sites. Look especially for "grass fed." Our Integral Collagen has close to 11 grams of protein per 1½ tablespoons, making it more budget friendly—that is, more collagen protein per tablespoon. (Can't resist including a "So there!")

PRISTINE WHEY PROTEIN — This makes all our smoothies and shakes creamy dreamy, and offers a fat-stripping form of protein to boot. Read about all of whey protein's health benefits in the "Specialty Food Stars" chapter of *Trim Healthy Mama Plan.* Whey protein is another "not absolutely necessary to do the plan" item. While many find it a wonderful helper, others with a "no special ingredient" mindset are quite happy using cottage cheese or 0% Greek yogurt as the creamy protein sources in their smoothies and shakes. If you would rather find a suitable whey protein locally, rather than buying online at our website, search for a CFM (cross-flow micro-filtered) whey protein isolate that is naturally lactose free and the least denatured form available. Second best is a basic micro-filtered whey protein isolate. Beware

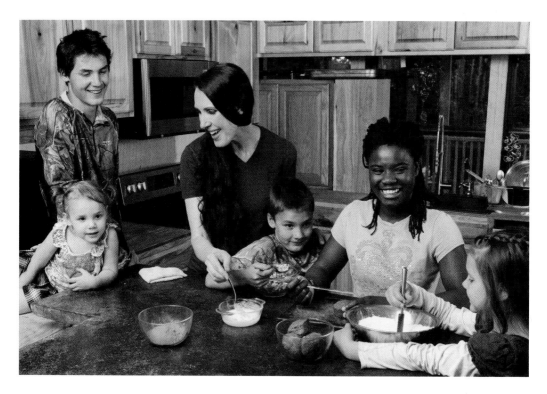

of cheap whey proteins flooding the market; these are harshly processed and use artificial sweeteners. Also, look for one with no more than 1 gram of carbohydrate per serving.

GLUCCIE – This is a natural thickener whose real name is glucomannan, but she became our kitchen buddy so we gave her a nickname that stuck. She might have a strange name, but Gluccie is simply the ground-up root of the konjac plant, and it has been used for centuries in Asian cuisine. Instead of using starchy, fattening thickeners to make your gravies, puddings, and shakes, Gluccie can do the job beautifully without any carbs or calories. She helps regulate your blood sugar and alkalize your body, and is a powerful weight-loss aid.

No, you can't buy Gluccie in stores at this time, but a 1-pound bag will last you months, perhaps a year. Only tiny amounts are needed, as she is a very powerful thickener. In all our recipes, we use the organic gray Gluccie available at www.trimhealthymama.com. It has not been bleached and is the most potent form. It thickens more effectively than other lesser grades of Gluccie. The key with Gluccie is to whisk or blend in very small amounts, and to stop adding any more right before your sauce or pudding is quite thick enough (put it in an empty salt shaker to help prevent lumps when sprinkling in). It will continue to thicken over the next 10 minutes or, in the case of a pudding, as it chills in the fridge. You don't want to overdo Gluccie amounts, as that can give your recipes a slightly strange texture. Of course, if you don't want to make the Gluccie purchase, no worries; you can use xanthan gum as a substitute. Xanthan does not have all the same health and slimming benefits, and it has a slightly different thickening texture, but it can do the job and is easily found at most grocery stores in little packets for less than a buck. Woot!

NOT NAUGHTY NOODLES – These noodles are made from Gluccie herself! They offer a wonderful filling factor without any carbs or calories. We're addicted to them, and we predict they're going to change your culinary world! If you're the type who does not like to purchase online, you can still make our yummy recipes that include them. Many grocery stores now carry some form of konjac noodles (including Walmart). They will be in the refrigerated section, usually close to the produce department. Look for the words "konjac root" on the ingredient list. Sadly, these store-bought options more often than not contain needless off-plan ingredients, like potato starch. But that doesn't mean you can't use them at all. The amount of off-plan ingredients is not so great that they'll destroy your meal or take it off plan. They might not be optimal, but they're not completely horrible, either.

Another problem with most store-bought konjac noodles is that they stink. Yes, you read it right: they have a strong fishy odor. This takes some rinsing in hot water to remove, but the smell will go away, we promise; it's just from the brine water they were packed in. Most store-bought konjac noodles are best rinsed well, then boiled for 2 to 3 minutes before cooking. Our Trim Healthy Mama Not Naughty Noodles don't have that strong smell, thankfully, and they don't have any added "fillers." They also don't need to be pre-boiled. But we don't want you to miss out on any of our noodle recipes because they're so good and so slimming! So go ahead and give these recipes a try, using what is available to you and your budget.

WHOLE-HUSK PSYLLIUM FLAKES – This is not a "rush out and buy straight away" ingredient, but at some point you might like to get around to making the Wonder Wraps (page 204). Aside from their deliciousness and our addiction to them, they can be a powerful trick to help you prepare ahead of time and stay on plan. You can find this inexpensive fiber/flour at www.trimhealthymama.com or at some natural grocery stores. Don't confuse it with that orange powder people drink to stay regular.

PRESSED PEANUT FLOUR – Yes, another specialty ingredient, but we're almost at the end of this list and we promise ('cause we know some of your heads are spinning) that you're going to find so many great recipes without any specialties. This defatted peanut flour gives wonderful peanutty taste without thousands of needless calories that can come with a peanut butter addiction. Natural, sugar-free peanut butter is certainly on plan, but the defatted flour version helps you not to overdo the butter form. You can do a little of both. Try our Shake Gone Nuts (page 411) or the fun Peanut Junkie Butter (page 481), which is actually a Fuel Pull! If you don't want to purchase our Trim Healthy brand online, you can buy defatted peanut flour in most grocery stores. Sadly, once again, the store-bought versions usually contain sugar, but the amounts are pretty minimal so while not perfectly optimum, they shouldn't mess with ya too much. We'll call them a second best that can do in a pinch.

NUTRITIONAL YEAST – You can find this in some grocery stores or at health food stores (bulk bins have it for the least expense). It has a delicious cheesy flavor and is full of minerals and vitamins. We use it to give flavor to soups and stews—just about anything that isn't sweet is made better with nutritional yeast. Our children can barely tolerate popcorn without it, and we could not bear to eat fried eggs without a sprinkle of it on top. But if you've lived your life this long without nutritional yeast, you'll be okay without rushing to buy it, even though it will liven up your food world. You've got a lifetime to slowly try some of these new foods.

SUNFLOWER LECITHIN – This is last on the list of ingredients you may not have heard of before. You'll notice it in just a few of the recipes. We only discovered this amazing substance in the last year, so don't think you have to immediately purchase it. But if you must be dairy free on plan, it can be an amazing bonus. It helps the Trimmaccino coffee (page 427) stay creamified and frothy to the last drop, and creamy shakes and smoothies are even smoother! You can read about its health-boosting abilities in the "Specialty Food Stars" chapter of *Trim Healthy Mama Plan.*

OUR BIG CHUNKY BOOK

Before we get to the recipes, we need to come clean about something. There is no official count for the recipes in this book. The reason is that we had to disguise some of the recipes from our publisher—yes, literally hide them. At the beginning of this project, we told our editor this cookbook would have about 200 recipes, so that is what the publishing team planned for. But that list kept growing, and we never realized by how much because we never kept track. We simply kept coming up with ideas for more recipes. We knew we needed to include lots

USEFUL INFORMATION

NSI = No Special Ingredients

DF = Dairy-Free (many dairy-intolerant people do well with Pristine Whey Protein because it is lactose free, but we couldn't in good conscience label recipes containing it as dairy-free)

Scoop of Integral Collagen = 1½ tablespoons

Scoop of Pristine Whey Protein = ¼ cup

Doonk = 1/32 teaspoon

Pinch of salt = roughly ¼ doonk (our pinches are small; we didn't realize this until Serene's husband followed one of our recipes (he was in the mood for a chocolate muffin). His pinches looked like five of ours. When it comes to following our pinches, you may want to go by your own tastes. (*If you ever see "half a pinch" in a recipe, blame Serene for that ridiculousness; I'm not owning up to that.* —Pearl)

NOTE

We did not include a gluten-free label for recipes, as most Trim Healthy Mama recipes are naturally gluten free, as are our products. We understand some people must be gluten free for health reasons; that will be easy on plan, but personally we do not despise gluten. It is a natural substance in ancient grains, and God put it there for a reason, we think. We simply steer away from most modern, hybridized wheat varieties, where the level of gluten is unnaturally elevated.

of family-friendly recipes, lots of single recipes, and lots of Purist recipes—but of course, the Drive Thru Sue's need their recipes, too! We wanted to have dairy-free recipes, and plenty that use no special ingredients, but we also knew Mamas have been waiting for lots of recipes using our Baking Blend and other products (like Just Gelatin and Integral Collagen).

We're not the most organized girls—in fact, just the opposite. We had recipes and chapters scattered everywhere. Every day for five months straight we just kept cooking up a storm. The day finally arrived when we put all the recipes together in one document, added

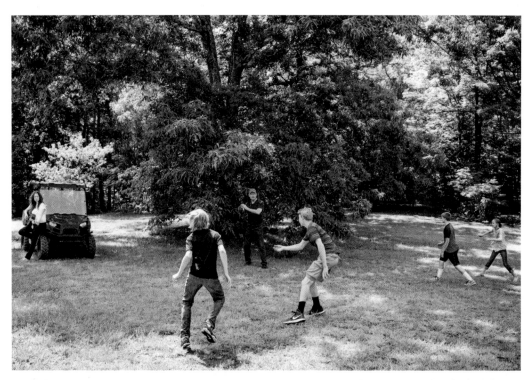

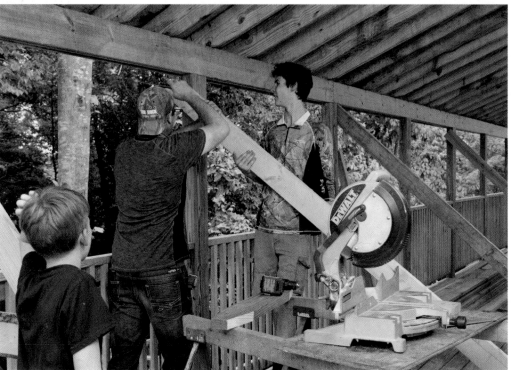

them up, and, gulp, there were more than 370 recipes! We couldn't part with them (well, we ditched just a couple), but we knew if we got rid of the quick and easy ones, somebody would miss out; if we nixed the puristy recipes, somebody else would miss out; if we dropped the dairy- or allergen-free ones, others would miss out. Trim Healthy Mama is not for one type of person—it's for all types. And we wanted this book to be a resource that will be a kitchen staple in your home for years to come.

So what did we do? We came up with a brilliant, crafty plan to make it look like certain variations of recipes were really just *one* recipe. That way the count would not look so ridiculously high to our publisher. (To our fellow church-going readers, don't look at this like a sinful deception; we were just softening the blow.) We're not really sure we fooled our publishing team, but they've been long suffering with us. We certainly know we've caused them a sleepless night or two. And they have had their hands full with us, in more ways than one. We don't "do" conventional well. Our first self-published book was all "Throw in this spice, then add that to taste." We left out baking times, dish sizes, and didn't bother to mention serving sizes. That's the way we cook, and we pretty much thought everyone else would just get it! Well, we've come a long way, but it's been hard to tame us—free spirits are not bridled easily. We are the "Go big or go home" type of Mamas who love to create recipes in a wild chaos of cooking joy. We're ferociously protective and proud of every one of the three hundred and sumpin' sumpin' recipes in this book. We know they are going to help revolutionize your health and deliciously trim your waistline. So, let's eat!

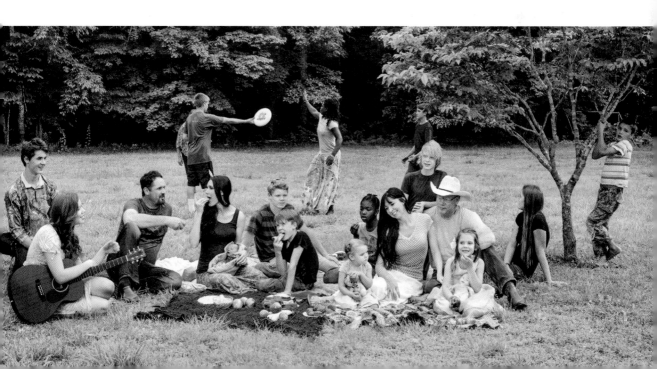

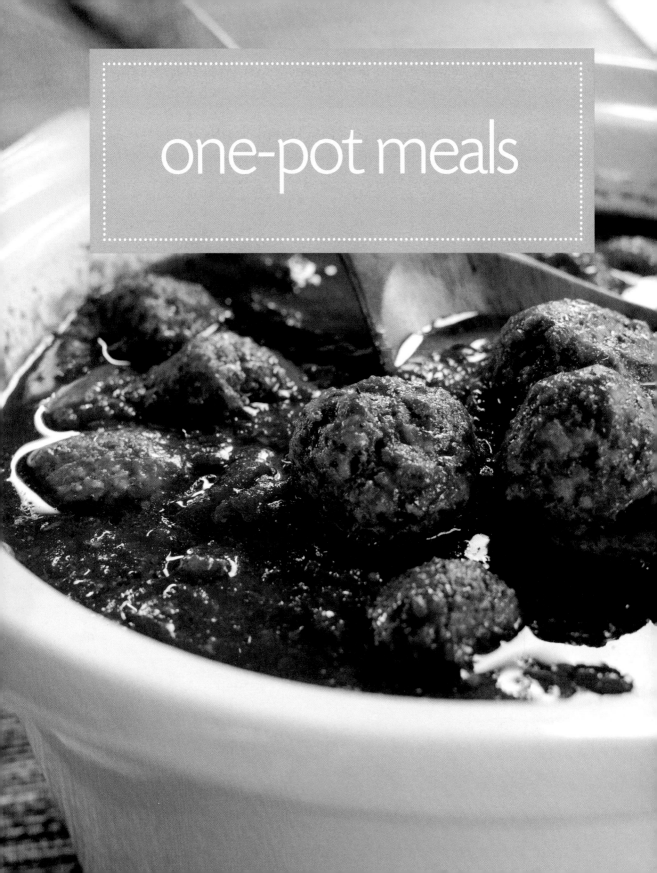

one-pot meals

● = S   ● = E   ● = FP   MORE THAN ONE DOT INDICATES OPTIONS

CROCKPOT MEALS

Trim Healthy Mama and the crockpot work wonderfully together. The following 15 recipes are loved by our families, and are well suited for freezer-to-crock preparations. Repeat each recipe as written just once, and you have a full month of trimming, healthy meals ready to go!

The poor old crockpot was sadly named, we think. It should be renamed the "destressor pot" because it can take so much stress out of your life. Just the knowledge that you have a nourishing meal simmering away in your kitchen all day, whether you are there or not, can bring those stress hormones way down. And it prevents the dreaded witching hour—you know, that time between 5:30 and 6:30 in the evening, when you are struggling to get dinner on the table. Your children are over-tired, over-hungry, and generally making it difficult for you to concentrate. Or, you're in the car in traffic, worrying about what on earth you'll pull together for dinner. Goodbye witching hour, hello crock sweet life!

Many crockpot recipes pride themselves on "dump" ingredients—you just dump them in the pot and forget about them. But sadly, most of those recipes are unhealthy collections of overly processed ingredients. Cans of cream-of soups, bottles of store-bought dressings with all sorts of crazy ingredients, and packets of taco or ranch seasoning laden with fake fillers—these are all the rage for crockpot cooking, but are not kind to your body. You won't find processed and unhealthy foods here, even though we have done our darnedest to keep it simple. Whether you are a Purist, a Drive Thru Sue, or even a Mama with multiple food sensitivities, check out all these recipes, as you are sure to find some that will suit your needs.

Many folks in the THM community love to have a "prep-cooking day," in which they assemble a couple weeks' to a full month's worth of slimming yet nourishing meals, nicely stored in their freezer and all ready to be slow-cooked to perfection. We have kept all the prep to an absolute minimum here so that task will be easier for you. For instance, there is no need to pre-cook anything; we find that pre-cooking takes the ease out of crockpot prep and slows it down too much.

All of the following recipes feed between 6 and 8 hungry people, so if your family is smaller (say, 2 adults and 2 small children), you can set aside just a few hours of your day to prep these recipes. Divide the contents for each recipe into two sturdy freezer bags and voilà!, you now have a full month's worth of healthy, yummy evening meals ready to go.

But, hey, if all that prep seems intimidating, there is no THM law that says you have to become a monthly freezer stocker. Simply enjoy these crockpot recipes whenever you desire. Or start the freezer stocking in baby steps; it's a big achievement to get even a week's worth of freezer-to-cooker meals prepared. Choose seven of these recipes that interest you the most, and give it a whirl! Grab a husband or older child to help, or get help from a friend. Make it a fun project.

Crockpot recipes make chicken breasts and other boneless meats lovely and tender, but in keeping with the Trim Healthy Mama approach to include glycine-rich meals, we've also included a couple of "bone-in, skin-on" dishes. Don't miss out on those. You'll notice those recipes use an acid medium of either lemons or limes to help extract all the nutrients from the bones.

TIPS FOR SUCCESS

We have had many trials and errors with crockpot preparations. We have found that putting thawed meat (especially chicken) into the crockpot, rather than frozen, is not only safer but also you can drain away the excess liquid before cooking. Crockpot dishes can be overly watery if the sauces are combined with frozen chicken, then returned to the freezer. If you want to do the freezer-to-cooker preparation, label the bags of meat and sauce separately for each recipe, with the reminder of which sauce bag it matches, then put them in the freezer. You will take out both the meat and sauce bags for your desired recipe twenty-four hours before cooking to thaw in the fridge. Once the meat is fully thawed, you can drain away all excess liquid from it before placing it in the crockpot, and then add the sauce. Most frozen bags of chicken breasts handily come in 2.5-pound bags, which is usually the amount our recipes call for, so no need to waste time transferring them to another freezer bag unless you have purchased chicken breasts in amounts other than 2.5 pounds, in which case you'll want to use a separate freezer bag for the meat. Of course our ultra-purist Mamas can use glass containers. (You *can* use frozen meat in your cooker; gotta be honest and say that we do that occasionally if we forget to thaw, but don't blame us for any trouble with it, 'kay?)

cajun cream chicken   Ⓢ

2½ pounds thawed and drained boneless chicken tenderloins, breasts, or thighs

2 (8-ounce) packages ⅓ less fat cream cheese

½ cup chicken broth or bone stock (pages 495–496)

1½ teaspoons MSG-free Creole seasoning

It cannot possibly get easier than this recipe, but the flavor and creaminess are a home run!

1. Place the chicken in the crockpot.
2. Blend the cream cheese, broth or stock, and seasoning in a blender, then add to the crockpot.
3. Cook on low heat all day or on high heat for 5 to 6 hours.
4. *For later:* 15 to 30 minutes before serving, break up the chicken with a fork and stir into the sauce.

SERVING IDEAS: Serve over Cauli Rice (page 225), Spaghetti Squash (page 224), or Not Naughty Noodles—or simply enjoy it on its own, with a side salad.

FOR FREEZER-TO-CROCK PREP: Label frozen bag of chicken breasts or tenderloins as "Cajun Cream Chicken – S" with a Sharpie. Blend all other ingredients and pour into another freezer bag. Label the freezer bag with recipe name and put both bags in freezer. The morning before cooking (24 hours prior), put the chicken and sauce bags in the refrigerator to thaw; the next morning, pour out excess fluid from the chicken and place the chicken in the crockpot. Add the sauce.

NSI

wicked white chili

2½ pounds thawed and drained
  boneless, skinless chicken breasts
  or tenderloins
4 (15-ounce) cans great northern
  beans, rinsed and drained, or
  6 cups soaked and cooked dried
  beans, drained
2 cups chicken broth or bone stock
  (pages 495–496)
2 (10-ounce) cans Rotel-style tomatoes
  and chilies (mild, medium, or hot)
1 (14½-ounce) can diced tomatoes
1½ cups Seasoning Blend
  (frozen diced onion, celery, and
  green pepper)
2 cups frozen corn kernels,
  or 1 (14½-ounce) can corn, drained
1 teaspoon Mineral Salt
2 teaspoons ground cumin
2 teaspoons chili powder
1 teaspoon onion powder
½ teaspoon garlic powder
½ cup plain 0% Greek yogurt
  (optional)

PEARL CHATS: While loading their bowls high, my teenage boys call this chili "wicked." Thankfully that happens to be a good word in their terminology, so I take it as a compliment. Hearty and filling, this meal fits a whole family's needs on any busy night. Since there is no browning of meat required for a white chili, it is a perfect match for the crockpot. Even though we're in solid E mode here, blending some of the beans with broth or stock gives a creamier, heartier base, which tricks your taste buds into thinking there is more fat in the sauce. Top with some Blendtons (page 476) or sprinkle on some baked blue corn chips, add plenty of grated cheese to the children's bowls to give them a crossover, and perhaps just a sprinkling garnish to your bowl to stay in E mode. You're all set!

1. Place the chicken in the bottom of the crockpot.
2. Blend 2 of the cans of beans with the broth in a blender and add to pot.
3. Add all the other ingredients (including remaining 2 cans beans) except the yogurt and stir.
4. Cook on low heat all day or on high heat for 5 to 6 hours.
5. *For later:* Thirty minutes before serving, take out the chicken and shred it with 2 forks, then return it to the cooker (or you can shred it in the pot). Combine well, then add the yogurt and mix well.

FOR FREEZER-TO-CROCK PREP: Label frozen bag of chicken breasts or tenderloins as "Wicked White Chili – E" with a Sharpie. Blend the beans with the broth, pour into another freezer bag, then add all other ingredients except the yogurt. Label the freezer bag with recipe name and put both bags in the freezer. The morning before cooking (24 hours prior), put the chicken and chili sauce bags in the refrigerator to thaw. Next morning, pour out excess fluid from the chicken and place the chicken in the crockpot. Add the sauce.

NSI DF (IF YOU OMIT THE YOGURT)

rich and tender stew

FAMILY SERVE – FEEDS 6 TO 8 (HALVE INGREDIENTS IF YOUR FAMILY IS SMALLER)

2½ to 3 pounds thawed and drained beef or venison (bone-in cuts can work here, too, but account for the bones in the total weight)

2 large green, yellow, or red bell peppers, cored, seeded, and cut into chunky pieces

8 celery stalks, cut into chunky pieces

2 medium onions, cut into chunky pieces

1 (16-ounce) bag radishes, cut into halves

1 (6-ounce) can tomato paste

2 cups beef broth

3 tablespoons Worcestershire sauce

2 teaspoons Mineral Salt

½ teaspoon black pepper

¼ teaspooon cayenne pepper

1 teaspoon onion powder

½ teaspooon garlic powder

1 teaspoon dried oregano

¼ cup nutritional yeast (optional)

¼ cup heavy cream or full-fat coconut milk

¼ to ⅓ teaspoon Gluccie or xanthan

This meal is perfect for rougher, less expensive cuts of meat, as the crockpot magically tenderizes them. Have a hunter in your family? You're in luck, as venison cuts work beautifully here. There is no need to pre-cut the meat into strips; bigger cuts will break up easily into smaller pieces once they are tender. Pre-cut stew meat works fine too, if that is what you have on hand.

1. Pour off any excess liquid from the meat, then place in the crockpot.
2. Add the veggies.
3. Blend the tomato paste, broth, and seasonings, then add to the pot.
4. Cook on low heat all day or on high heat for 5 to 6 hours.
5. *For later:* Fifteen minutes before serving, turn the cooker off. Add the cream or coconut milk and stir, then slowly shake in the Gluccie while whisking well. Stop adding Gluccie before you think the stew is thick enough. You shouldn't need much Gluccie, as this stew is not meant to have a thick consistency. Allow the Gluccie to create just a slightly thicker broth.

FOR FREEZER-TO-CROCK PREP: Label package of meat as "Rich and Tender Stew – S" with a Sharpie. Blend the tomato paste with the broth and seasonings. Pour into another freezer bag, then add the vegetables. Label the freezer bag with recipe name and put both bags in the freezer. The morning before cooking (24 hours prior), put the meat and stew sauce bags in the refrigerator to thaw. Next morning, pour out excess fluid from the meat and place in the crockpot. Add the stew sauce.

NSI (IF USING XANTHAN)   DF (IF MADE WITH COCONUT MILK INSTEAD OF CREAM)

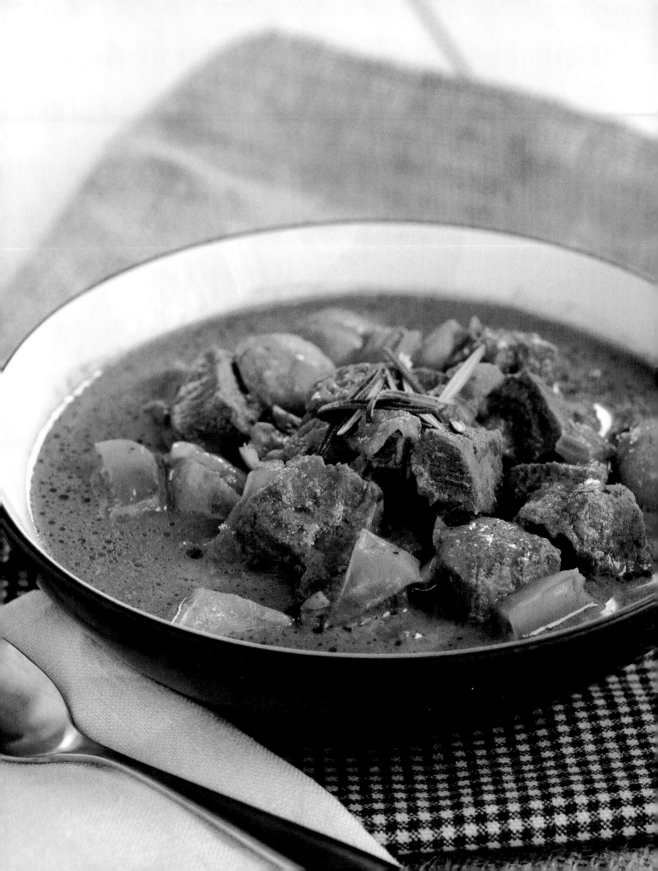

ridiculous meatballs and spaghetti

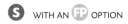

FAMILY SERVE – FEEDS 6 TO 8 (HALVE INGREDIENTS IF YOUR FAMILY IS SMALLER)

2½ pounds thawed ground Italian-style
    sausage meat (we use turkey or
    chicken, and sometimes venison,
    but you can use pork if you'd prefer)
1 (28-ounce) can crushed tomatoes
1 tablespoon Italian seasoning
1 teaspoon onion powder
1 teaspoon garlic powder
¼ teaspoon Mineral Salt
¼ teaspoon black pepper
3 doonks Pure Stevia Extract, or
    2 teaspoons Super Sweet Blend
2 (14½-ounce) cans petite diced
    tomatoes
1 family package Not Naughty Noodles
    (optional)

This meal is so crazy, stupid, easy that it's ridiculous! The meatballs hold together perfectly in the sauce without any fuss of having to pre-mix them with eggs or flour. If you've got picky little ones who need a night off from having to eat their onions, they'll be in kid heaven with this recipe (feel free to add 1 large chopped onion to the sauce if your entire family is onion loving).

1. Break off small hunks of ground sausage and press into meatballs (you may have to cut through casing if using link sausage). Place each ball carefully in the cooker. You can layer them if your cooker is small.

2. Blend all the other ingredients except 1 can of diced tomatoes and the Not Naughty Noodles (if using). Pour the sauce over the meatballs, then add the remaining can of tomatoes. If deciding to use Not Naughty Noodles, rinse and drain noodles, snip smaller, then place over the sauce.

3. Cook on low heat all day or on high heat for 5 to 6 hours.

SERVING IDEAS: The family pack of Not Naughty Noodles is not necessary here if you've got a tight budget. But the noodles do become wonderfully tender after cooking in the sauce all day, and children usually love them. If you'd rather use whole-grain noodles for your children to save a few dollars, that's perfectly fine. For your own noodles, you can choose from Troodles (page 222), Spaghetti Squash (page 224), or an individual package of Not Naughty Noodles. Occasionally, Drive Thru Sue's may want to choose Dreamfields pasta, but you can assess your own reaction to that pasta.

NOTE: This could easily be a Fuel Pull if you use ultra-lean turkey sausage and keep your meat portion to between 3 and 4 ounces. We are only classifying this as an **S** here to give you the option of using any type of sausage—and because this dish is divine topped with grated cheese. However, topping it with a sprinkle of Parmesan will still leave you in **FP** mode if you'd rather keep this meal a lighter option.

FOR FREEZER-TO-CROCK PREP: Here's a recipe that can all go in one large freezer bag. Label the bag with a Sharpie. Break off small pieces of sausage (you may have to cut through casing if using link sausage) and roll into meatballs. Place all the meatballs in a large freezer bag. Blend all the ingredients except one can of tomatoes. Pour the sauce into that same freezer bag, add 1 can of tomatoes, and put the bag in the freezer. The morning before cooking (24 hours prior), put the bag in the refrigerator to thaw. Next morning, pour the contents of the bag in the crockpot. Then add Not Naughty Noodles (if using).

NSI (WITHOUT NOT NAUGHTY NOODLES) DF (WITHOUT THE GRATED CHEESE; YOU CAN USE GRATED HELLO CHEESE, PAGE 487)

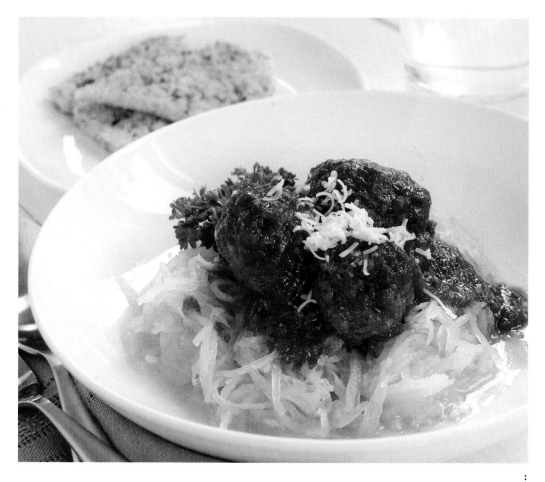

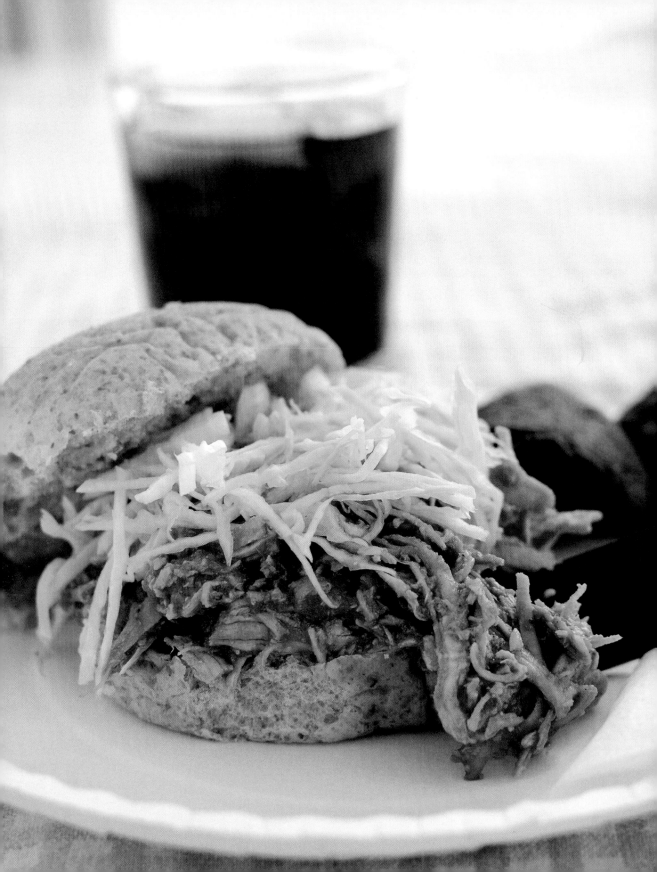

wipe your mouth bbq Ⓔ

2½ pounds thawed and drained boneless, skinless chicken breasts

1 (14½-ounce) can diced tomatoes

4 teaspoons onion powder

2 teaspoons garlic powder

1 tablespoon tomato paste

3 tablespoons prepared yellow mustard

3 tablespoons apple cider vinegar

3 tablespoons paprika

1 teaspooon cayenne pepper (or to taste; this makes a spicy BBQ, try ¼ teaspoon if you have children who can't abide heat)

3 to 4 teaspoons Mineral Salt

1 teaspoon black pepper

2 teaspoons Liquid Smoke

2 teaspoons blackstrap molasses

1 cup drained pineapple chunks

4 teaspoons Super Sweet Blend, or 4 doonks Pure Stevia Extract

This is a smack-your-lips, sweet heat, wipe-that-mouth saucy BBQ! It's perfect on sprouted rolls or over brown rice with Light and Lovely Coleslaw (page 231) on the side. Or, simply throw some finely cut cabbage in with your sandwich if you want less fuss. If you don't have any sprouted rolls or bread handy, and are hankering for a BBQ sandwich, whip up some Swiss Bread rolls (page 196) and then have a Mangosicle (page 367) for dessert to get more E fuel into your meal.

1. Place the chicken in the crockpot.
2. Place all other ingredients in a blender and process until smooth.
3. Add the sauce to the crockpot and cook on low heat all day or on high heat for 5 to 6 hours.
4. Once the chicken is cooked, shred it and mix it into the sauce. Let sit in the sauce (to soak up the BBQ sauce) for 10 to 15 minutes, then serve.

FOR FREEZER-TO-CROCK PREP: Label frozen bag of chicken breasts or tenderloins as "Wipe Your Mouth BBQ – E" with a Sharpie. Blend all the other ingredients and pour into another freezer bag. Label the freezer bag with recipe name and put both bags in freezer. The morning before cooking (24 hours prior), put both bags in the refrigerator to thaw. Next morning, pour out excess fluid from the chicken and place the chicken in the crockpot. Add the sauce.

NSI (IF USING FAVORITE HANDY ON-PLAN SWEETENER) DF

smarty-pants stroganoff

2½ pounds boneless thawed beef or venison (cut into strips)

¼ cup Trim Healthy Mama Baking Blend or almond flour

1 very large onion, or 2 medium onions, sliced

3 garlic cloves, minced

1 cup beef broth or bone stock (pages 495–496)

1½ teaspoons Mineral Salt

¾ teaspoon black pepper

1 teaspoon onion powder

3½ tablespoons Worcestershire sauce

1 (16-ounce) package sliced button mushrooms

1 family package Not Naughty Noodles, rinsed and drained (optional)

⅓ to ½ teaspoon Gluccie

1 cup sour cream

This classic dish oozes comfort and flavor. Sadly, it is usually a waistline exploder because the rich, creamy sauce is traditionally paired with starchy white noodles. You won't miss a thing when you make this the smarty-pants way. It is still ultra-flavorful and ultra-comforting; you'll simply choose from your favorite on-plan noodle option. Also, the mushrooms help build your immune system because they are packed with the powerful cancer fighter vitamin D. Stroganoff is usually an involved recipe preparation, but it doesn't have to be. We've taken out the many, multiple steps of this recipe, since like us, you probably don't have time for all that. No precooking. Just throw the ingredients into your crockpot. And don't buy expensive meat for this recipe—get the cheapest cuts you can find. The slow, long cooking time tenderizes the meat beautifully. If you have hunters in your family, as we do, don't be afraid of using venison here.

1. Lay the beef in the crockpot, then sprinkle the Baking Blend over the meat. Add the onions, garlic, broth, and seasonings.

2. Put the mushrooms on top. If using, lay the Not Naughty Noodles over the mushrooms.

3. Cook on low heat all day or on high heat for 5 to 6 hours.

4. Fifteen minutes before serving, whisk in Gluccie, then add sour cream.

SERVING IDEAS: Not Naughty Noodles become lovely and soft in the crockpot and work well with this dish, but a less expensive alternative is to serve it over Troodles (page 222). This is also wonderful over creamy Mashed Fotatoes (page 219).

FOR FREEZER-TO-CROCK PREP: Label 2 freezer bags as "Smarty Pants Stroganoff – S," using a Sharpie. Place the meat in one bag. Blend the broth or stock with all the seasonings and the Baking Blend, then place in the second freezer bag. Add the onion. Write "needs mushrooms" on that bag as a reminder. Place both bags in the freezer. The morning before cooking (24 hours prior), put the meat and sauce bags in the refrigerator to thaw. Next morning, pour off excess fluid from the meat and place the meat in the crockpot. Add the mushrooms, then add the sauce.

NSI (WITHOUT NOT NAUGHTY NOODLES OR IF USING XANTHAN INSTEAD OF GLUCCIE)

coconut thai chicken   Ⓢ

2½ pounds thawed and drained boneless chicken thighs or breasts

1 (15-ounce) can full-fat coconut milk

1 cup chicken broth or bone stock (pages 495–496)

½ cup Pressed Peanut Flour, or ¼ cup sugar-free, natural-style peanut butter

4 teaspoons red curry paste

2 teaspoons fish sauce

¼ to ½ teaspoon cayenne pepper (reduce if you have children who cannot tolerate spicy)

½ teaspoon ground ginger

1 teaspoon Super Sweet Blend

2 teaspoons Mineral Salt

1 (12-ounce) bag frozen stir-fry veggies (avoid broccoli)

2 cups Seasoning Blend (frozen diced onion, celery, and pepper)

1 teaspoon red pepper flakes

1 family package Not Naughty Noodles

Here's tender chicken in a rich and tasty broth that sends you to Thai heaven! The Not Naughty Noodles become lovely and soft, cooked all day until they take on the delicious chicken flavor. You should be able to find fish sauce and red curry paste in the international aisle of your grocery store; if not, any Asian market will have them. (If your family is small, make only half this recipe as written, as the Not Naughty Noodles do not freeze well; leftovers, of course, are great for lunches.)

1. Add the chicken to the crockpot.
2. Blend the coconut milk, broth, peanut flour or peanut butter, and all the seasonings except the red pepper flakes in a blender and pour over the chicken.
3. Add the frozen veggies, seasoning blend, and red pepper flakes.
4. Rinse and drain the Not Naughty noodles, then snip into smaller pieces with scissors and add to the crockpot.
5. Cook on low heat all day or on high heat for 5 to 6 hours. Break up the chicken with 2 forks and combine all the ingredients well before serving.

FOR FREEZER-TO-CROCK PREP: Label frozen bag of boneless chicken thighs or breasts as "Coconut Thai Chicken – S" with a Sharpie. Put all the veggies in another freezer bag. Blend the coconut milk, broth, peanut flour or peanut butter, and seasonings except red pepper flakes and add to the second bag, then add the pepper flakes. Label bag with name of recipe and write "Needs Not Naughty Noodles" as a reminder, then put both bags in the freezer next to each other. The morning before cooking (24 hours prior), place both bags in the refrigerator to thaw. Next morning, pour out the excess fluid from the chicken and add the chicken to the crockpot. Add the bag of sauce and veggies, and the Not Naughty Noodles.

DF

chicken florentine

FAMILY SERVE – FEEDS 6 TO 8 (HALVE INGREDIENTS IF YOUR FAMILY IS SMALLER)

2 (10-ounce) packages frozen chopped spinach

2½ pounds thawed and drained chicken breasts or tenderloins

2 (8-ounce) packages ⅓ less fat cream cheese

1 cup finely grated Parmesan cheese (green can kind is fine)

1 teaspoon Mineral Salt

½ teaspoon black pepper

1½ teaspoons onion powder

¾ to 1 teaspoon garlic powder

1 large onion, chopped

1½ cups chicken broth or bone stock (pages 495–496)

Cayenne pepper to taste (optional)

This is reminiscent of spinach dip. It's easy-peasy and gives you a nice dose of healthy greens.

1. Place the frozen spinach at the bottom of the crockpot.
2. Add the thawed, drained chicken breasts.
3. Blend the cream cheese with the seasonings (except the cayenne) and add to the cooker.
4. Add the onion and broth.
5. Cook on low heat all day or on high for 5 to 6 hours.
6. Break up the chicken, and combine with the sauce before serving. Season to taste with the cayenne (if using).

SERVING IDEAS: Enjoy with Troodles (page 222) or Cauli Rice (page 225).

FOR FREEZER-TO-CROCK PREP: Label frozen bag of chicken breasts as "Chicken Florentine – S" with a Sharpie. Blend the cream cheese with the broth and seasonings, pour into a freezer bag, and add the onion and frozen spinach. Label bag with name of recipe. Put both bags in the freezer next to each other. The morning before cooking (24 hours prior), put the chicken and sauce bags in the refrigerator to thaw. Next morning, pour off any excess fluid from the chicken and place the chicken in the crockpot. Add the sauce.

NSI

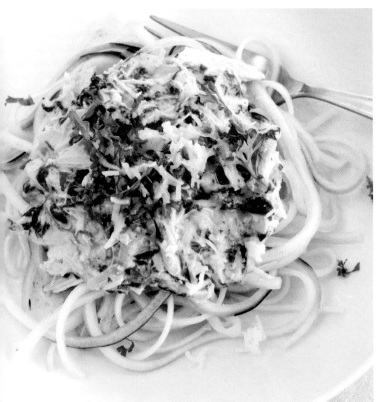

wacha want mexican chicken

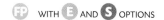
FAMILY SERVE – FEEDS 6 TO 8 (HALVE INGREDIENTS IF YOUR FAMILY IS SMALLER)

2½ pounds thawed and drained
  boneless, skinless chicken breasts
  or tenderloins
1 (24-ounce) jar salsa of choice

This versatile, easy meal asks the question of whether your body wants an S or an E meal, or whether you want to stay in FP mode. Have you not had enough E meals lately? Pair this dish with two half E servings of beans and rice, or choose ½ cup of rice—then have a Mangosicle (page 367) for dessert. Or, craving cheese and sour cream? Top your bowl with grated cheese, sour cream, and a garnish of diced avocado for S mode. Have stubborn pounds and realize it's time for a Fuel Pull? Keep the meat to between 3 and 4 ounces and enjoy over Cauli Rice (page 225) or Not Naughty Rice and top with a little Greek yogurt. Finish your meal with a Strawbsicle (page 367) or Lemonade Slushy (page 372).

1. Place the chicken in the crockpot.
2. Add the salsa and cook on low heat all day or on high heat for 5 to 6 hours.

FOR FREEZER-TO-CROCK PREP: Label frozen bag of chicken breasts as "Wacha Want Mexican Chicken – FP" with a Sharpie. Write on bag "needs jar of salsa." Place the bag in the freezer. The morning before cooking (24 hours prior), put the bag in the refrigerator to thaw. Next morning, pour off any excess fluid from the chicken and place the chicken in the crockpot. Add the salsa.

NSI DF (IF OMITTING THE CHEESE AND SOUR CREAM; SUBSTITUTE HELLO CHEESE, PAGE 487)

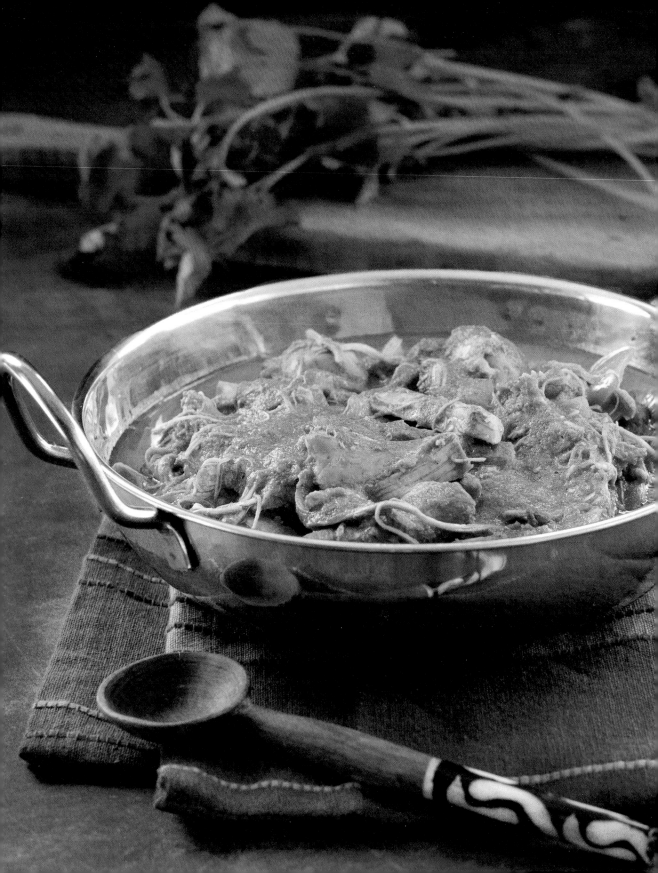

buttah chicken

FAMILY SERVE – FEEDS 6 TO 8 (HALVE INGREDIENTS IF YOUR FAMILY IS SMALLER)

2½ pounds thawed and drained
  boneless chicken thighs
1 (28-ounce) can crushed tomatoes
1 tablespoon plus 1 teaspoon garam
  masala
1 teaspoon onion powder
2½ teaspoons Mineral Salt
1 doonk Pure Stevia Extract
½ teaspoon cayenne pepper
3 tablespoons butter or coconut oil
1 large onion, diced, or 1½ cups
  Seasoning Blend (frozen diced onion,
  celery, and pepper)
2 teaspoons minced garlic
1 (24½-ounce) can petite diced
  tomatoes, drained
½ cup plain 0% Greek yogurt
¼ cup heavy cream

This is our favorite Indian dish, partly because we love the blend of Indian spices and partly because we love BUTTAH! Three cheers for butter! Even if you are not a fan of Indian food, we urge you to give this a try. Oh my, it's so delish! If you are not a hot and spicy fan, take the cayenne pepper down to ⅛ to ¼ teaspoon, or leave it out altogether; but we love the kick and use even more than listed here. Sadly, butter-chicken recipes are often complicated, time-consuming, and contain cup after cup of heavy cream. Don't deny yourself the cream, but don't abuse it, either. We have simplified the preparation to level 1 expertise—even Drive Thru Sue is going to think this is a cinch.

1. Place the chicken thighs in the bottom of the crockpot.
2. Blend the crushed tomatoes with the seasonings and butter, then add to the crockpot.
3. Add the onion, garlic, and the diced tomatoes.
4. Cook on low heat all day or on high heat for 5 to 6 hours.
5. Just before serving, break up the chicken with 2 forks, then mix in the yogurt and cream.

SERVING IDEAS: Serve over your choice of Cauli Rice (page 225) or Not Naughty Rice. Or enjoy over a bed of sautéed spinach—or eat just by itself in a bowl!

NOTE: If you are dairy intolerant, you can use a can of full-fat coconut milk instead of the cream and yogurt.

FOR FREEZER-TO-CROCK PREP: Label a frozen bag of boneless chicken thighs as "Buttah Chicken – S" with a Sharpie. Blend the crushed tomatoes, all the seasonings, and the butter and pour into another freezer bag, then add onion, garlic, and diced tomatoes. Label bag with name of recipe, write "needs cream and yogurt" on the bag as a reminder of the fresh ingredients needed, then put both bags in the freezer next to each other. The morning before cooking (24 hours prior), place both bags in the refrigerator to thaw. Next morning, open chicken bag and pour out the excess fluid from the chicken. Add thawed chicken and sauce to the crock.

NSI DF (IF USING COCONUT MILK INSTEAD OF CREAM AND YOGURT)

pot roast with radishtoes and gravy (S)

3- to 3½-pounds boneless chuck beef roast (thawed)

2 (16-ounce) bags fresh radishes, larger ones cut in half

8 celery stalks, chopped into 1-inch pieces

2 large onions, cut into large wedges

1½ teaspoons Mineral Salt, plus more for sprinkling

1 teaspoon onion powder

½ teaspoon black pepper, plus more for sprinkling

3 tablespoons nutritional yeast

1 to 2 squirts Bragg liquid aminos (optional)

About 1 teaspoon Gluccie to thicken (amount used will depend on how much liquid is being turned into gravy)

Cayenne pepper to taste

Whether your family knows these radishes aren't potatoes full of starch or whether you keep that a secret is up to you. We don't say a thing about it in our homes, and nobody has ever complained. Once cooked, the radishes lose their bite and soften beautifully in the crockpot. They look just like little red potatoes. There's no need to peel them, but it is best to cut the bigger ones in half.

1. Put the meat in the crockpot and sprinkle with salt and pepper. Add the vegetables, then add enough water to just cover the ingredients. (It is okay if the top of the meat peeks through the water.)

2. Cook on high heat all day.

3. *For later:* Thirty minutes before serving, scoop out the veggies and lift out the meat, and transfer temporarily to a large bowl. Ladle or pour out some of the liquid so you are left with roughly 3 cups in the crockpot.

4. Add the 1½ teaspoons salt, onion powder, ½ teaspoon pepper, Nutritional Yeast, and liquid aminos (if using) to the liquid, then whisk a little Gluccie in slowly from a shaker; stop just before the gravy is as thick as you would like it.

5. Return the meat to the gravy and break into smaller pieces but don't shred it. Return the veggies to the cooker as well, and let everything sit in the gravy for 15 to 30 more minutes.

6. Taste and adjust the seasonings, adding the cayenne to suit. Note: It is common to need more salt, liquid aminos, or pepper because the Gluccie can mask the flavors a little bit.

FOR FREEZER-TO-CROCK PREP: Label package of meat as "Pot Roast with Radishtoes and Gravy – S" with a Sharpie. Put the veggies in another freezer bag and label bag with recipe name; write additional ingredients needed for gravy on bag as a reminder. Put both bags in the freezer next to each other. The day before cooking (24 hours prior), place both bags in the refrigerator to thaw. Next morning, pour off any excess fluid from the meat, add the meat to the crock, and sprinkle with some salt and pepper. Add the veggies and water to cover. After cooking, follow steps 3 to 6 for making the gravy.

NSI (IF USING XANTHAN TO THICKEN) DF

lemon herb drummies

⑤

6 to 8 pounds thawed and drained
chicken drumsticks or mini drums
(wing portions)

½ cup chicken broth or bone stock
(pages 495–496)

Juice of 2 or 3 lemons

¼ cup coconut oil or butter, melted

2 cups Seasoning Blend (frozen diced
onion, celery, and pepper)

2 to 2½ teaspoons Mineral Salt

¼ teaspoon black pepper

2 teaspoons onion powder

1 teaspoon garlic powder, or 2 garlic
cloves, minced

1 teaspoon crumbled dried rosemary

1 teaspoon paprika

2 tablespoons dried parsley

1 family package Not Naughty Rice
(optional)

It is unusual to find crockpot recipes for bone-in meats unless the meat is browned first. This recipe (and the Cilantro Lime-Burst Chicken Thighs, page 54) requires no browning, yet it works beautifully in the crockpot. Your body will receive all the healing goodness of the glycine and proline that's inside the bones and skin of the chicken pieces, released slowly all day as it cooks with the help of the citrus acid in the broth. Bones take up quite a bit of weight, so to feed 6 to 8 hungry people you'll need 1½ or 2 bags of chicken drums or thighs (most bags are 4 pounds each). Thankfully, these bone-in meat pieces are the least expensive parts of chicken.

1. Put the thawed, drained drumsticks in the crockpot.
2. Blend the broth with the lemon juice and add to the chicken. Add the coconut oil, Seasoning Blend, and seasonings. Add the Not Naughty Rice (if using) last.
3. Cook on high heat for 6 to 8 hours.

SERVING IDEAS: The Not Naughty Rice is wonderful in this recipe but optional if your budget is tight. As a healthy Cross-over, your children will love this over brown rice to help sop up all the tasty broth. You can also use an individual pack of NNR (heated up separately) or quickly whip up some Cauli Rice (page 225), or simply enjoy this on its own in a bowl with some buttered Swiss Bread (page 196) on the side.

FOR FREEZER-TO-CROCK PREP: Label freezer bags of chicken drums as "Lemon Herb Drummies" with a Sharpie. Blend the lemon juice and broth and pour into another freezer bag. Add the coconut oil and all other seasonings to the bag. Label the bag with name of recipe, and if you intend to use Not Naughty Rice, write "needs NNR" as a reminder. Put the meat and sauce bags in the freezer next to each other. The morning before cooking (24 hours prior), place both meat and sauce bags in the refrigerator to thaw. Next morning, pour out any excess fluid from the chicken, add the chicken to the crock, then add the sauce, and optional NNR.

NSI (IF OMITTING THE NOT NAUGHTY RICE) DF

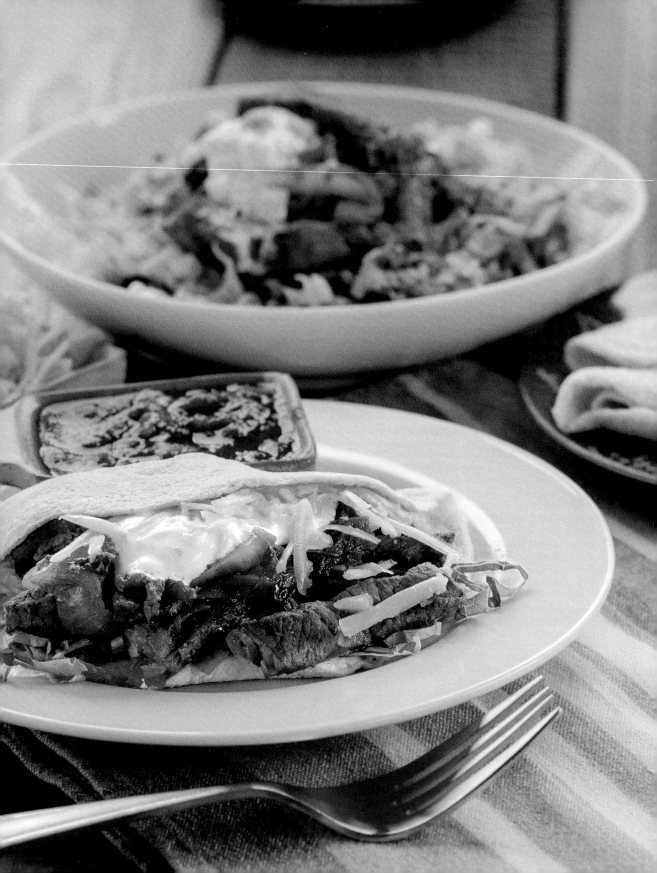

slow fajitas

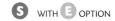 **S** WITH **E** OPTION

2 to 2½ pounds thawed and drained boneless beef or venison strips, or boneless chicken breasts cut into strips (try a combination of chicken and beef)

3 large green bell peppers, cut into strips

2 large onions, cut into strips

2 (14½-ounce) cans diced tomatoes, drained

2 teaspoons ground cumin

2 teaspoons chili powder

1¾ teaspoons Mineral Salt

1 teaspoon onion powder

½ teaspoon garlic powder, or 2 garlic cloves, minced

¼ teaspoon cayenne pepper (optional)

2 tablespoons coconut oil or butter

1. Put the meat and/or chicken in the cooker.

2. Add the peppers, onions, and tomatoes; add all the seasonings and coconut oil or butter, then stir gently to combine.

3. Cook on low heat all day or on high heat for 5 to 6 hours.

SERVING IDEAS: Use a slotted spoon to scoop out the meat, chicken, and veggies onto a bed of finely shredded lettuce (from the bag is fine for Drive Thru Sue's). Top with sour cream, grated cheese, and salsa with some optional diced avocado. You could also choose to roll up the mixture in store-bought low-carb tortillas or Wonder Wraps (page 204). Caution, however: this makes a lot of liquid when cooked in the crockpot, so you'll need to use that slotted spoon and even press out a lot of the liquid from the meat if using with bread or wrap items.

NOTE: For an **E** version, omit the coconut oil or butter, use the chicken breast option only, and enjoy with half **E** servings of both brown rice and refried beans. Top with salsa.

FOR FREEZER-TO-CROCK PREP: Cut thawed meat into strips and place in freezer bag and label as "Slow Fajitas – S" with a Sharpie. Put all the other ingredients into another large freezer bag. Label the freezer bag with recipe name and put both bags in the freezer. The morning before cooking (24 hours prior), put the bags in the refrigerator to thaw. Next morning, pour off any excess fluid from the meat or chicken, and place the meat or chicken in the crockpot. Add the other bag of ingredients.

NSI DF (IF OMITTING CHEESE; YOU CAN USE SUBSTITUTE HELLO CHEESE, PAGE 487)

cilantro lime-burst chicken thighs Ⓢ

6 to 8 pounds thawed and drained chicken thighs with skin and bone

1 bunch fresh cilantro

1 medium onion, diced

4 to 6 large mixed-color bell peppers, cored, seeded, and julienne sliced

1 family package Not Naughty Rice (optional)

1 cup frozen diced okra

½ to ¾ cup fresh lime juice

2 teaspooons Mineral Salt

½ teaspoon black pepper

½ teaspoon garlic powder, or 1 to 2 garlic cloves, minced

Not only is this meal rich in the gelatin that is released from the chicken bones, which helps heal and nourish your gut, but the okra here also does its own healing magic on your stomach. The okra is undetectable in this dish, so we've never felt the need to mention it to our children or husbands. Some things are better left unsaid.

1. Place the chicken thighs in the crockpot.
2. Remove the leaves from the cilantro and chop half of them (save stems for blending). Add the chopped cilantro, diced onion, julienned peppers, and Not Naughty Rice (if using) on top of the chicken.
3. Blend the remaining cilantro (stems and remaining leaves) with the okra, lime juice, and seasonings. Pour over the chicken and veggies.
4. Cook on high heat for 6 to 8 hours.

NOTE: If you choose not to use the Not Naughty Rice, this dish is delicious served over Cauli Rice (page 225) for those needing to stick to a single fueling or over brown rice for growing children as a Crossover.

FOR FREEZER-TO-CROCK PREP: Label frozen bags of chicken thighs as "Cilantro Lime-Burst Chicken Thighs" with a Sharpie. Blend half the cilantro with the lime juice, okra, and seasonings and pour into freezer bag. Add the peppers and chopped cilantro and label the bag with name of recipe. If you intend to include the Not Naughty Rice, write "needs NNR" as a reminder. Put the chicken and sauce bags in the freezer next to each other. The morning before cooking (24 hours prior), place both bags in the refrigerator to thaw. Next morning, pour off any excess fluid from the chicken and add the chicken to the crock, then add the bag of sauce and veggies, and the optional NNR (if using).

NSI (IF OMITTING THE NOT NAUGHTY RICE) DF

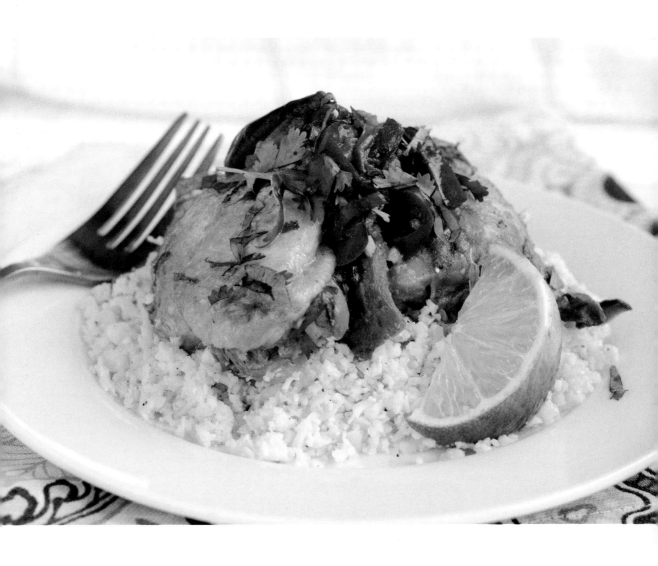

balsamic chicken

FAMILY SERVE – FEEDS 6 TO 8 (HALVE INGREDIENTS IF YOUR FAMILY IS SMALLER)

2½ pounds thawed and drained boneless, skinless chicken breasts or tenderloins

2 large onions, sliced into long strips, or 1 (16-ounce) package frozen pearl onions

2 (14½-ounce) cans diced tomatoes

1½ tablespoons Italian seasoning

½ teaspoon onion powder

1 teaspoon garlic powder, or 3 or 4 garlic cloves, minced

½ teaspoon Mineral Salt

1 to 2 doonks Pure Stevia Extract

¼ cup balsamic vinegar

½ cup chicken broth or bone stock (pages 495–496)

1. Put the thawed and drained chicken breasts in the crockpot.

2. Lay the onions and tomatoes on top of the chicken, and then add the seasonings.

3. Add the vinegar and broth, and stir gently to blend.

4. Cook on low heat all day or on high heat for 5 to 6 hours.

SERVING IDEAS: This dish lends itself perfectly to **E** mode. The chicken, veggies, and yummy broth are perfect over a bed of brown rice or quinoa. For **S** mode, serve over any on-plan noodles, like Not Naughty Noodles or Troodles (page 222), or Spaghetti Squash (page 224), then top with some grated mozzarella cheese—perfection! To stay in Fuel Pull mode, keep the meat portion to between 3 and 4 ounces, and wrap the chicken in Wonder Wraps (page 204) or have over Cauli Rice (page 225) or Not Naughty Rice.

FOR FREEZER-TO-CROCK PREP: Label frozen bag of chicken breasts or tenderloins as "Balsamic Chicken – S" with a Sharpie. Pour all other ingredients into another freezer bag. Label the freezer bag with recipe name and put both bags in the freezer. The morning before cooking (24 hours prior), put the chicken and sauce bags in the refrigerator to thaw. Next morning, pour off any excess fluid from the chicken and place the chicken in the crockpot. Add the sauce.

NSI (IF USING YOUR FAVORITE HANDY ON-PLAN SWEETENER) DF (IF NOT USING MOZZARELLA CHEESE)

FAMILY SKILLET MEALS

Grab your big ol' iron skillet, just like Grandma used to use. We have two weeks worth of the tastiest, fillingest, no-fuss Trim Healthy Mama skillet meals right here for you and your family. These will work even if you've got less than half an hour to get the evening meal on the table—no worries. You got this!

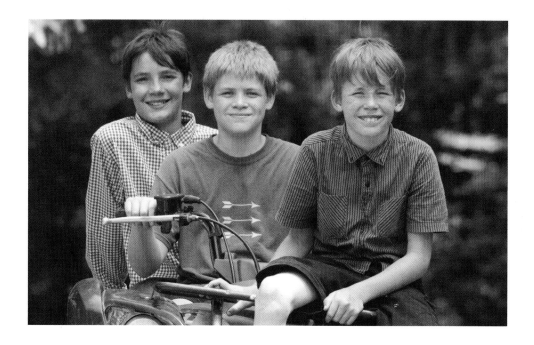

cabb and saus skillet

⑤

Coconut oil cooking spray

1½ pounds smoked sausage, sliced

3 tablespoons butter

1 very large cabbage, cored and sliced

½ cup chicken broth or bone stock
(pages 495–496)

¾ teaspoon Mineral Salt

¼ teaspoon black pepper

2 tablespoons nutritional yeast
(optional)

Dash of onion powder and garlic
powder (optional)

PEARL CHATS: This is a favorite in my home. It's so stinking quick and painless to make that I always relax a little when I know it is on the menu. My teenage boys love this with a side of Deviled Eggs (page 228). Cabbage is one of the most inexpensive veggies you can buy, yet it is a potent cancer fighter. The more cabbage you eat, the more you protect yourself and your family against many diseases.

For this recipe, we use jalapeño turkey or beef sausage, but you can use any type of pre-cooked sausage of your preference, and it does not need to be smoked.

1. Spray a large skillet with coconut oil, turn the heat to medium high, and brown the sausage pieces for a few minutes, flipping all the pieces a few times so they don't burn. Remove the sausage from the skillet and set aside.

2. Melt the butter in the same skillet, then add the cabbage, tossing for a minute in the butter, then add the broth and seasonings and cover the skillet. Cook for 3 to 4 minutes.

3. Uncover, toss the cabbage again, re-cover, and cook for another 5 to 7 minutes, tossing occasionally.

4. Return the sausage to the skillet, toss all together, then serve.

NOTE: Many smoked sausage meats are in the 5 to 6 carb range. These needless carbs are sugar or other fillers. Try to keep your net sausage carbs to 2 or less, but 3 can still slip by.

NSI (WITHOUT THE NUTRITIONAL YEAST) DF

cowboy grub

FAMILY SERVE – FEEDS 6 TO 8 (HALVE INGREDIENTS IF YOUR FAMILY IS SMALLER)

2 pounds ultra-lean ground meat (turkey or venison are great)

3 cups Seasoning Blend (frozen diced onion, celery, and pepper), or 2 large onions and 3 green bell peppers, chopped

2 cups cooked brown rice, or 2 cups parboiled "instant brown rice" plus 1¾ cups water

2 (14½-ounce) cans diced tomatoes, or 3 (10-ounce) cans mild Rotel-style tomatoes and chilies

1 (15-ounce) can pinto beans, rinsed and drained, or 1½ cups cooked pinto beans, drained

1 (14½-ounce) can corn kernels, or 1½ cups frozen corn kernels (drained)

1½ tablespoons chili powder

1½ teaspoons garlic powder

1½ teaspoons ground cumin

1½ teaspoons Mineral Salt

¼ teaspoon black pepper

¼ teaspoon cayenne pepper (optional)

This is a thick, hearty hash that is easy on your budget because it can be stretched a long way, especially if your kids stuff it into whole-grain tortillas with cheese and sour cream as a hearty Crossover. Our teenage boys love this stuff! To stay in clean E mode, you can serve yours in a bowl topped with Greek yogurt, a small sprinkling of skim-milk mozzarella, and a few crumbled blue corn chips or Blendtons (page 476) or Joseph's Crackers (page 453).

We have Stephanie Copeland to thank for this recipe. You can read more about her THM story in the "Heads Up: Turtle Losers!" chapter of *Trim Healthy Mama Plan*. Stephanie came to Trim Healthy Mama from a lifetime of dieting. She'd been afraid of carbs most of her adult life, losing and gaining the same 50 pounds over and over on her low-carb diets. Owing to a damaged metabolism, it took Stephanie a few months to see any weight loss with Trim Healthy Mama, but it started once she got over her fear of E meals and began to add in healthy carbs! She remembered this recipe that her grandma used to make when Stephanie was a child. It fits the THM plan perfectly as a filling E meal.

1. Brown the meat in a large skillet. If the meat is not at least 96% fat free, rinse under very hot water after cooking, then return it to the skillet.

2. Add the Seasoning Blend and stir until the peppers and onions start to tenderize, about 2 minutes.

3. If you are using parboiled rice, add both the rice and the water, stir, cover the pan, and simmer for 5 minutes.

4. Stir in the remaining ingredients (including the cooked rice, if you are using that) and continue to heat, stirring, until all is cooked through and the rice is no longer crunchy.

NOTE: Instant brown rice should not be confused with instant oatmeal, which is not as kind to your blood sugar. Instant brown rice has simply been partially cooked and has no higher glycemic effect. If you can fit another can of pinto beans into your skillet without it overflowing, feel free to do so. Leftovers of this meal are always devoured.

NSI DF (IF NOT TOPPING WITH ANY CHEESE)

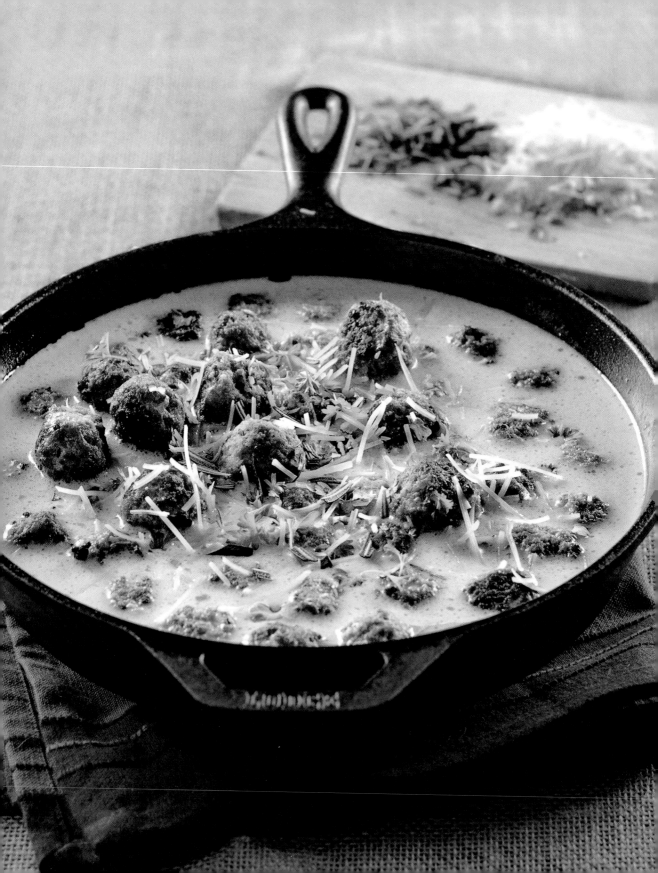

swedish meatballs in cream sauce

FOR THE MEATBALLS

2 pounds ground meat (beef or turkey work well)

1 large egg plus 2 egg whites (⅓ cup from carton)

6 tablespoons Trim Healthy Mama Baking Blend

¾ teaspoon Mineral Salt

1 teaspoon onion powder

1 teaspoon garlic powder

2 tablespoons butter or coconut oil

FOR THE CREAM SAUCE

4 tablespoons (½ stick) butter

¼ cup Trim Healthy Mama Baking Blend

3½ cups chicken broth

1 teaspoon Mineral Salt

¼ teaspoon black pepper

½ teaspoon onion powder

2 tablespoons nutritional yeast

Up to 1 teaspoon Gluccie

½ cup sour cream

Watch out—your family is going to gobble this up!

1. Make the meatballs. Combine the ingredients except the butter and mix well. Form into small meatballs (they cook faster than large ones). Figure on each person getting about 5 meatballs (except for little tykes, of course).

2. Sauté the meatballs in the butter until cooked through and crispy, about 7 minutes. They will be squished tight into your skillet, but it is faster to get them all cooked at once if you can manage that; they will shrink and create more room as they cook. Turn the meatballs to brown on all sides, then transfer to a paper towel–lined plate.

3. Make the sauce. Melt the butter in the same skillet, leaving all the crispies from the meat, and add the Baking Blend; whisk well until thickened. Add the broth and seasonings, then whisk well and bring to a simmer.

4. Put 1 teaspoon of Gluccie in an empty salt or spice shaker, and shake over the sauce in the pan, whisking well at the same time. Simmer until the sauce becomes thickened somewhat, then add the sour cream and whisk well again.

5. Return the meatballs to the skillet and simmer until they are cooked through (about 10 minutes). The sauce will thicken even more as it simmers. Add more broth if it gets too thick.

SERVING IDEAS: Enjoy over Troodles (page 222), Spaghetti Squash (page 224), or with rinsed and drained Not Naughty Noodles or Not Naughty Rice. Now-and-then Drive Thru Sue's may want to enjoy this over Dreamfields pasta; however, don't opt for that choice every time you make this.

egg roll in a bowl

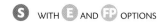

FAMILY SERVE – FEEDS 6 TO 8 (HALVE INGREDIENTS IF YOUR FAMILY IS SMALLER)

2 pounds thawed ground meat

2 medium (or 1 large) onions, chopped

2 to 3 tablespoons toasted sesame oil (or oil of your choice if you don't have sesame, but the sesame really makes the dish!)

4 garlic cloves, minced

2 teaspoons ground ginger

⅓ cup soy sauce, or 1 to 2 generous squirts Coconut aminos or Bragg liquid aminos

1 very large head of cabbage, cored and thinly sliced, or 2 to 3 (16-ounce) bags coleslaw mix

4 green onions, finely chopped

Mineral Salt and black pepper

1 teaspoon red pepper flakes (optional)

Same great taste you get in an egg roll, minus the deep-fried wrapper! Unbelievably easy to make, SUPER quick, and extremely budget friendly! Diana Rodbourn posted this recipe in the main Trim Healthy Mama Facebook group and it has been a runaway hit ever since. Diana uses pork for this recipe, but we have great success with beef or turkey.

1. Brown the meat in a large skillet over medium heat until fully cooked.

2. Turn up the heat to medium high and add the chopped onions and sesame oil, and lightly brown the onions.

3. In a small bowl, mix the garlic, ginger, and soy sauce and add to the skillet, then immediately add the cabbage and stir well (cabbage will threaten to spill out of the pan but it will soon shrink and fit). Cook for several more minutes, until the cabbage is tender and wilted, stirring often.

4. Turn off the heat, and add the green onions and salt and black pepper to taste. Stir one last time, sprinkle with the red pepper flakes (if using), and serve.

NOTE: To make this an **E** meal, enjoy it over rice or quinoa. Make sure to use extra-lean meat (at least 96% lean) or brown the meat and then rinse well under hot water to remove fat before returning to the skillet. Use no more than 2 tablespoons of oil. Owing to a lack of juiciness (fat) in the meat, add ¼ cup of fat-free chicken broth or water. To make this a Fuel Pull, follow same directions for **E,** but enjoy over Cauli Rice (page 225) or Not Naughty Rice.

NSI DF

slim sloppy joes

FAMILY SERVE – FEEDS 6 TO 8 (HALVE INGREDIENTS IF YOUR FAMILY IS SMALLER)

2 pounds ground beef or venison

2 cups Seasoning Blend (frozen diced onion, celery, and pepper)

1 (6-ounce) can tomato paste

1 (8-ounce) can tomato sauce

¾ cup water

3 to 4 tablespoons prepared yellow mustard

1 teaspoon Mineral Salt

1 teaspoon onion powder

½ teaspoon garlic powder

1 teaspoon chili powder

1½ teaspoons Super Sweet Blend, or 2 doonks Pure Stevia Extract

1½ tablespoons apple cider vinegar

Dash of cayenne pepper

PEARL CHATS: My family is crazy about this meal. If it's not on the menu every week or so, they start asking for it. Most of my children are still growing like weeds, so they have their joes with lots of grated cheese in between buttered slices of whole-grain toast. My husband loves this open face, on thin slices of Swiss Loaf (page 198) or on the single-serve Swiss Bread made in the muffin tins (page 196) for a more traditional approach—it's quicker, too. I love this meal not only for the flavor but also for its ease of preparation. You don't even have to chop anything when you use the handy frozen Seasoning Blend. Sweet Creamy Coleslaw (page 230) or Light and Lovely Coleslaw (page 231) are the perfect pairings for this meal.

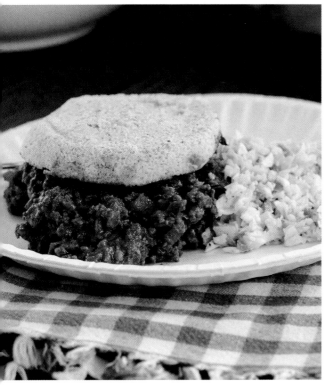

1. Brown the meat in a large skillet, then briefly remove the meat and drain most of the fat (keep some in for flavor); return the meat to the skillet. (If your meat is lean, there is no need to drain the fat, so you can save time.)

2. Add the Seasoning Blend and sauté for a few minutes, stirring with the meat.

3. Add the remaining ingredients, stir well, and simmer for 10 minutes.

4. Serve on plan-approved bread or make sandwiches with it, adding some grated cheese.

NOTE: You can easily convert this into an **E** meal by using ultra-lean meat (at least 96% lean) or by rinsing the browned meat very well under hot water to release any extra fat. Use a sprouted roll or two pieces of sprouted bread or Artisan Sourdough Bread (page 206).

NSI (IF USING YOUR FAVORITE HANDY ON-PLAN SWEETENER) DF (IF NOT TOPPING WITH GRATED CHEESE; CAN USE GRATED HELLO CHEESE, PAGE 487)

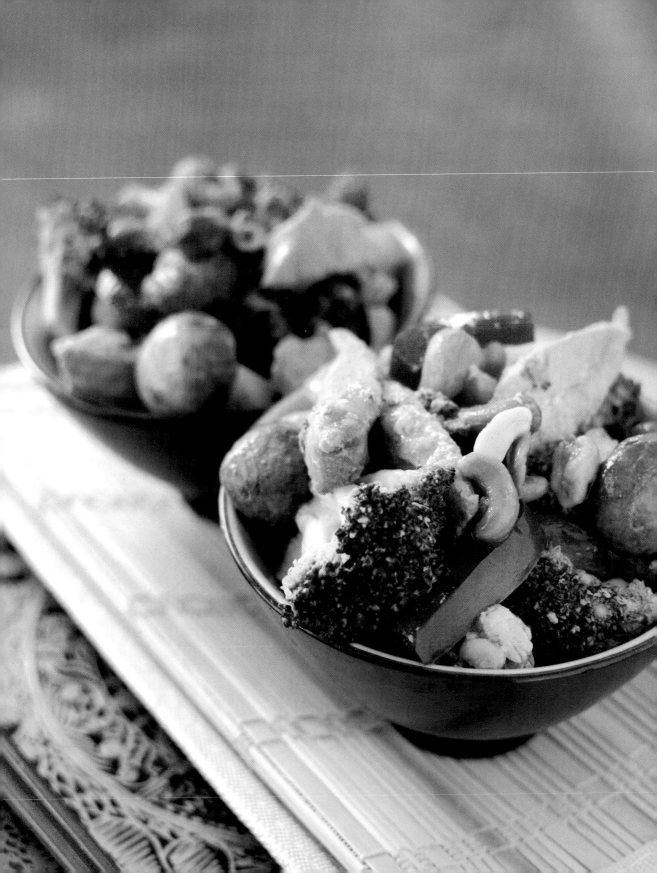

cashew chicken

FOR THE CHICKEN

1 tablespoon coconut oil or butter

2½ pounds boneless chicken breasts, tenderloins, or thighs, thawed, cut into bite-size pieces

FOR THE SAUCE

⅓ cup soy sauce, or 1 to 2 generous squirts Bragg liquid aminos

⅓ cup rice vinegar

2½ tablespoons minced fresh ginger

2½ tablespoons fish sauce

2½ tablespoons toasted sesame oil

1½ teaspoons Super Sweet Blend

½ to ¾ teaspoon red pepper flakes

2 garlic cloves, minced

About ½ teaspoon Gluccie

FOR THE VEGGIES

1½ heads of broccoli, cut into florets

2 red or yellow bell peppers, cored, seeded, and sliced

12 ounces button or baby portbello mushrooms

⅔ cup roasted cashews, chopped small (see Note)

1. Make the chicken. Heat a large skillet over medium-high heat and add the coconut oil. Add the chicken and let the pieces begin to sear, turning the pieces when they brown. Remove the chicken and set aside.

2. Make the sauce. Put all the ingredients in a blender and blend well for a few seconds.

3. Finish the dish. Turn the heat down to medium, and add the sauce from the blender and the broccoli, peppers, and mushrooms. Cook for 10 minutes, or until the veggies are almost cooked. Add the chicken, stir well, and cook 5 minutes more, or until the chicken is cooked through. The Gluccie should cause the sauce to thicken a little more as it simmers, but you could shake in a little more if it's too thin for your liking or add more chicken broth if it's too thick.

4. Just before serving, sprinkle on the cashews.

SERVING IDEAS: Eat this flavorful dish on its own or over Not Naughty Noodles or Cauli Rice (page 225). Kids or those at maintenance stage will enjoy this dish over brown rice.

NOTE: Peanuts or slivered almonds may be used instead. Cashews are a little on the higher side of carbs when it comes to nuts, so keeping them chopped small means you get a little of their goodness in most bites. If you like, you can make the sauce ahead of time (minus the Gluccie) and marinate the chicken in it all day or overnight. This increases the flavor.

NSI (IF USING XANTHAN INSTEAD OF GLUCCIE) DF

2½ pounds thawed and drained chicken tenderloins, can leave as tenderloins or cut into smaller pieces

Mineral Salt, black pepper, garlic powder, chili powder, and ground cumin, for blackening

Coconut oil cooking spray

1 tablespoon butter

2½ cups frozen mango chunks

2½ cups Seasoning Blend (frozen diced onion, celery, and pepper)

1 (15-ounce) can black beans, rinsed and drained

Juice of ½ lime

¼ teaspoon black pepper

1½ teaspoons Super Sweet Blend

¼ teaspoon red pepper flakes (optional)

Sweet and tangy with a little bit of heat, this is another great E meal that won't leave you hungry afterward. If you work outside the home, leftovers make for a yummy lunch rolled up into a low-carb tortilla or Wonder Wrap (page 204). If your little children aren't too keen on the mango–black bean sauce, they'll love the cooked chicken pieces, so set some aside for them—more sauce for you!

1. Lightly sprinkle the top sides of the chicken pieces with the salt, pepper, and garlic powder, then generously sprinkle with the chili powder and cumin to fully cover for a blackening effect.

2. Heat a large skillet over medium-high heat and spray lightly with coconut oil spray, then add the butter. Once the skillet is hot and the butter has melted, add the chicken, blackened side down. While the underside is browning, blacken the tops by sprinkling on more seasonings as before. Turn the pieces once after about 5 minutes, and continue until the pieces are cooked through. Remove the chicken and set aside on a plate.

3. Put the mango chunks in a food processor and pulse until they are in small pieces but not broken down to a puree. You'll want thumbnail-size pieces.

4. Add the Seasoning Blend, beans, mango, lime juice, and spices to the skillet and cook, stirring, for a few minutes.

5. Return the chicken to the skillet and heat through with the other ingredients for another minute or two.

SERVING IDEAS: Serve over small amount of cooked brown rice or quinoa (less than ½ cup) since you have the **E** fuels of beans and mango already, or enjoy on its own.

NSI DF

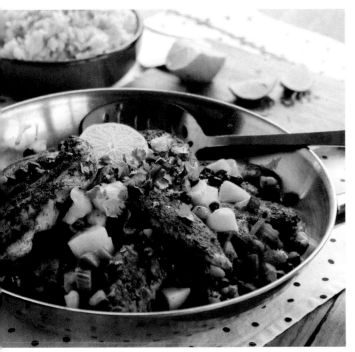

chicken alfredo

2½ pounds thawed and drained boneless chicken breasts, tenderloins, or thighs, cut into bite-size pieces

Mineral Salt, black pepper, and garlic and onion powder, for seasoning chicken

2 tablespoons butter

FOR THE SAUCE

4 tablespoons (½ stick) butter

½ cup heavy cream

1 cup finely grated Parmesan cheese (green can kind is fine)

¾ to 1 teaspoon black pepper

¼ teaspoon Mineral Salt

2½ cups chicken broth

½ to 1 teaspoon Gluccie

½ cup grated part-skim mozzarella cheese

1 family package Not Naughty Noodles (optional)

We Trim Healthy Mamas love butter and cream, and refuse to deny ourselves the indulgence. But this does not mean we should take an opposite extreme and abuse those calories. You can make a creamy Alfredo sauce without having to use two sticks of butter and 2 whopping cups of cream! This is the sensible way to eat Alfredo—still all the taste of the good stuff but cut with some chicken broth and thickened with the help of Gluccie (or xanthan). Don't be weirded out by the Gluccie and think that your sauce will be slimy; you'll use just enough to thicken the sauce as it reduces.

1. Sprinkle the chicken with the salt, pepper, and garlic and onion powders. Place in a large skillet and sauté all at once in the butter over medium-high heat. Sear on all sides, then transfer the partly cooked chicken to a plate and set aside.

2. Make the sauce. Put all the ingredients except the Gluccie and mozzarella in the skillet and place over medium heat. Slowly whisk in ½ teaspoon Gluccie. Simmer the sauce for several minutes; it should thicken somewhat as it cooks and reduces. If after 5 minutes it is not thick enough, add another ¼ to ½ teaspoon Gluccie, whisking well. Simmer for a couple more minutes, then add the grated cheese and stir to combine.

3. If using the Not Naughty Noodles, add them to the saucepan and simmer so they take on the flavor of the sauce, 2 to 3 more minutes.

4. Add the chicken to the skillet and simmer for another 5 minutes, until cooked through. Taste and adjust the seasonings, then serve to your liking—"own it"!

SERVING IDEAS: If your budget does not allow for the Not Naughty Noodles, you can serve the chicken and sauce over Troodles (page 222) or Spaghetti Squash (page 224). Growing children may enjoy their portion over whole-grain noodles.

NSI (WITHOUT NOT NAUGHTY NOODLES OR IF USING XANTHAN IN PLACE OF GLUCCIE)

taco time

FAMILY SERVE – FEEDS 6 TO 8 (HALVE INGREDIENTS IF YOUR FAMILY IS SMALLER)

2 pounds thawed ground beef, venison, or turkey

2 large onions, or 2½ cups Seasoning Blend (frozen diced onion, celery, and pepper)

2 garlic cloves, minced, or ½ teaspoon garlic powder

2 tablespoons chili powder

2 teaspoons ground cumin

2½ teaspoons paprika

1¾ teaspoons Mineral Salt

¼ teaspoon black pepper

¼ teaspoon cayenne pepper, or to taste

1½ teaspoons onion powder

1 (8-ounce) can tomato sauce

1 (15-ounce) jar salsa

½ cup refried beans (see Note)

2 cups grated cheddar cheese (dairy-free can use grated Hello Cheese, page 487)

1. Brown the meat in a large skillet over medium to medium-high heat. Pour off any grease that's been released if you're using store-bought fatty beef; keep any juices in the pan if using lean meat, or grass-fed source of beef.

2. Add the onions or Seasoning Blend and stir until the veggies start to tenderize.

3. Add the remaining ingredients except the cheese. Combine well and allow to simmer for 10 minutes or so.

4. Top with the cheese and allow it to melt on top. Don't stir anymore. Serve.

SERVING IDEAS: Enjoy this mix in romaine lettuce leaves that serve as slimming taco shells or fold into Wonder Wraps (page 204), or even low-carb wraps for a now-and-then option. Top with your choice of the following items: sliced avocado, sour cream, shredded lettuce, chopped ripe tomatoes, chopped fresh cilantro.

NOTE: The refried beans give a lovely hint of bean flavor in this dish without causing any major clashing problems with the **S** fuel per serving.

NSI DF (IF USING GRATED HELLO CHEESE, PAGE 487)

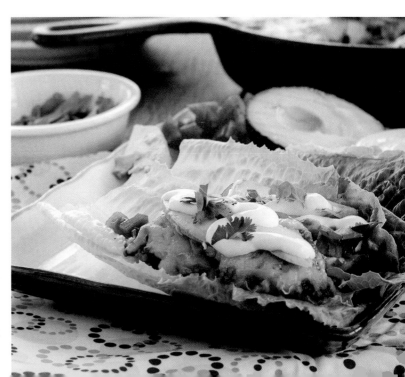

quinoa goes cajun

FAMILY SERVE – FEEDS 6 TO 8 (HALVE INGREDIENTS IF YOUR FAMILY IS SMALLER)

1½ to 2 pounds thawed, ultra-lean ground turkey, or diced pre-cooked chicken breast

3 cups Seasoning Blend (frozen diced onion, celery, and pepper), or 1 large green bell pepper, 5 celery stalks, and ½ medium onion, diced

4 garlic cloves, minced

1 tablespoon butter or coconut oil

3¾ cups chicken broth or water

3 tablespoons dried parsley

2 to 2½ teaspoons MSG-free Creole seasoning (such as Tony Chachere's Original Creole Seasoning)

1½ teaspoons ground sage

1½ cups quinoa, rinsed

1 (15-ounce) can red beans, drained and rinsed

We love quinoa for its nutritional profile. It is full of magnesium and iron, both important for pregnant and nursing women and also for those who suffer from headaches. Eat a quinoa-based meal if you feel a headache coming on; there is evidence it can help relieve headaches due to its favorable effect on the dilation of blood vessels. We also love quinoa because it is gentle on blood sugars, is gluten free (for our sensitive Mamas), and cooks up super quick.

The idea for this recipe was inspired by Amanda Coers, who is a Trim Healthy Mama with an awesome blog full of great on-plan recipes and Trim Healthy tips. She and her husband have dropped 100 pounds together on THM, and they are both healthier, at goal weight, and filled with a lot more energy for their big, beautiful family. There is Cajun blood in their family, so Amanda is always looking for ways to THM-ify Cajun foods. She came up with a Dirt–E rice recipe that was a big hit in the community. We've tweaked her idea to include quinoa, but it has the same great flavor. Visit Amanda's blog at www.thecoersfamily.com for more recipes.

1. If the turkey is at least 96% lean, put the turkey, Seasoning Blend, and garlic in a large skillet with a tight-fitting lid and add the butter and ¾ cup broth. If your ground turkey is not that lean, brown it first before adding the Seasoning Blend, butter, and water. Once browned, rinse it well under very hot water, return it to the skillet, then add those other ingredients. Cook over medium heat until the vegetables are tender.

2. Add the seasonings and stir well. If your skillet has a tight lid that does not allow steam to escape, add the quinoa and remaining 3 cups broth to the skillet. Bring to a quick boil then immediately turn the heat to low, cover the skillet, and simmer for 15 minutes. If your skillet does not properly seal with a lid, put the quinoa and broth in a saucepan with a tight-fitting lid, bring to a boil, then simmer for 12 to 15 minutes.

3. Once quinoa is cooked and fluffy, add the beans, toss everything together in the skillet, and serve in lettuce shells or in a bowl as one big tasty mess!

NSI DF

tilapia veracruz

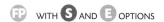
FAMILY SERVE – FEEDS 6 TO 8 (HALVE INGREDIENTS IF YOUR FAMILY IS SMALLER)

2 pounds thawed tilapia fillets

¾ to 1 teaspoon Mineral Salt, plus more for sprinkling over fish

Black pepper and chili powder, for sprinkling over fish

4 teaspoons butter

1 large onion, or 1½ cups Seasoning Blend (frozen diced onion, celery, and pepper)

2 to 3 garlic cloves, minced

2 poblano chilies, seeded and diced (or jalapeño peppers, if you like a lot of heat)

5 large ripe tomatoes, 2 diced and 3 left whole

15 sliced green olives

Juice of 2 limes

Chopped fresh cilantro (optional)

We first tasted this dish at a Mexican restaurant in Dallas just last year, when we were speaking at a conference. We both ordered it the first night of the weekend conference and loved it so much we went back the second night just so we could eat it again. We came home, played with the ingredients, and now get to enjoy it whenever we like.

It is often difficult to find wild-caught tilapia, and while most farm-raised fish is not optimal, according to Dr. Nicholas Perricone, author of *Ageless Skin, Ageless Mind,* farm-raised tilapia is a safe and healthy fish option. We buy frozen fillets, as they are much more affordable for big families like ours. Put the fillets in the fridge in the morning, and they should be thawed by late afternoon. If you forget to do that, though, keep them in their plastic packet wraps and thaw in a big pot of lukewarm water for a couple of hours.

1. Pat the tilapia fillets dry and lightly sprinkle the salt, pepper, and chili powder over them.

2. Melt 2 teaspoons butter in a large skillet over medium heat. Once hot, add half the tilapia (you may have to cut some of the fillets smaller to fit them in the pan). Brown the fillets for 2 minutes on each side (they do not have to be cooked through and it doesn't matter if they break apart somewhat). Remove from the pan and keep warm.

3. Melt the remaining 2 teaspoons butter in the skillet and repeat with the remaining fish. Remove and keep with first batch of fillets.

4. Put the onion, garlic, and poblanos in the skillet and sauté for a few minutes, tossing often.

5. Put the 3 whole tomatoes in the blender and puree. Once blended, add the tomato puree to the skillet along with the ¾ to 1 teaspoon salt and more pepper to taste. Allow the sauce to simmer for a few minutes.

6. Add the fish back to the skillet and allow to heat through and become fully cooked. You can break the pieces of fish up smaller, if desired.

7. Turn off the heat and add the diced tomatoes, olives, lime juice, and cilantro (if using).

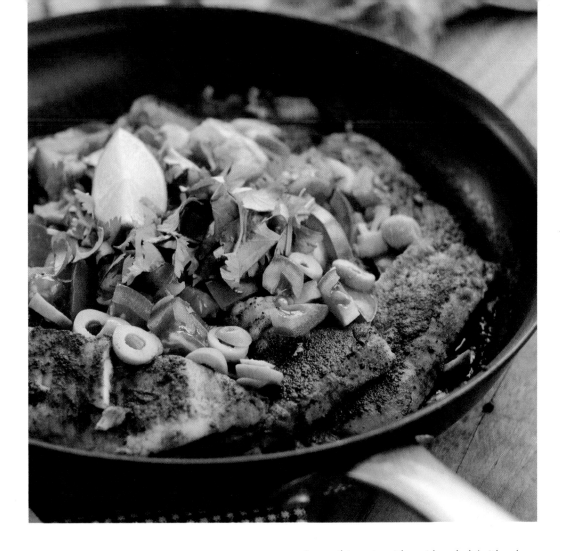

SERVING IDEAS: Serve this as is with a side salad (with a lean dressing) to stay in .**FP** mode or enjoy over Not Naughty Rice (sautéed in coconut oil spray in another small pan). Have over ¾ cup brown rice or quinoa for **E**. This recipe can easily be modified to **S** by using more fat during the cooking of the fish and then adding more butter before sautéing the veggies. You can also up the number of green olives in an **S** version. As appears here, we keep the number of olives well within fat guidelines for **FP** and **E**.

NOTE: Drive Thru Sue's can use two 14-ounce cans of petite diced tomatoes in place of the fresh tomatoes to make life easier, but the fresh tomato taste is amazing in this dish.

NSI DF

orange chicken

FAMILY SERVE – FEEDS 6 TO 8 (HALVE INGREDIENTS IF YOUR FAMILY IS SMALLER)

FOR THE CHICKEN

2½ to 3 pounds thawed and drained boneless chicken thighs or breasts, cut into bite-size pieces

¾ cup Trim Healthy Mama Baking Blend

1 teaspoon Mineral Salt

½ teaspoon black pepper

1 teaspoon Super Sweet Blend

5 to 6 tablespoons coconut oil

FOR THE SAUCE

½ cup soy sauce

2 garlic cloves, minced

1 teaspoon grated fresh ginger

4 teaspoons Super Sweet Blend

3 tablespoons rice vinegar

4 tablespoons water

½ teaspoon red pepper flakes

2 tablespoons toasted sesame oil

3 green onions, diced

2 teaspoons orange extract

⅓ to ½ teaspoon Gluccie

½ head green cabbage, very finely sliced, or use some packaged coleslaw mix

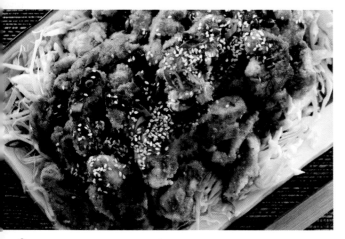

"Oh, boy," or should we say, "Oh, Mama!" We're so excited to give you and your family this recipe. All the sweet, spicy goodness of Chinese food is now Trim Healthy Mama–fied! This dish sits perfectly on angel hair sliced cabbage, so there's no need for extra time spent on cooked sides—or even a side salad unless you really wanna. Since this chicken is breaded, you may need to cook it in a couple of batches to get it properly browned, so we do cheat a little here and use one extra little saucepan to make the sauce separately. But don't worry; this is still a quick, simple meal. If you truly want to keep this to a strict one pot-to-wash meal, cook the chicken first in your skillet, remove it and set to the side, then make the sauce in your skillet, too—with all those little crispy bits of goodness left in! Even tastier! Open a bag of angel hair cabbage, and you have a meal ready that's fit for a dynasty!

1. Prepare the chicken for cooking. Place chicken pieces in a large bowl or 9 × 13-inch pan. Mix the Baking Blend, salt, pepper, and Super Sweet Blend in a small bowl, and sprinkle the chicken with the mixture. Stir to evenly coat the chicken pieces with the breading mix.

2. Mix all the sauce ingredients except the Gluccie in a medium saucepan, and bring to a simmer. Sprinkle in the Gluccie while whisking vigorously to almost the desired thickness. The sauce will thicken a little more the longer it simmers.

3. Cook the chicken. Heat the oil in a large skillet over medium heat and add the chicken pieces. You may need to cook it in two batches, so make sure to divide the coconut oil appropriately. Cook the chicken, turning once to cook evenly on both sides, for approximately 10 minutes. Cut a piece open to check for doneness.

4. Spread the cabbage on serving plates and divide the chicken among them, then drizzle the sauce over the top.

DF

reuben in a bowl

FAMILY SERVE – FEEDS 6 TO 8 (HALVE INGREDIENTS IF YOUR FAMILY IS SMALLER)

1 very large head of green cabbage,
cored and sliced, or 2 to 3 (16-ounce)
bags coleslaw mix

2 tablespoons butter

2 to 3 (14½-ounce) cans sauerkraut,
drained

2 pounds turkey pastrami or beef
pastrami (sliced)

3 to 4 cups shredded Swiss cheese

FOR THE DRESSING

½ cup plus 2 tablespoons mayonnaise
(Body-Burn Mayonnaise, page 470,
or store bought)

5 tablespoons sugar-free ketchup
(Trim Healthy Ketchup, page 482,
or store bought)

6 dashes hot sauce of choice

6 tablespoons dill relish

1 teaspoon Super Sweet Blend, or
2 teaspoons Gentle Sweet,
or to taste

Carol is an active Mama in the THM community. She shared this recipe and made thousands of other Mamas and their families very happy by doing so. If you love the flavors of Thousand Island dressing and pastrami, you're going to love this.

1. Place the cabbage in a large skillet with the butter and cook over medium heat until tender.

2. Add the sauerkraut and heat through.

3. Add the pastrami slices and continue to heat until all the flavors have blended, about 10 minutes.

4. Add three-fourths of the cheese and stir. Layer the rest of the cheese on top and heat until melted. Spoon the mixture into bowls.

5. Mix the ingredients for the dressing. Spoon the dressing over the pastrami-sauerkraut mixture and serve.

NSI

blt frittata

S

6 ounces bacon slices, diagonally cut
into large bite-size pieces

12 large eggs

2 cups grated cheese of choice

1 (8-ounce) package baby tomatoes,
sliced in half

½ medium onion, diced (optional)

¼ teaspoon Mineral Salt

¼ teaspoon black pepper

1 teaspoon dried parsley

Busy weeknight dinners can be saved as long as you have some bacon, veggies, and eggs in your house. A frittata is basically a crustless quiche cooked in a skillet and then finished in the oven. It's super quick and inexpensive. You'll need an oven-safe skillet for this. By the way, "BLT" here stands for "bacon loves tomato." The two really are a perfect match. Pair this frittata with a side salad and you'll have your lettuce, if you'd rather go with the traditional meaning.

Owing to our religious beliefs, we use turkey rather than pork bacon here, but that is totally your choice. But, say that you have a picky eater or two in your home—one doesn't like tomato, the other doesn't like bacon. Hold on—doesn't like bacon? Like that's going to happen? Just in case it does, though, this basic recipe can be the foundation for your own creation. Once you have your eggs, cheese, and seasonings, use or don't use the frittata ingredients as you wish—whatever your heart desires. Some additions are spinach, mushrooms, yellow squash, asparagus, or sausage.

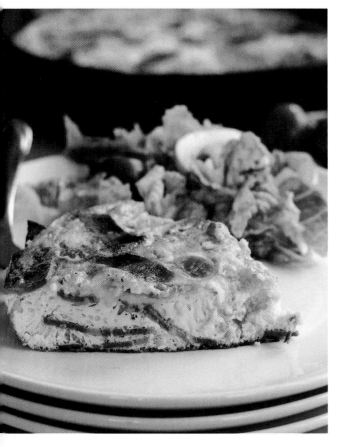

1. Preheat the broiler. Cook the bacon pieces in a large oven-safe skillet until slightly crisp (if using pork bacon, drain off most of the grease after cooking), then remove from the heat.

2. Whisk the eggs in a large mixing bowl until light, then add the cheese, tomatoes, and onion (if using). Stir in the salt, pepper, and parsley, and combine well. Pour the egg mixture into the skillet with the bacon, then put the skillet back over medium heat. Cover and cook for about 5 minutes, or until the egg mixture is just setting around the sides.

3. Place the skillet in the oven, uncovered, and broil for 3 to 5 minutes, until lightly browned on top. Keep a good eye on it because these few minutes go fast and you don't want to end up with a dark brown frittata.

NSI

QUICK SINGLE SKILLET MEALS

The following recipes make tasty, quick lunches if you're home during the lunch hour but they're also great to pre-cook, pack, and go if you (or your hub) work outside the home and have access to a refrigerator and—close your eyes, Serene—a microwave. Or, they make ultra-speedy single-serve dinners. If you've got between 5 and 15 minutes, you've got a meal!

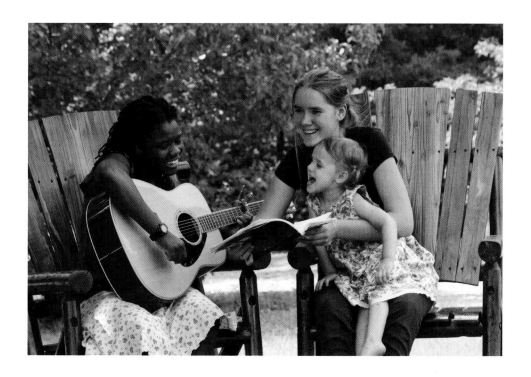

1 sweet potato, peeled and diced small

1 large tomato, diced finely

½ medium onion, diced finely

¼ cup chicken broth (or water with a pinch of Mineral Salt)

½ teaspoon Mineral Salt

⅛ teaspoon cayenne pepper, or ¼ teaspoon black pepper

1 tablespoon nutritional yeast

1 teaspoon apple cider vinegar

⅛ teaspoon garlic powder

¼ teaspoon ground cumin

1 or 2 sprinkles Creole seasoning (optional)

3 to 6 ounces cooked (or quick pouch or canned) **E** protein meat, like chicken breast or tuna

1 teaspoon extra-virgin coconut oil

Grated pecorino romano or finely grated Parmesan cheese (or Hello Cheese, page 487), for sprinkling

This sweet potato is pumped up! Some Mamas find they get hungry soon after an E meal. Keeping to just one sweet potato for safe blood sugar's sake can sometimes seem like there is not enough food on your plate. This recipe makes one sweetie grow volumes larger and it fills your bowl to the tippy top. When you need an E meal but you also want something that will stick to your ribs, you got this! And did we mention that it is scrumptulicious? There is nothing dry and stingy about it. Dig in and get full!

1. Place the sweet potato, tomato, and onion in a medium saucepan. Add the broth and bring to a boil over high heat. Tightly cover and simmer on lowered heat until tender.

2. Uncover the saucepan and turn up the heat a bit to allow the liquid to start to evaporate while you add the seasonings.

3. Start to smash everything with the back of a fork until nearly smooth. Add the cooked meat and toss all until heated.

4. Add the coconut oil and taste, adjusting the flavors to "own it." Garnish with a small amount of the cheese.

NOTE: If you are not a fan of spices like we are, you can always use more simple flavors. Stick to the salt and pepper and the cooking type of coconut oil or butter. You can also use a leftover baked sweetie. Reduce the broth to 2 tablespoons and cook the veggies without the 'tater. When the veggies are tender, add the baked sweetie, skin and all, and smash. Finish up following the directions and you are set for a yummy meal.

NSI DF (WITHOUT THE CHEESE OR SUBSTITUTING GRATED HELLO CHEESE, PAGE 487)

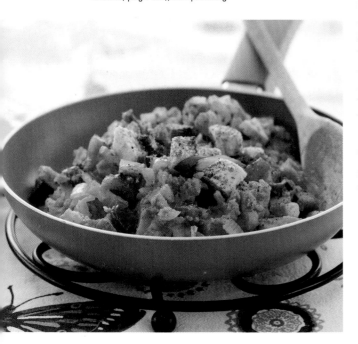

chicken chicken bang bang

SINGLE SERVE

Seasoning mixture of Mineral Salt, black pepper, and garlic powder

1 tablespoon Trim Healthy Mama Baking Blend, or 1 tablespoon coconut flour

3 to 6 ounces cooked chicken, cut into bite-size pieces

Coconut oil cooking spray

1 tablespoon coconut oil or butter

1 garlic clove, minced

¼ red bell pepper (sliced) or any other veggie like broccoli (optional)

2 teaspoons apple cider vinegar

1½ teaspoons Super Sweet Blend

⅛ to ¼ red jalapeño pepper (or more if you like a lot of heat)

⅓ cup water or chicken broth

⅛ teaspoon Gluccie

¼ teaspoon Mineral Salt

1 tablespoon mayonnaise (or 1 tablespoon plain Greek yogurt)

Dash of Sriracha sauce (optional)

1 single-serve package Not Naughty Noodles, rinsed and drained, or cooked Troodles (page 222)

This is a feisty, sweet heat sauce that shoots bursts of flavor into your mouth. We have Cindy Young to thank for this idea. She is a 62-year-old Trim Healthy Mama who had given up on any hope of ever finding her trim body again after menopause. But she surprised herself and went all the way to goal weight on plan and is now happily maintaining her new weight. She shared this combination of flavors with us, which is a healthy twist on a popular restaurant-chain dish. Cindy pairs the sauce with shrimp, but we decided to try it with leftover cooked chicken. We tweaked the recipe just a bit and absolutely love it this way. You can stick to peeled and deveined shrimp, if you prefer, but the quick breaded chicken option we do for a speedy lunch is wonderful—and sprouted tofu works just as well, too.

1. Add the seasoning mixture to the Baking Blend and mix.

2. Put the chicken in a bowl, spray with coconut oil, then toss with the Baking Blend mixture.

3. Melt the coconut oil in a medium skillet over medium-high heat. Add the chicken and garlic, and sauté until lightly brown, 3 to 4 minutes. Remove and set aside. If using other veggies (like red pepper or broccoli), cook them on medium-high for a few minutes in the skillet.

4. Blend all the remaining ingredients except the noodles in a blender on high until the jalapeño is pureed. Pour the sauce into the skillet and cook, whisking well, over medium heat until it is reduced a little and starts to thicken.

5. Add the Not Naughty Noodles or Troodles and chicken to the skillet, and stir.

NOTE: Can be made **FP** by reducing butter to 1 teaspoon, not going over 4 ounces of meat and using Greek yogurt in place of mayo.

NSI (IF USING XANTHAN OR TROODLES AND YOUR FAVORITE ON-PLAN SWEETENER)

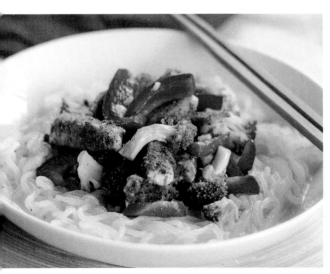

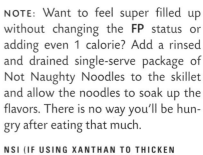
3 large handfuls of ultra-thin-sliced
   cabbage or coleslaw mix

⅓ to 1 cup chicken broth

1 to 2 light Laughing Cow cheese
   wedges, or 1 to 2 tablespoons
   Laughin' Mama Cheese (page 484)

3 to 4 pinches Mineral Salt

¼ teaspoon black pepper

¼ teaspoon onion powder

¼ teaspoon garlic powder

1 tablespoon finely grated Parmesan
   cheese (green can kind is fine)

Cayenne pepper to taste

1 to 2 squirts Bragg liquid aminos or
   dash or 2 of soy sauce

3 to 4 ounces diced cooked chicken
   breast

⅛ teaspoon Gluccie (optional)

There's no cream to be found in this recipe, but you wouldn't know it. This is a fast, filling Fuel Pull lunch (or even a supper, if you are on your own). Quadruple or more the recipe and feed the whole family this lovely dish, but make sure the children get some whole grains or fruit for some carbs (children don't need Fuel Pull suppers).

1. Put the cabbage in a small skillet with ⅓ to ½ cup broth. Cook over high heat until tender, stirring occasionally.

2. Reduce the heat to a simmer. Add the cheese and all the seasonings except the Gluccie. Stir until the cheese breaks down and melts into the broth. Simmer for about 1 minute, then add the chicken.

3. Decide if you want more sauce or not. If so, add the remaining ½ cup broth. Sprinkle in the Gluccie (if using) and whisk well until somewhat thickened. Taste and adjust the flavors.

NOTE: Want to feel super filled up without changing the **FP** status or adding even 1 calorie? Add a rinsed and drained single-serve package of Not Naughty Noodles to the skillet and allow the noodles to soak up the flavors. There is no way you'll be hungry after eating that much.

NSI (IF USING XANTHAN TO THICKEN INSTEAD OF GLUCCIE) DF (IF USING LAUGHIN' MAMA CHEESE, PAGE 484)

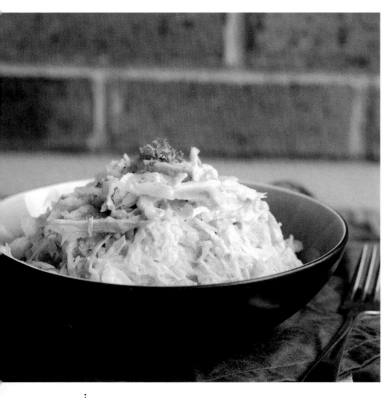

two-minute nutty noodles

SINGLE SERVE

1 to 2 teaspoons coconut oil

1 single-serve package Not Naughty Noodles, rinsed and drained

1 generous tablespoon crunchy natural-style peanut butter (no sugar added, we prefer crunchy style for this)

2 tablespoons soy sauce

Squeeze of fresh lime juice or lime juice from concentrate, about 1 tablespoon

Dash of hot sauce of choice

3 to 6 ounces diced or shredded cooked chicken or quick pouch salmon (optional)

1. Put the coconut oil in a medium saucepan and turn the heat to medium-high.

2. Add the noodles and toss for a minute or two in the oil.

3. Add the remaining ingredients and toss until combined.

NOTE: If you leave out the chicken or salmon, end your meal with something that contains protein like a Baby Frap (page 421), Collagen Tea (page 436), or a Healing Trimmy (pages 427–433), or have a few Lemon Pucker Gummies, Berry Yummy Gummies (pages 387–388), or Superfood Chocolate Chews (page 383).

NSI (IF USING STORE-BOUGHT KONJAC NOODLES) DF

lightly nutty noodles

SINGLE SERVE

1 teaspoon coconut oil

1 single-serve package Not Naughty Noodles, rinsed and drained

2 to 3 tablespoons Pressed Peanut Flour

2½ tablespoons soy sauce

Squeeze of fresh lime juice or lime juice from concentrate, about 1 tablespoon

Dash of hot sauce of choice

3 to 4 ounces diced or shredded cooked chicken or canned salmon

Same great flavor, just a Fuel Pull variation on the previous recipe.

Same as preparation for Two-Minute Nutty Noodles (above), substituting the peanut flour for the peanut butter.

DF

crispy salmon siesta

SINGLE SERVE

2 heaping tablespoons coconut oil
  or butter
1 salmon fillet, thawed (best with skin
  on, but still good without)
Mineral Salt, black pepper, chili
  powder, nutritional yeast, red pepper
  flakes, and sesame seeds, for
  sprinkling on fish
1 large yellow squash or zucchini,
  finely diced

Salmon lies down on a comfortable bed of succulent buttery yellow squash in this recipe. It may just want to take that nap, but you'll eat it before it can get too comfortable. Lunch is the perfect time to get healthy salmon into your life (or you can make it for a quick single dinner). We buy inexpensive frozen wild-caught fillets from budget grocery stores. Fish is quick to cook, and this recipe can turn you from being on the fence about salmon to diving over and loving it!

1. Place the coconut oil in a medium skillet and heat over medium heat.
2. Sprinkle one side of the fillet with the seasonings and lay the fillet seasoned side down in the skillet on one side of the pan.
3. Add the squash to the other side of the skillet and season the top side of the fish while the bottom is crisping and gently toss the squash occasionally in the pan juices.
4. Turn the salmon over to crisp the other side and to cook through, about 7 to 10 minutes total cooking. The squash may be ready a couple minutes before the salmon.
5. Put the squash on a plate and top with the salmon—you're done!

NSI DF

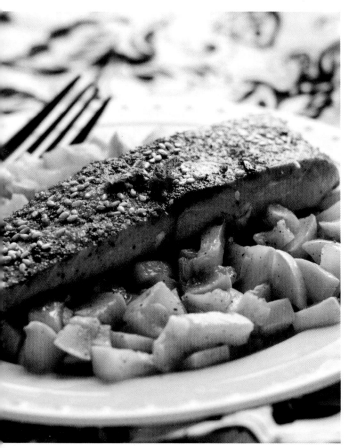

avo bacon noodle toss

4 bacon slices (turkey or other), cut into smaller pieces

1 teaspoon coconut oil (if using leaner turkey bacon)

1 to 2 garlic cloves, minced

½ green or red bell pepper, cored, seeded, and finely sliced

1 single-serve package Not Naughty Noodles, rinsed and drained

2 to 3 tablespoons soy sauce, or 1 to 2 squirts Bragg or Coconut liquid aminos

2 teaspoons toasted sesame oil

½ medium avocado, diced

Red pepper flakes

1. If using turkey bacon, cook it in the coconut oil in a small skillet along with the garlic and pepper until the bacon is crisp, about 5 minutes. If using pork bacon, simply sauté it in the skillet without the extra fat.

2. Add the noodles, soy sauce, and sesame oil. Stir to heat the noodles for a couple of minutes, then taste and adjust the seasonings.

3. Put the contents of the skillet in a bowl, add the avocado, and sprinkle with the red pepper flakes and enjoy.

NSI (IF USING STORE-BOUGHT KONJAC NOODLES) DF

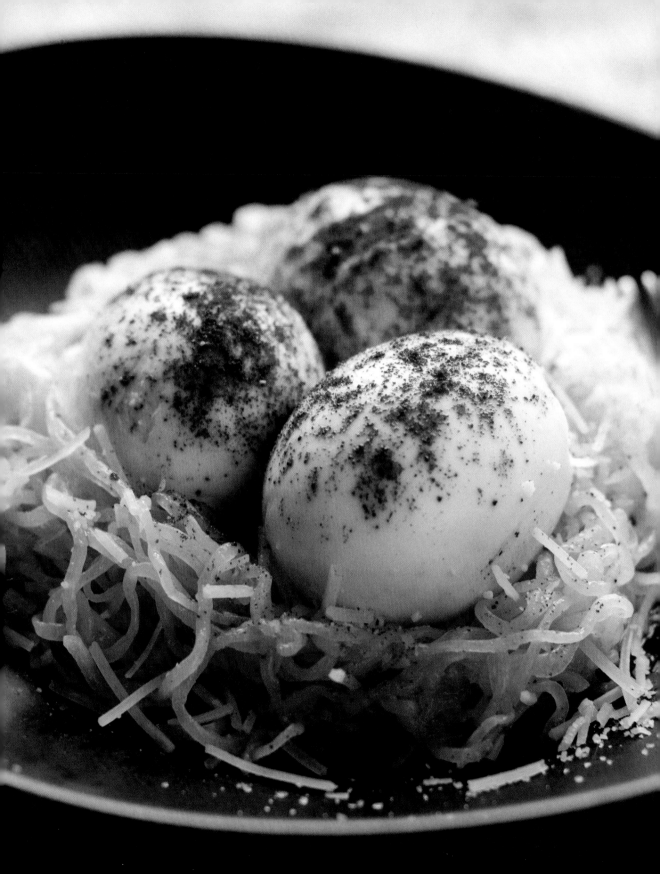

eggs in a nest

S

SINGLE SERVE

1 tablespoon butter or ghee
  (clarified butter)
1 single-serve package Not Naughty
  Noodles, rinsed and drained
Mineral Salt and black pepper to taste
½ teaspoon onion powder
⅛ to ¼ teaspoon garlic powder
1 to 2 tablespoons finely grated
  Parmesan cheese (green can kind is
  fine) or grated light sheep's cheese,
  like pecorino romano
1 tablespoon nutritional yeast
2 or 3 hard-boiled large eggs, peeled
  and still hot
Smoked or regular paprika

Weird name? The eggs sit in a tasty nest of Not Naughty Noodles. This recipe is super quick, super simple, and super delicious, and it looks like you are being served at one of those fancy-shmancy gourmet restaurants where food is for art's sake but you go home hungry. Well, this meal is beautiful and artsy, but it's also a real tummy filler.

1. Heat the butter in a medium skillet over medium-high heat. Add the noodles and toss in the butter. Add the salt and pepper, plus the onion powder, garlic powder, cheese, and nutritional yeast and toss well until warmed through.

2. Make a nest of the noodles on a dinner plate or in a large pasta bowl, then place the eggs in the center. Sprinkle with the paprika and a pinch of extra salt.

NSI (IF USING STORE-BOUGHT KONJAC NOODLES AND LEAVING OUT YEAST) DF (IF USING HELLO CHEESE, PAGE 487)

spiced eggy noodles

S

SINGLE SERVE

Coconut oil cooking spray
1 single-serve package Not Naughty
  Noodles, rinsed and drained
2 to 3 hard-boiled large eggs, chopped
3 tablespoons sour cream or Greek
  yogurt
¾ teaspoon curry powder
3 pinches Mineral Salt
Black pepper
Thinly sliced green onion (optional)

Another quick-as-a-flash lunch idea using eggs—or perhaps you're alone for dinner and don't want to fuss. If you have any boiled eggs in the fridge and a package of Not Naughty Noodles, you have your meal! If you don't have boiled eggs handy, boil several up and you'll have a few more for easy snack options.

1. Spray a medium skillet with coconut oil and place over medium-high heat.

2. Add the noodles, stir to coat with the oil, then add the remaining ingredients and toss until combined and hot.

SINGLE SERVE

¾ cup chicken broth

6 to 8 ounces (or half a 16-ounce bag) frozen stir-fry veggies

2 tablespoons Pressed Peanut Flour, or 1 teaspoon natural-style peanut butter

2 to 3 tablespoons soy sauce, or 1 to 2 squirts Bragg or Coconut liquid aminos

½ teaspoon Super Sweet Blend or 1 teaspoon Gentle Sweet

Several pinches of cayenne pepper, up to ⅛ teaspoon

¼ teaspoon onion powder

¼ teaspoon garlic powder

¼ teaspoon Gluccie (or enough to thicken sauce)

3 to 4 ounces cooked chicken breast or ultra-lean steak

Single-serve package Not Naughty Noodles, rinsed and drained (optional)

1. Put the broth and veggies in a medium skillet over medium-high heat, and cook until almost tender, stirring occasionally, about 5 to 8 minutes. (You can cover the skillet if you want to speed the process.)

2. Add the peanut flour, soy sauce, Super Sweet Blend, and the seasonings. Whisk well, then push the veggies to the side to make some room. Slowly whisk the Gluccie into the sauce. Simmer over low heat, allowing the sauce to thicken for a few more minutes (add only enough Gluccie to thicken to your own preference).

3. Taste and adjust the seasonings to "own it"—it may need more salt, or sweetness, or spice. Then add the chicken or steak and stir.

4. If using the Not Naughty Noodles, add them to the skillet and stir to heat through.

NOTE: You can make this an **E** meal by serving it with ¾ cup cooked brown rice or quinoa instead of the noodles.

NSI (IF USING STORE-BOUGHT KONJAC NOODLES, PEANUT BUTTER, AND YOUR FAVORITE ON-PLAN HANDY SWEETENER) DF

FAMILY SOUPS

Gather the family around—it's soup night! Down with small portions of flavorless diet broth. Let's eat hearty, delicious comfort food and get our bellies filled. The following recipes are not sides or starters to a meal—they *are* the meal! And you'll only have one pot to wash. The crowd goes wild! Eat these soups (and chili) alone or pair them with a side salad or on-plan bread option that suits the fuel of your meal. Blendtons (page 476) and crumbled Mad Melbas (page 454) or Swiss Crackers (page 455) are always fabulous with these recipes, too.

If you have children who don't yet eat as much as adults, you'll have leftovers for the next day's lunch, which deserves a very dorky happy dance.

trim zuppa toscana

(S)

2 pounds thawed ground sausage meat (spicy works great)

1 large onion, or 1½ cups Seasoning Blend (frozen diced onion, celery, and pepper)

2 tablespoons butter

2 quarts chicken broth

2 cups water

½ cup heavy cream

2 (16-ounce) bags frozen cauliflower florets

2 cups frozen diced okra

6 cups fresh kale or spinach

1¾ teaspoons Mineral Salt

¼ teaspoon black pepper

½ teaspoon onion powder

¼ teaspoon garlic powder

½ to 1 teaspoon red pepper flakes

Generous handful or two of real bacon crumbles or turkey bacon crumbles, optional

The Olive Garden restaurant made this soup famous. People who had previously never been kale fans suddenly changed their minds about that veggie with one slurp of this soup. There are many copycat recipe versions out there floating around in cyberspace, but this is our trimming version—and it's easy enough for any Drive Thru Sue!

The soup is a solid S, but thankfully it's not ridiculously loaded with abusive amounts of heavy cream; there's just enough to give a delicious and satisfying mouth feel when it's blended with the cauliflower and okra. You won't miss the potatoes that were in the original, either. We've subbed those out with cauliflower florets. (We've heard of people using water chestnuts or radishes as S potato subs, so you might have fun experimenting with those, but we are happy with our cauli.) We use venison sausage here because we have plenty of that in our freezers, thanks to the hunters in our families, but feel free to make this with pork, turkey, beef, or chicken sausage.

1. Brown the sausage with the onion (or seasoning blend) and butter in a large soup pot. Once the sausage is cooked through, transfer the meat and veggies to a bowl and set aside.

2. Pour the broth, water, and cream into the soup pot. Add the cauliflower and okra, cover the pot, turn the heat to high, and bring to a quick boil. Turn the heat down and simmer the veggies until tender (takes just a few minutes).

3. Using a slotted spoon, transfer about half the cauliflower and all the okra to a blender. Add 1 cup of the soup broth to the blender. Blend until smooth, then return the puree to the pot and stir to incorporate.

4. Return the sausage and sautéed veggies to the soup pot as well, then add the kale, seasonings, and bacon crumbles (if using), then simmer the soup for another 15 or so minutes. Taste and adjust the seasonings to "own it."

NSI

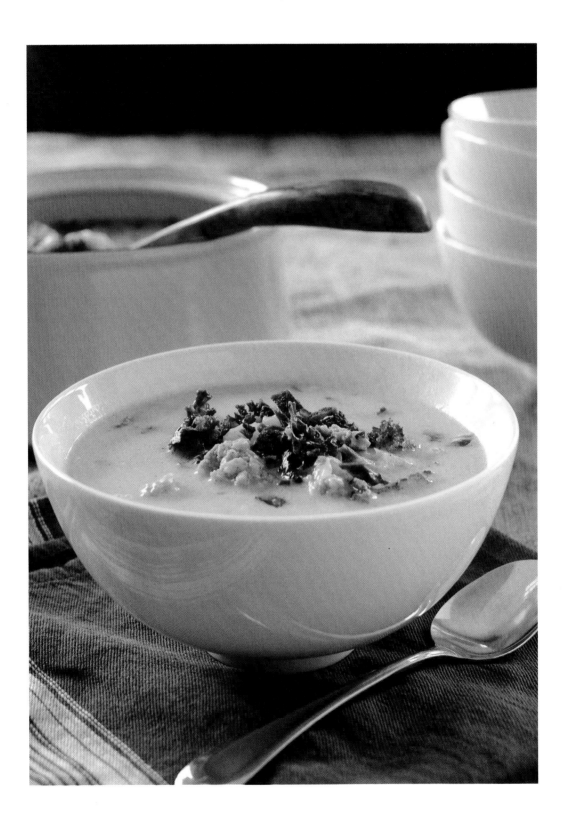

cheapskate soup

1 medium onion, or 1 cup Seasoning Blend (frozen diced onion, celery, and pepper)

1 tablespoon butter

12 cups water

2 pounds split peas, soaked and drained

4 teaspoons Liquid Smoke

3½ to 4 teaspoons Mineral Salt

¾ teaspoon black pepper

3 teaspoons onion powder

1 to 2 squirts Bragg liquid aminos (optional)

2 tablespoons nutritional yeast (optional)

⅓ cup turkey bacon crumbles (optional)

PEARL CHATS: Budgeting Mamas, this one's for you! Split peas are ridiculously inexpensive. You'll feed a hungry crowd for less than five bucks, and likely have leftovers. You'll want to soak your dried peas to avoid gassy problems (after all, this is not Trim Tooting Mama). Start that process early in the morning. Put dried peas in a bowl, cover with warm water, and add 1 tablespoon apple cider vinegar. Soak for approximately 7 hours, then drain and rinse. Once soaked, the peas will take less than 1 hour to be fully cooked and creamy. I like to start cooking this soup by mid-afternoon and simmer it long and slow. You can also cook it in the crockpot all day after soaking overnight.

This soup does contain some protein, but not as much as most of your other Trim Healthy Mama meals. If you want to up the protein content here, add some diced cooked chicken breast to the soup as your most budget-friendly E option or stir some Just Gelatin into your soup.

1. In large soup pot, sauté the onion in the butter, until translucent, about 3 minutes. Add the water and peas to the pot with all the seasonings. Cover the pot, turn the heat to high, and bring to a quick boil. Then turn the heat to low and simmer for a few hours (or cook a bit faster on medium heat for 1 hour or so).

2. Thirty minutes or so before serving, ladle some of the soup into a blender and puree (or use a stick blender in the pot). Add the puree back to the pot and stir. This helps create a creamier texture, but you want to keep some of the split peas in their whole state, too.

3. Add the bacon crumbles (if using). Taste and adjust the seasonings to "own it."

SERVING IDEAS: You can enjoy this soup with a piece or two of Swiss Bread (page 196) with just a small smear of butter, or there is still fuel room for a piece of **E** sprouted or sour dough toast. Or nix the bread and enjoy this with a side salad with lean dressing. Children will want to top theirs with lots of grated cheese for a Crossover effect.

NSI (WITHOUT NUTRITIONAL YEAST) DF

lentil soup

2 pounds brown lentils

4 cups chicken stock or bone broth (pages 495–496)

8 cups water

1 large onion, or 1½ cups Seasoning Blend (frozen diced onion, celery, and pepper)

3 teaspoons Mineral Salt

Black pepper

Cayenne pepper

2 teaspoons onion powder

1 teaspoon garlic powder

3 tablespoons nutritional yeast (optional)

2 to 3 generous squirts Bragg or Coconut liquid aminos (optional)

Chicken breast or Just Gelatin for added protein (optional)

This meal is cheap, cheap, cheap! It's tasty, too, not to mention being fantastic for your health. Let's hope you'll have enough left over for a bowl for lunch the next day, but beware: children go nuts over this as a yummy Crossover with grated cheese and whole-grain bread to dunk.

All beans and lentils are easier on the digestive system after they have been soaked in water for 7 hours, but lentils don't require the soaking as much. If you do want to soak them, put the lentils in a bowl, cover with water, and add 1 tablespoon apple cider vinegar; do this early in the morning, so you can start cooking your soup mid-afternoon (about 3 p.m.), as this soup is better cooked long and slow. Or, soak the lentils overnight and cook in the crockpot on high heat all day.

1. Put all the ingredients except the chicken (if using) in a large soup pot. Bring to a simmer over low heat and cook on low for several hours, until the lentils are extremely soft. Add more water if the soup is getting too thick for your liking.

2. Add the chicken or Just Gelatin (if using). Before serving, taste and adjust the seasonings to "own it."

SERVING IDEAS: Serve with a dollop of Greek yogurt and garnish with a smattering of grated skim-milk mozzarella for **E** or full-fat grated cheddar for a Crossover.

NSI (WITHOUT THE NUTRITIONAL YEAST) DF

chicken jalapeño popper soup

S

FAMILY SERVE – FEEDS 6 TO 8 (HALVE INGREDIENTS IF YOUR FAMILY IS SMALLER)

6 to 8 jalapeño peppers

1 large onion, chopped

2 red bell peppers, cored, seeded, and sliced

3 garlic cloves, minced

2 tablespoons butter

2 (16-ounce) bags frozen cauliflower florets

4 cups chicken broth or bone stock (pages 495–496)

8 ounces cream cheese

2 (14-ounce) cans diced tomatoes with juice

1 cup black beans, soaked and drained

2 to 2 ½ pounds cooked chicken breast, diced (see Note)

1 (12-ounce) jar salsa

4 teaspoons chili powder

2 teaspoons ground cumin

1 teaspoon Mineral Salt (or more to taste)

This soup went viral in the Trim Healthy Mama community. Carol Layman and Kara Reising are a mother-daughter team doing Trim Healthy Mama together. They came up with this recipe and want to share the love with you.

1. Remove the seeds and veins from the jalapeños and dice small.

2. In a large soup pot, sauté the onion, peppers, jalapeño, and garlic in the butter until golden, 3 to 5 minutes. Remove the veggies from the pot and set aside.

3. Put the cauliflower and broth in the soup pot, turn the heat to high, and bring to a quick boil. Reduce the heat to medium-high and cook until tender (takes just a few minutes).

4. Blend the cauliflower with the cream cheese in the pot using a stick blender or transfer all the cauli and cream cheese to a blender along with some of the broth and blend until smooth (you may have to do this in two batches if your blender is small).

5. Return the puree to the soup pot, add the sautéed veggies, then stir in the tomatoes, beans, chicken, salsa, and seasonings. Simmer until all the ingredients take on the great flavors.

SERVING IDEAS: Kara and Carol like to serve this soup topped with crumbled cooked bacon, shredded cheese, or diced fresh cilantro.

NOTE: You can use leftover chicken from Super Prepared Roasted Chicken (page 168). The 1 cup of beans in this large amount of soup still enables you to stay in **S** mode because it will be well less than ¼ cup beans per serving.

NSI

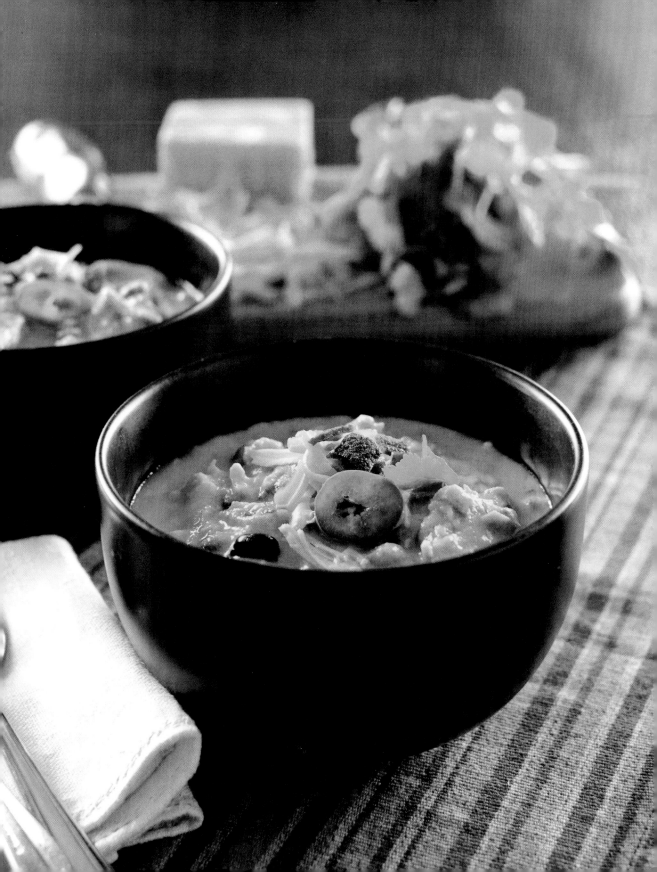

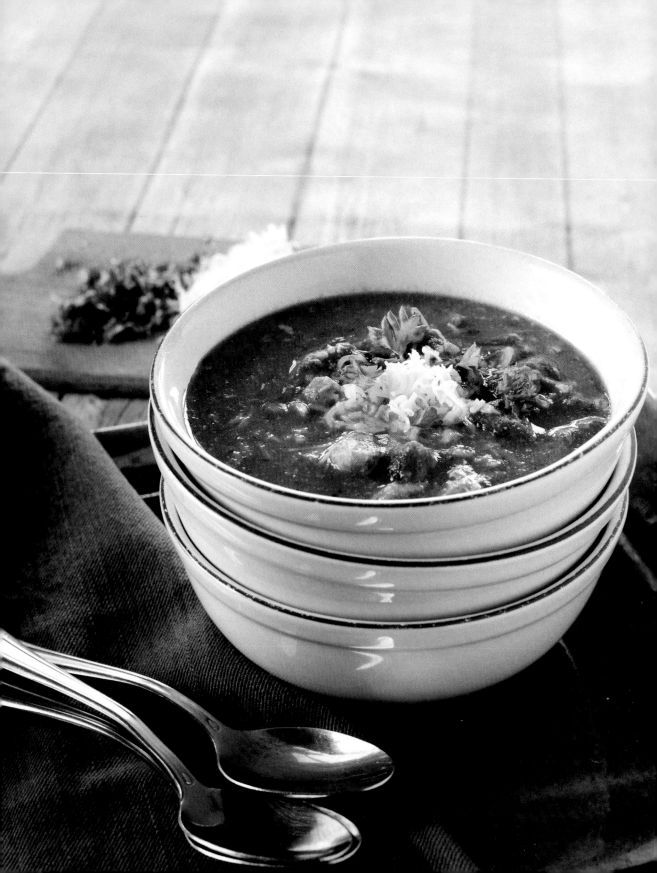

tomato chicken bisque

FAMILY SERVE – FEEDS 6 TO 8 (HALVE INGREDIENTS IF YOUR FAMILY IS SMALLER)

2 to 2½ pounds cooked chicken
breasts, diced

2 (14½-ounce) cans diced tomatoes
(purists can use 3½ cups of home
preserved or freshly stewed toms)

½ (15-ounce) can full-fat coconut milk

1½ (6-ounce) cans tomato paste

1 tablespoon Mineral Salt

¼ teaspoon black pepper

¼ teaspoon cayenne pepper (optional)

1 teaspoon onion powder

½ teaspoon garlic powder

¼ cup nutritional yeast

½ cup finely diced destalked parsley,
or 1 tablespoon dried parsley

5 to 6 cups hot (not quite boiling) water

2 generous tablespoons extra-virgin
coconut oil

2 tablespoons Just Gelatin (optional)

2 cups frozen diced okra

SERENE CHATS: *As a busy mom of nine children still living at home—and one currently on the way—I need ultra-fast dinner (and if I'm to make it through to the deadline of having this book ready without too many major meltdowns, I have to keep it simple). This soup is my easiest dinner of them all! It is so nutritious, healing to the gut, tasty, and a winner with my whole family. I make a triple batch to feed my huge hungry crowd and to ensure that I have leftovers for lunch the next day. My children love it with piece after piece of buttered homemade Artisan Sourdough Bread (page 206). My children are all lean, so they need their Crossovers.*

I have one picky ten-year-old boy who is completely icked-out by the thought of okra in anything. He loves this soup, and you can bet I am not about to tell him it is in there! Okra is the special friend of pregnant women. It is full of folate, which is such a necessary nutrient during pregnancy; I know I'm doing my baby and myself a favor every time I eat it.

1. Place the chicken, tomatoes, coconut milk, and tomato paste, and seasonings in a large soup pot but don't turn the heat on yet.

2. Put 3 cups of the hot water, the coconut oil, gelatin, and okra in a blender and blend well until completely smooth. Pour the puree into the soup pot, turn the heat to medium-high, and add 2 more cups hot water. Stir well and heat through. You can simmer for a few minutes, but you don't have to; as soon as the soup is hot, it is ready.

3. Taste and adjust the seasonings to "own it."

SERVING IDEAS: Enjoy this soup garnished with grated raw sheep's cheese, such as pecorino romano (or other cheese of your choice) and with the optional addition of a scoop of collagen to your personal bowl for a powerhouse boost.

DF (IF NOT USING CHEESE FOR GARNISH)

comfy cozy chicken dumpling soup Ⓢ

FOR THE DUMPLING DOUGH

1½ cups chicken broth

2 tablespoons oat fiber

2 tablespoons Gluccie

1 scoop Integral Collagen

1 teaspoon dried sage

½ teaspoon Mineral Salt (add another
   ¼ teaspoon if using homemade stock
   or broth)

¼ teaspoon black pepper

1 egg

1 tablespoon nutritional yeast

2 teaspoons light colored miso
   (optional: use another ½ tablespoon
   nutritional yeast if you don't have
   miso)

2 teaspoons ghee or butter

1 teaspoon aluminum-free baking
   powder

FOR THE SOUP

1 quart chicken broth

3 cups water

1 medium onion, diced

6 celery stalks, diced

1 cup frozen peas

1 large daikon radish, diced, or
   1 (16-ounce) bag frozen cauliflower
   florets

1 teaspoon Mineral Salt

¼ teaspoon black pepper

¼ teaspoon turmeric

1 to 2 teaspoons dried sage

½ teaspoon garlic powder, or 2 garlic
   cloves, minced

1 teaspoon onion powder

4 to 5 cups diced cooked chicken
   pieces

½ cup regular heavy or raw pastured
   cream (or if not using cream, add
   1 more tablespoon butter, ghee, or
   MCT oil to dumpling broth)

Let the stress of the world roll off you with every soothing spoonful of this soup. Bless your tummy with the gelatin-rich broth. Be soothed by the aroma of roasted meats and herbs. This is a heart warmer and a body healer.

If you love dumplings and think that now you are trying to reclaim your health and trim, they should be banished from your life, then *think again*! And don't be intimidated by the idea of making dumplings from scratch—there's nothing too complicated here. It does look a bit overwhelming at first, but once you've made this soup once or twice, it will feel like a cinch.

While these dumplings are not "healthy tasting," they are very healthy for you. It took us weeks of crazy Mad Scientist experiments to come up with a batch of dumplings that we didn't want to throw against the kitchen wall. Instead, we wanted to nestle them in our tummies. They plump up in the soup broth—they actually Plump! Oh, the joy! So, enjoy the goodness and turn an unhealthy favorite meal into a health renewer, the comfy, cozy way.

1. Make the dumpling dough. Place 1 cup of the broth in a blender. Add the oat fiber and Gluccie, and turn the blender on for 10 seconds, just to disperse the powders and avoid later problematic lumps. Turn blender off. Add all other dumpling ingredients except the baking powder and the remaining broth, then turn blender on again on the lowest possible speed for a full minute. Let the blender rest a full minute, then add ¼ cup more broth and blend for another full minute on the lowest setting. Let blender rest again for 2 minutes. Finally, add the last ¼ cup broth and blend for a final full minute on low speed. During the last 15 seconds, drop in the baking powder and make sure it gets dispersed.

2. Transfer the dumpling dough to a bowl, put in the fridge, and let sit while you begin making the soup. (Or you can make the dumpling dough earlier in the day, or the day before, and let it sit covered in the fridge.)

3. Make the soup. Put the chicken broth plus the water in a large soup pot along with all the veggies, and seasonings. Bring to a swift boil, cover, and simmer on medium-low heat until the veggies are almost tender, about 10 minutes, then turn heat to the lowest setting and add diced, precooked chicken.

FOR THE DUMPLING BROTH
1 quart chicken broth
2 tablespoons butter or ghee (clarified butter) or MCT oil
2 tablespoons Just Gelatin
¾ to 1 teaspoon Sunflower Lecithin (optional)

4. Finish the dumplings. Dig teaspoon-size balls out of the dough. Place each between your palms and roll to form a compact ball; roll without your fingers touching the balls. You should have 30 to 35 dumpling balls.

5. Put the dumpling broth ingredients in a blender and blend well. Transfer to a large saucepan and bring to a quick boil over high heat. Reduce the heat enough to tame the liquid to a gentle boil (but not a simmer). Use a spoon to carefully lower the dumplings into the saucepan, then quickly cover the saucepan and do not lift the lid for 10 minutes. The dumplings will steam to perfection.

6. Carefully add the dumplings and remaining liquid to the soup pot. Avoid actively stirring at this point or you will break up the dumplings.

7. Turn off the heat and add the cream. Move the pot carefully around with a few swirls by the handles to get the liquids blended, or ever so carefully give a slow, gentle stir. Taste and adjust the seasonings to "own it."

NOTE: These dumplings are very delicate, with 1½ cups broth in the dough. This is the way we prefer them, but if you would like a firmer, less delicate dumpling, then use only 1¼ cups broth. For a more foodie, puristy version of this soup, you can cook a whole chicken in the soup pot earlier in the day. Add 2 quarts plus 3 cups water and the chicken. Add 1 tablespoon apple cider vinegar, bring to a boil, and then cover and simmer long and slow until the chicken is tender. This takes more time, but fills the house with a nostalgic aroma. Remember to remove any scum that bubbles up on the top of your liquid. When done, remove the chicken and set aside. You'll return some of the meat to the soup.

DF (IF USING MCT OIL IN PLACE OF CREAM)

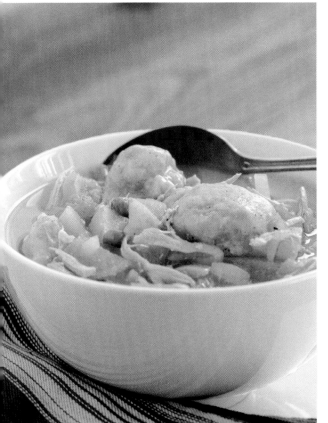

pink salmon chowder

1 medium or large onion, diced

6 large celery stalks, diced

1 cup frozen peas

1 to 2 tablespoons butter

1 pound radishes

1 (16-ounce) bag frozen cauliflower florets or 2 to 3 cups cut fresh florets

6½ cups chicken broth or bone stock (pages 495–496)

2 teaspoons Mineral Salt

½ teaspoon black pepper

1 teaspoon onion powder

2 garlic cloves, minced, or ½ teaspoon garlic powder

2 tablespoons dried parsley, or 1 cup chopped fresh parsley

¼ teaspoon cayenne pepper

2 (15-ounce) cans salmon, drained, with skin and bones

½ cup heavy cream (pastured raw or store-bought, depending on your purism standards)

This soup has a lovely pink hue that comes from the radishes, which lose all bitterness when cooked. They harmonize beautifully with the delicate pink color of salmon and are a super low-calorie, nutrient-packed "nonstarchie." The inclusion of the canned salmon with very soft bones (you would never notice, as they dissolve) makes this meal nutrient dense and rich with glycine, the amino acid that is lacking in our modern diet. If you really are icked-out by bones, buy canned salmon without bones and we'll try to forgive you.

Our families love this hearty but simple soup with its yummy veggies swimming in the soothing, creamy base reminiscent of traditional chowder. It actually has a double veggie punch since most of the veggies are blended into the cream and disappear, so you won't be hearing any fuss from children—a great secret way to get a giant dose of vegetables into little ones who have decided they don't LOVE veggies.

1. In a large soup pot set over medium-high heat, sauté the onion, celery, and peas in the butter for a minute or two, then add ¼ cup water and continue to cook the veggies until almost tender. Remove from the pot and set aside.

2. Put the radishes, cauliflower, and broth in the pot, cover, bring to a boil over high heat, then reduce the heat and simmer until tender (takes just a few minutes). Using a slotted spoon, scoop out the radishes and cauliflower, and put in a blender along with some of the liquid. Blend the veggies until smooth, then return to the pot.

3. Add back the sautéed veggies and all of the seasonings. Add the salmon, using your fork to break it into pieces. Simmer the soup for several more minutes, so the flavors meld.

4. Right before serving, add the cream and stir well. Taste and adjust the seasonings to "own it."

SERVING IDEAS: This is delicious with toasted Swiss Bread (page 196) for dunking for single fueling, or children can use whole-grain or sprouted toast for a Crossover.

NOTE: Sautéing your veggies in a separate small skillet while the radishes and cauliflower cook in the soup pot may save time.

NSI DF (IF YOU SUBSTITUTE FULL-FAT COCONUT MILK FOR THE CREAM)

mother hubbard soup

FAMILY SERVE – FEEDS 6 TO 8 (HALVE INGREDIENTS IF YOUR FAMILY IS SMALLER)

1 dozen large eggs (or about 2 eggs per person)

1 head green cabbage, cored and sliced

1 (16-ounce) bag frozen green beans, or 1 pound fresh

1 (15-ounce) can full-fat coconut milk (if you don't have this, then just add 5 tablespoons coconut oil or butter instead of 2)

7 cups hot (not quite boiling) water

2 teaspoons mild curry powder

1 tablespoon Mineral Salt

1 teaspoon onion powder

½ teaspoon garlic powder, or 3 to 4 garlic cloves, minced

2 tablespoons extra-virgin coconut oil or butter

OPTIONAL INGREDIENTS
(FOR NOT-QUITE-BARE CUPBOARDS)

¼ teaspoon Gluccie OR 2 tablespoons Just Gelatin OR ¼ cup okra to create a slight thickening of the broth, which is nice but not crucial

1 or 2 squirts soy sauce or Bragg liquid aminos

1 medium onion, diced (added with the other veggies)

1 tablespoon dried parsley

¼ cup nutritional yeast

SERENE CHATS: *This soup came about years ago, when it had been way too long since I'd gone grocery shopping. I felt like Mother Hubbard in that nursery rhyme. I'd run out of meat, had no fresh veggies or cheese, and the last can of beans had been used up—my fridge and cupboards were mostly bare. Then I realized we usually have a half decent-looking cabbage in the bottom of the fridge. Score! I pulled the outer leaves off and hoped for the best. I still had a dozen eggs left, so that meant protein—and yes, one bag of frozen green beans in the freezer. My children had been playing stack the cans the day before and sure enough—I found a can of coconut milk that had rolled under the couch. Dinner was born!*

At first this may look like an odd soup, with the whole eggs floating like little boats on top, but what started as odd has now become a family favorite. My children ask for this because they think it is fun to get their own two eggs in their bowls. The flavors are mild and child friendly, so add more spice to your own bowl if you want. But that night I couldn't chance a dud meal with my children so I made the flavors very five-year-old friendly.

1. Hard-boil the eggs, then put them aside to cool and peel. (We usually boil them in the early afternoon, well before making the soup.)

2. In a large soup pot, combine the cabbage and green beans, add the coconut milk and 5 cups of the hot water, and sprinkle in the seasonings. Cover and bring to a rapid boil, then turn down to a simmer.

3. Meanwhile, put the coconut oil, remaining 2 cups hot water, and the optional Gluccie or Gelatin or okra in a blender and puree. Transfer to the soup pot. If using the soy sauce, parsley, and nutritional yeast, add those now as well.

4. Peel and add the eggs, and simmer until heated through. Taste and adjust the flavors to "own it."

SERVING IDEAS: This soup is great served with buttered toasted sourdough or sprouted bread for children as a Crossover, and buttered Swiss Bread (page 196) for you for a clean **S**. Of course, if you don't have any Swiss Bread, then it is super yummy and satisfying just as is (or you can use toasted Joseph's pitas).

NSI DF

kai sai ming

3 pounds ground beef or venison

1½ heads green cabbage, cored and thinly sliced

2 medium onions, sliced

4 cups water, beef broth, or bone stock (pages 495–496)

1½ teaspoons Mineral Salt

½ teaspoon black pepper

1 to 2 teaspoons onion powder

2 to 3 tablespoons nutritional yeast

Garlic powder

Cayenne pepper

1 to 2 generous squirts Bragg liquid aminos or soy sauce

We grew up with this recipe, and are so thrilled to hear how Trim Healthy Mamas from all over the globe have now adopted it as a family staple. It is inexpensive, tasty, and super easy.

1. Brown the beef in a soup pot over medium-high heat. If you are using beef that is not grass fed, drain off most of the fat.

2. Add the cabbage and onions, cover, and simmer until the cabbage wilts.

3. Add the water and seasonings. Cover again and simmer, stirring now and then, until the cabbage is soft and well cooked, 30 to 45 minutes.

NSI DF

FAMILY SERVE – FEEDS 6 TO 8 (HALVE INGREDIENTS IF YOUR FAMILY IS SMALLER)

2 pounds chana dal, soaked and
  drained
4 cups chicken stock or bone broth
  (pages 495–496)
6 to 8 cups water
1 large onion, finely diced, or 1½ cups
  Seasoning Blend (frozen diced onion,
  celery, and pepper)
3 teaspoons Mineral Salt
Black and cayenne pepper to taste
2 teaspoons curry powder
½ teaspoon turmeric
2 teaspoons onion powder
1 teaspoon garlic powder
1½ teaspoons garam masala (optional)
3 tablespoons nutritional yeast
1 to 2 generous squirts Bragg liquid
  aminos
Diced cooked chicken breast or Just
  Gelatin to boost protein content
  (optional)

Anybody with blood sugar issues, such as diabetes, pre-diabetes, or hypoglycemia, should use chana dal, an Indian legume, as a frequent option for E meals. Its healthy carbs burn extremely slowly in the body. Incredibly, chana dal has a rating of only 8 on the glycemic index. (Most other beans and legumes have a glycemic index in the 30s or 40s.) It has three times the fiber of most other legumes, yet has a beautiful creamy texture.

Chana dal looks a bit like a small chickpea or lentil, but should not be confused with them. You can easily find it online, or at international food stores, but even more general stores like Walmart carry it as well. Soaking is a must for chana dal. You'll want to start cooking your soup mid-afternoon, as it is better cooked long and slow. Start your soak early in the morning, as you'll want the dal to soak for seven hours. Place the dal in a bowl, cover with water, and sprinkle in 1 tablespoon baking soda. The baking soda helps break down the hard shell of the dal so it can soften; if you're cooking the soup in a crockpot all day, though, there is no need to add the baking soda.

1. Put all the ingredients except the chicken or Just Gelatin (if using) in a large soup pot. Bring to a simmer over medium-high heat, then reduce the heat to low and and cook for several hours, until the dal is very soft.

2. Lightly blend the soup with a stick blender in the pot or transfer a few cups to a blender and puree. Add back to the soup and stir.

3. If the soup is too thick for your preference, add a bit more water. If using chicken breast, add some (any amount) or a few tablespoons Just Gelatin to boost protein, but you can just leave the soup as is, if preferred. Taste and adjust the seasonings to "own it."

SERVING IDEAS: Serve with a dollop of Greek yogurt and garnish with a sprinkling of skim-milk mozzarella for **E** or with a grated full-fat cheese like cheddar for a Crossover.

NSI (IF NOT USING THE NUTRITIONAL YEAST) DF
(WITHOUT THE YOGURT OR CHEESE GARNISH)

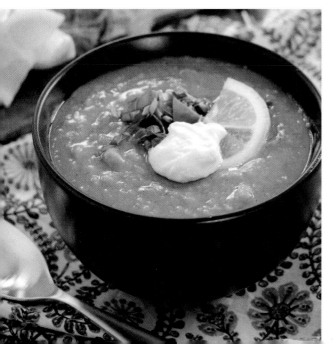

2 (16-ounce) bags frozen cauliflower florets, or 1 large head of fresh cauliflower, cut into florets

2 ½ quarts chicken broth

3 to 4 cups chopped carrots

3 to 4 cups chopped celery

1 large onion, diced or sliced, or 1½ cups Seasoning Blend (frozen diced onion, celery, and pepper)

¾ cup wild rice

3 teaspoons Mineral Salt

1 teaspoon black pepper

1½ teasoons dried thyme

3 ounces ⅓ less fat cream cheese

4 to 5 cups diced cooked chicken

Here's a wonderful recipe from Rohnda Monroy, our very clever and creative friend who has taken all the wonderful pictures in this book. She's a flat-out Trim Healthy Wizard in the kitchen.

1. Put the cauliflower and broth in a soup pot over high heat and bring to a quick boil. Turn the heat down a little and simmer until the cauliflower is tender (takes just a few minutes). Scoop out the cauliflower with a slotted spoon or strainer. Put the cauliflower into a blender with 2 cups of the broth and set aside.

2. Add the carrots, celery, onion, and wild rice to the soup pot along with the salt, pepper, and thyme and simmer for 45 minutes to 1 hour. You want the veggies to be tender and the wild rice to begin breaking open.

3. Add the cream cheese to the blender and puree for 1 minute or until smooth. Transfer to the soup pot, stirring well.

4. Add the chicken and simmer the soup for another 15 to 20 minutes. The rice will break apart and soak up all the flavor and more of the liquid. Combine all ingredients well and heat through. (You can simmer for a few minutes but you don't have to. As soon as soup is hot, it is done.) Check the seasonings and serve.

NSI

pearl's chili

FAMILY SERVE – FEEDS 6 TO 8 (HALVE INGREDIENTS IF YOUR FAMILY IS SMALLER)

3 pounds ground beef or venison

1 large onion, diced

2 (10-ounce) cans Rotel-style tomatoes and chilies or just 1 can of the Rotel and 1 (14.5-ounce) can of diced tomatoes

1 (8-ounce) can tomato sauce

2 (15-ounce) cans beans of any kind, rinsed and drained

2 to 4 cups water (depending on how broth-y you like your chili)

2 teaspoons Mineral Salt

1½ tablespoons chili powder

1 teaspoon onion powder

Garlic powder to taste

1 to 2 squirts Bragg liquid aminos (optional)

PEARL CHATS: I'm trying not to get too big a head about the fact that, in our first book, my chili was more popular than Serene's. Nah, that's a lie—I'm loving it! Hey, she invented the Fat-Stripping Frappa (page 418), and I'll never be able to compete with that, so I'll take what I can get. If you want to keep this in a safe S mode, go light on the beans for your serving and save more of them for your children. You should be okay with up to ¼ cup beans in the occasional S meal.

1. Brown the meat with the onion in a large skillet over high heat, about 5 minutes. If the meat is fatty, brown alone first, drain off the fat, then brown the onions with the cooked meat.

2. Add all other remaining ingredients and simmer for 30 minutes to 1 hour. Check the seasonings and serve.

SERVING IDEAS: Top the chili with Blendtons (page 476) or crumbled Mad Melbas (page 454) or Swiss Crackers (page 457), add a dollop of sour cream, and sprinkle on grated cheese.

NSI DF (IF OMITTING THE SOUR CREAM AND SUBSTITUTING HELLO CHEESE, PAGE 487)

2 medium onions, diced

1½ tablespoons coconut oil or butter

4 garlic cloves, minced

6 celery stalks, chopped

4 sweet potatoes, peeled and cubed

2 quarts chicken broth

2 cups water

1½ cups old-fashioned rolled oats

2½ teaspoons Mineral Salt

Generous pinch of black pepper

3 to 4 cups diced cooked chicken
breast (4 to 5 breasts)

4 cups chopped fresh kale

Oatmeal is not just for breakfast—it also makes a wonderful thickener for soups! This soup could not be more packed with nutrition. It will nourish your whole family with vital nutrients. Kale, sweet potatoes, and oats are all powerhouse whole foods that are easy on your budget but are powerful disease fighters. This energizing meal is also easy to make.

The soup calls for cooked chicken; if you're a Drive Thru Sue, just use the breast meat from a grocery-store rotisserie chicken for this E meal. Or, quickly poach some chicken breasts in water while you sauté the onions.

1. In a soup pot over medium-high heat, sauté the onions in the coconut oil until soft. Add the garlic, celery, sweet potatoes, broth, water, oats, salt, and pepper. Simmer on low heat for 30 minutes, or until the vegetables are soft and the oats are swelled and cooked.

2. Add the chicken and kale. Heat another 10 minutes, or until the kale is wilted.

NSI DF

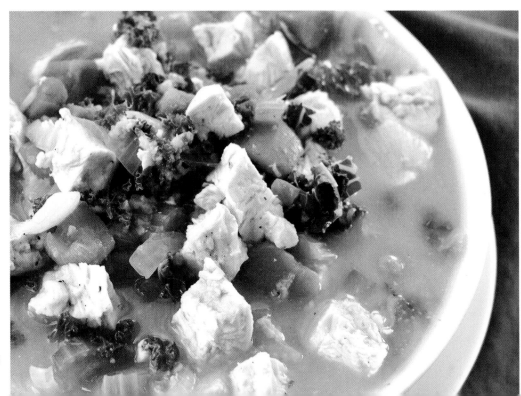

mulligan soup

FAMILY SERVE – FEEDS 6 TO 8 (HALVE INGREDIENTS IF YOUR FAMILY IS SMALLER)

3 pounds ground venison or ground beef

8 cups hot (not quite boiling) water

1½ (6-ounce) cans tomato paste

1 head green cabbage, cored and sliced

1 large onion, sliced

1 (1-pound) bag frozen ultra-thin green beans, or 1 pound fresh, trimmed

1 bunch fresh parsley, diced

4 garlic cloves, minced, or ½ teaspoon garlic powder

2 cups frozen diced okra

2 tablespoons Just Gelatin

2 to 3 tablespoons of healthy fat . . . tahini (sesame paste) is my favorite but other yummy options are coconut oil, red palm oil, organic pastured butter, or ghee

1 tablespoon Mineral Salt

½ to 1 teaspoon black pepper

1 teaspoon onion powder

¼ teaspoon cayenne pepper (optional)

2 tablespoons hot sauce of choice

¼ cup nutritional yeast

2 teaspoons miso or Bragg liquid aminos to taste

SERENE CHATS: *Funny name? It comes from a book our mother read to us while we were in the car, traveling across the wild Yukon along the northern border between Canada and Alaska during that first year when we arrived in America (1991). The book was called* Nothin' Too Good for a Cowboy, *and it had a hilarious description of a cowboy cook named Mulligan and this soup. The soup contained everything he could get his hands on—there was nothing he wouldn't throw in the pot, even whole cabbages. The cowboys would eat the soup until they were so stuffed they couldn't even hear the word "Mulligan" without rolling over on their stomachs and groaning, "seeeeeek" from all that soup. But in a day or two, it was Mulligan Soup that they craved, above all else.*

Our rendition of Mulligan Soup is, we hope, a bit more civilized—no whole cabbages but plenty hearty with a garden load of veggies and lots of meat. It's cheap, quick, and satisfies. The recipe makes a very large pot because, in keeping with the spirit of traditional Mulligan, there should always be second helpings available (which you don't have to eat until you are "seeeeek"). I actually triple this recipe in my HUGE cauldron of a soup pot, and this soup feeds my large family for days.

1. Brown the meat in a large soup pot over high heat. If using store-bought beef that is not grass fed, drain the fat (if I don't have grass-fed meat, I rinse the browned meat under hot water to release all the fat, which is where the toxins are stored). While the meat is browning, heat up the water in a kettle, as the hot water helps get things cooked more quickly and allows the oil to break down in the blender.

2. Return the meat to the pot, add 5 cups of the hot water along with the tomato paste, cabbage, onion, beans, parsley, and garlic. Bring the ingredients to a rapid boil over high heat, then turn the heat down, cover, and simmer.

3. Meanwhile, blend the okra with the remaining 3 cups hot water, the gelatin, and the tahini or other healthy fat until smooth. Transfer contents of blender to pot, add the salt, pepper, onion powder, and cayenne, then stir in the hot sauce, nutritional yeast, and miso. Once veggies are tender, your soup is ready. Taste and adjust seasonings to "own it."

DF

popeye's power soup

1 (32-ounce) package frozen chopped
  spinach

2 cups frozen diced okra

3 cups hot (not quite boiling) water

2 heaping tablespoons extra-virgin
  coconut oil (if you don't want the
  coconut flavor, you can use MCT oil)

2 rounded tablespoons Just Gelatin

4 tablespoons grated pecorino romano
  or finely grated Parmesan cheese
  (dairy-free Mamas can use
  4 tablespoons Hello Cheese,
  page 487)

1 tablespoon miso (optional; if not
  using, add ½ to 1 teaspoon salt)

1 tablespoon Mineral Salt

½ teaspoon black pepper

Pinch of cayenne pepper (optional)

¼ cup nutritional yeast

¼ teaspoon garlic powder

1 teaspoon onion powder

1 tablespoon rice vinegar, or
  ½ tablespoon apple cider vinegar

This soup is a fun way for children to learn to love spinach. Who doesn't want to be as strong as Popeye? Serve your children power-packed green meals like this one from a young age and you'll be arming them with good health and an adventurous palate.

1. Place the frozen spinach in a large soup pot, cover by 2 inches with water, bring to a boil over high heat, then turn the heat to low and simmer until cooked (takes just a few minutes).

2. Place half of the spinach in a blender and puree until smooth, using a little of the pot liquid if necessary to blend well. Stir spinach puree back into the soup pot.

3. Blend the frozen okra, hot water, coconut oil, gelatin, cheese, and miso until smooth. Transfer to the pot and stir to blend.

4. Add the salt, pepper, cayenne (if using), nutritional yeast, garlic and onion powders, and vinegar to the pot. Stir to blend and simmer for a few more minutes, until flavors are melded.

5. Taste and adjust the seasonings to "own it."

SERVING IDEAS: Serve the soup garnished with a small amount of grated pecorino romano cheese to stay in **FP** mode. For a protein boost, add a scoop of Integral Collagen to your personal bowl. As you can tell, this soup does not have meat protein—nothing beyond the gelatin and a little cheese. Your children can grate more cheese into their bowls to up the protein a bit (and because they love it), or you can add a little shredded cooked chicken. But having a lower-protein meal now and then won't hurt you because most of your meals have ample protein. Your call. Our children love to eat this with lots of buttered light rye Wasa crackers.

DF (IF USING 4 TABLESPOONS OF HELLO CHEESE, PAGE 487, INSTEAD)

tangy tato soup

4 medium sweet potatoes, peeled and cubed

1 cup frozen green beans, peas, or diced okra (this won't be blended, so make sure you love okra if you choose that option)

1 medium onion, sliced

7 cups hot (not quite boiling) water

2 tablespoons Just Gelatin (optional)

2 tablespoons coconut oil or butter

2 tablespoons light miso, or
   1 tablespoon red miso

1 tablespoon drained capers

2 to 3 garlic cloves, minced, or
   1 teaspoon garlic powder

2 teaspoons dried dill

1 teaspoon onion powder

1½ teaspoons ground cumin

1 tablespoon apple cider vinegar

Juice of ½ lime, or 1 tablespoon bottled lime juice concentrate

1 tablespoon Mineral Salt

¼ cup nutritional yeast

2½ pounds chicken breast, cooked and diced small

1. Put the sweet potatoes, green beans, peas, or okra, and onion in a soup pot and add 5 cups of the hot water, cover, and bring to a rapid boil. Reduce the heat and simmer until the sweet potatoes are tender.

2. Put the gelatin (if using), coconut oil, miso, and capers in a blender with the remaining 2 cups hot water and puree. Stir into the soup pot, then add the garlic, dill, onion powder, cumin, vinegar, lime juice, salt, and nutritional yeast.

3. Simmer for just a couple more minutes, then stir in the chicken and heat through.

4. Stir, taste for seasoning, and adjust to "own it."

SERVING IDEAS: This is delicious topped with a tablespoon of grated lower fat sheep's milk cheese, like pecorino. You also have the option of placing a scoop of Integral Collagen in your personal bowl for a Mama protein boost.

NSI (IF MADE WITHOUT THE GELATIN) DF (WITHOUT THE CHEESE)

nummy umami

FAMILY SERVE – FEEDS 6 TO 8 HUNGRY PEOPLE (HALVE INGREDIENTS IF YOUR FAMILY IS SMALLER)

2½ pounds boneless chicken breasts
or thighs, or 2½ to 3 pounds ground
venison or beef

8 baby bok choy, roughly chopped;
or 1 large head green cabbage,
cored and finely sliced; or
1½ (16-ounce) bags coleslaw mix

1 medium onion, diced, or 1 teaspoon
onion powder

4 to 6 garlic cloves, minced, or
1 teaspoon garlic powder

1 (16-ounce) bag frozen cauliflower
florets or 3 to 4 cups fresh-cut florets

½ to 1 cup diced baby portobello
mushrooms, or ½ cup dried shiitake
mushrooms, reconstituted

2 cups roughly chopped radishes

8 cups hot (not quite boiling) water,
for blending

4 tablespoons light miso, or
2½ tablespoons red miso

2 tablespoons soy sauce

¼ cup nutritional yeast

2 tablespoons rice vinegar

¼ teaspoon black pepper

2 to 3 teaspoons fish sauce

2 teaspoons toasted sesame oil

1 doonk Pure Stevia Extract

1 tablespoon dried parsley, or ¼ cup
chopped fresh parsley

2 tablespoons extra-virgin coconut oil
or ghee (clarified butter)

2 tablespoons Just Gelatin (optional)

¼ to ½ cup raw pastured cream or
regular heavy cream for Pearl and
her Drive Thru Sue peeps (optional)

SERENE CHATS: *Umami is a fifth basic taste, and just as important in gourmet food creations as sweet, salty, bitter, and sour. Umami provides a rounded taste experience that has been enjoyed for centuries, as far back as Ancient Rome. Humans develop a taste for umami through breast milk, which is rich in natural glutamate.*

Different cultures have used various methods of releasing the bound glutamic acid to impart that beloved umami taste. For instance, boiling, steaming, simmering, roasting, braising, drying, aging, and marinating free the umami flavors locked in natural foods. Of all methods, fermentation is the most effective.

This soup uses fermented and aged miso and soy sauce, nutritional yeast, and veggies that are rich in natural umami. All my fellow Purist and Foodie Mamas are going to have a blast with this one! But even if you are a Drive Thru Sue, you'll find it quick and easy.

1. Simmer the chicken until tender in water to cover in a soup pot set over medium heat. Once the chicken is cooked, discard the water, take the meat out, and dice the chicken into small chunks. (If using ground meat, brown it and, if not grass-fed, then drain and rinse under hot water to remove excess fat.) Set aside.

2. Put the bok choy, onion, garlic, cauliflower, mushrooms, and radishes in the soup pot. Add 5 cups hot water, then add the miso, soy sauce, nutritional yeast, vinegar, pepper, fish sauce, sesame oil, stevia, and parsley. Reduce the heat and simmer until the vegetables are tender, about 8 minutes.

3. Blend the remaining 3 cups of just off the boil water with the coconut oil and gelatin. Add this to the pot, return the chicken to the pot as well, and add the cream (if using). Stir to blend.

4. Taste and adjust the seasonings until you "own it."

SERVING IDEAS: Garnish with seasoned toasted nori and grated sheep's milk cheese (aged cheese has lots of umami), if desired. Add a scoop of Integral Collagen to your personal bowl for a healthy Mama protein boost.

NSI (WITHOUT THE JUST GELATIN) DF (WITHOUT THE CREAM AND GRATED CHEESE)

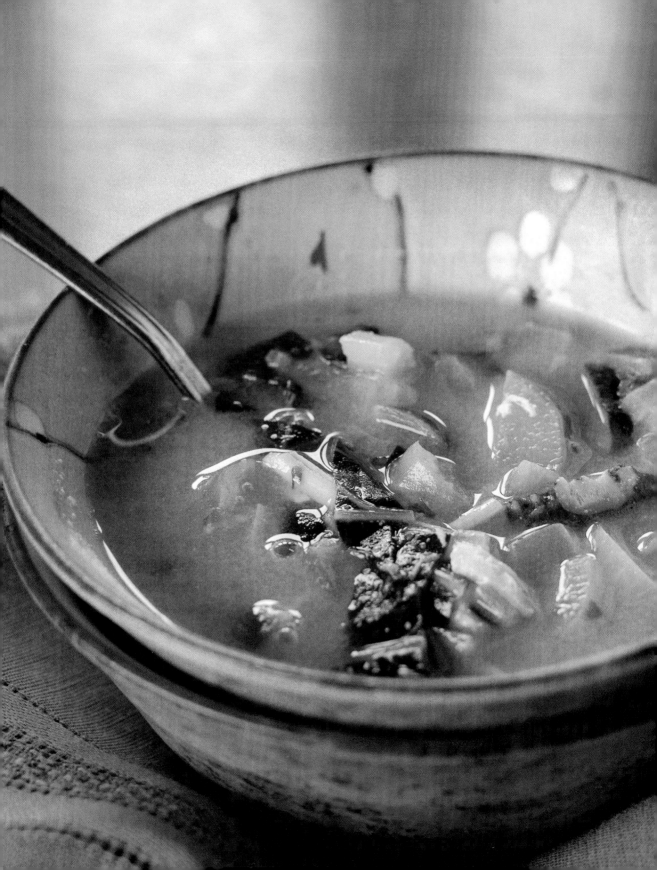

QUICK SINGLE SOUPS

When it comes to lunchtime, we like *big, hearty, filling* bowls of soup that don't take *big* chunks of time out of our day to make. Get filled up fast for lunch (or use these for a quick single-serve dinner), and allow the healing ingredients to work their health-promoting, slimming powers in your body.

Out of the home at lunchtime? Make your soup ahead, pour it into a thermos to stay hot or carry it in a cooler, then use your workplace microwave to heat it when it's time. (You-know-who just wrote that line—Serene is none too happy about it!) You can pair these soups with a side of on-plan bread or salad if desired, but they're big and mighty enough to stand alone.

The following 16 soups (plus 2 broth options) are speedy enough for any Drive Thru Sue to get excited about, yet our purist Mamas will love their purity and superfood ingredients. That's three weeks of Monday-to-Friday soups without having to repeat. How are you going to ever get to try them all? Life is always an adventure as a Trim Healthy Mama!

You'll notice okra is used in a few of these soups, as it is in some of the family soups. Not only does okra help to heal gut and blood sugar problems, but we delightfully discovered that it also acts as a wonderful thickener. Don't be afraid of it—you won't notice any strange slimy okra-ness in these soups, it is very well disguised. And please don't eyeball the okra amounts when cooking—shock and horror! We spent lots of time perfecting the amounts to use in each soup so they can work their magic but stay under the taste and texture radar. We used frozen diced okra for the family soups, but found we could get more exact amounts using frozen whole okra pods in the single-serve recipes. Purchase frozen whole okra pods in bags in your grocer's frozen veggie section, and you'll have the right amounts called for here.

bean boss soup

¾ cup cooked beans, drained (black beans work well)

1½ cups water

3 frozen whole okra pods

3 to 5 generous pinches Mineral Salt

¼ teaspoon onion powder

⅛ teaspoon garlic powder

1 or 2 squirts Bragg liquid aminos

1 tablespoon nutritional yeast

2 tablespoons salsa of choice

2 tablespoons frozen corn kernels (look for organic to avoid GMO, but if you can't afford that, hey, you'll survive!)

PEARL CHATS: Do E meals have you stumped? You're going to make an E meal like a Boss in less than 5 minutes with this recipe. This soup is an insanely inexpensive meal that does not require even one special ingredient—happy dance!

We Drive Thru Sue's will opt for canned beans in this recipe. Why do extra steps when you don't have to, right? Just make sure to drain the beans first, and it is best to find canned beans without BPA. Purists like Serene and her peeps will probably want to soak and cook their own beans. More power to ya!

The ¾ cup beans in this soup still leaves you room for a slice of sprouted or sourdough toast on the side with a small smear of butter, if you wish (but I'm a store-bought sprouted bread kinda gal). Or have a piece of Swiss Bread (page 196) and a side salad with a lean dressing, if your blood sugar does better with one E fuel at a time.

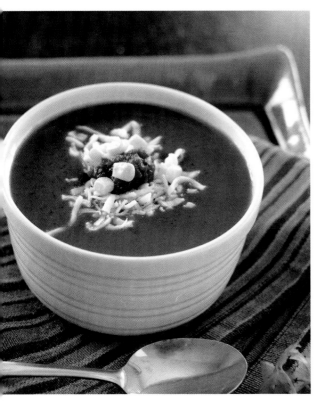

1. Place all the ingredients in a blender except the salsa and corn. Blend well for a couple of minutes, until smooth.

2. Transfer the puree to a small saucepan, add the salsa and corn, and heat over low heat until hot.

3. Taste and adjust the seasonings to "own it."

SERVING IDEAS: Top with a dollop of 0% Greek yogurt and garnish with a sprinkling of skim-milk mozzarella (to keep fat contained within **E** settings); however, this soup is so flavorful the cheese is not really needed.

NOTE: The beans offer some protein, but you can up the protein with either a scoop of Integral Collagen or some diced cooked chicken. Alternatively, you can enjoy some Lemon Pucker Gummies (page 387) or Berry Yummy Gummies (page 388), or a couple of Superfood Chocolate Chews (page 383) for a treat-like protein boost after your meal.

NSI (WITHOUT THE LIQUID AMINOS AND YEAST) DF (WITHOUT THE YOGURT AND CHEESE TOPPING)

cream of mushroom soup

SINGLE SERVE

1 tablespoon butter

4 ounces fresh button mushrooms, sliced

2 tablespoons finely diced onion

1½ cups chicken broth or bone stock (pages 495–496)

2 tablespoons finely grated Parmesan cheese (green can kind is fine)

4 generous pinches Mineral Salt

⅛ teaspoon black pepper

¼ teaspoon onion powder

2 tablespoons heavy cream

The humble mushroom has recently been found to hold powerful immune-boosting and cancer-fighting properties. A study published in a recent issue of *International Journal of Cancer* revealed that frequent consumption of mushrooms (approximately 1 button mushroom per day) has been linked to a 64 percent decrease in the risk of developing breast cancer. This delicious soup will make you want to get more mushrooms in your belly, not because you should but just because you wanna!

1. Melt the butter in a small saucepan over medium heat. Add the mushrooms and onion and sauté for 3 to 4 minutes, until well coated in butter and starting to release a pleasing aroma.

2. Transfer most of the mushrooms and the onion to a blender, leaving just a few mushrooms in the pan to continue cooking. Add the remaining ingredients except the cream and blend well.

3. Break apart the larger mushrooms in the pan, then add the blender puree and stir well. Simmer for a few minutes to heat through, then add the cream, and serve.

NSI

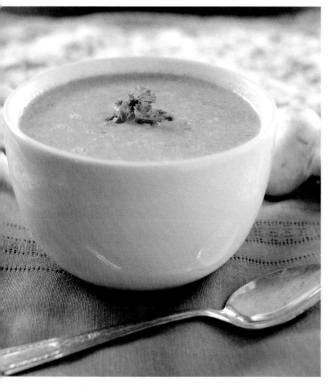

creamy broccoli and cheese soup

SINGLE SERVE

1¾ cups chicken broth or bone stock
  (pages 495–496)

1 cup frozen or fresh broccoli florets

5 frozen whole okra pods

4 to 5 generous pinches Mineral Salt

⅛ teaspoon onion powder

⅛ teaspoon black pepper

Cayenne pepper to taste

1 tablespoon nutritional yeast

1 ounce ⅓ less fat cream cheese

1 to 2 tablespoons heavy cream

Real or turkey bacon bits (optional)

The hidden okra in this soup acts as a gentle thickener but is also healing to your gut and pancreas. If you think you dislike okra, here's a way to get it into your diet with only sheer yumminess detected.

1. Put the broth, veggies, and seasonings in a small saucepan, cover, turn the heat to high, and bring to a quick boil. Reduce the temperature to medium-high and simmer the veggies until they are tender (takes just a few minutes).

2. Transfer the mixture to a blender and add the cream cheese. Make sure the lid is secure, and blend well for a few seconds. Turn the blender off, vent the hot air, then continue to blend until it's a smooth puree.

3. Pour the puree into the saucepan, bring back to a simmer over low heat, then add the cream. Stir to warm through and taste to adjust the seasonings. Top with bacon bits (if using).

SERVING IDEAS: Top with just a bit of grated cheese; you don't have to overdo the cheese, as this soup is already ultra-creamy from the magic of okra blended with the small amount of dairy.

NOTE: You can up the protein content of your meal by either adding some leftover chicken breast, stirring in a scoop of Integral Collagen, or enjoying some Superfood Chocolate Chews (page 383) or gummies (pages 387–388) for dessert.

NSI

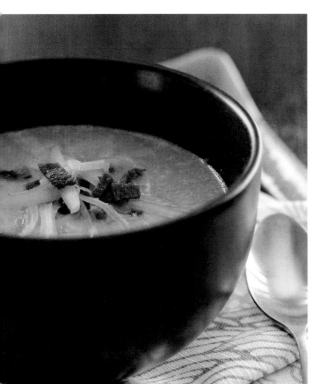

just like campbell's tomato soup

(S)

SINGLE SERVE

1 (8-ounce) can tomato sauce

1 cup chicken broth, water, or bone
   stock (pages 495–496)

¼ teaspoon Super Sweet Blend, or
   ½ doonk Pure Stevia Extract

3 generous pinches Mineral Salt

Black pepper to taste

Cayenne pepper to taste (optional)

1 tablespoon nutritional yeast

2 to 3 tablespoons heavy cream

This is comfort food at its best. Pair it with a grilled cheese sandwich made with Swiss Bread (page 196) or a Joseph's pita, and sit down to bliss.

1. Put all the ingredients except the cream in a small saucepan set over medium-high heat, and whisk while heating. When the soup is hot enough to serve, stir in the cream; taste and adjust the seasonings to "own it."

SERVING IDEA: Top with a sprinkling of grated cheddar cheese, if desired.

NSI (IF USING YOUR FAVORITE ON-PLAN SWEETENER OF CHOICE AND IF NOT USING NUTRITIONAL YEAST)

curry in a hurry soup

SINGLE SERVE

1¾ cups hot (not quite boiling) water

2 to 3 teaspoons coconut oil or MCT oil

1 scoop Integral Collagen

2 tablespoons plain Greek yogurt

¾ teaspoon curry powder

¼ teaspoon Super Sweet Blend, or
   ½ doonk Pure Stevia Extract

5 to 6 generous pinches Mineral Salt

⅛ teaspoon black pepper

Cayenne pepper to taste

2 teaspoons nutritional yeast

½ to 1 teaspoon hot sauce of choice

¾ cup frozen or fresh cauliflower
   florets

¼ cup frozen peas

Pressed for time but want good flavor and filling factor? We've got you covered here.

1. Put all the ingredients except the cauliflower and peas in a blender and puree. Transfer to a small saucepan and add the veggies. Cover and simmer until the cauliflower and peas are tender, about 5 minutes.

NOTE: With the yogurt and collagen, there is sufficient protein here, but there is still room for more, if desired. Add either diced cooked chicken or 2 teaspoons Just Gelatin during blending process.

DF (IF USING 1 TO 2 TABLESPOONS COCONUT CREAM OR MANNA IN PLACE OF THE YOGURT)

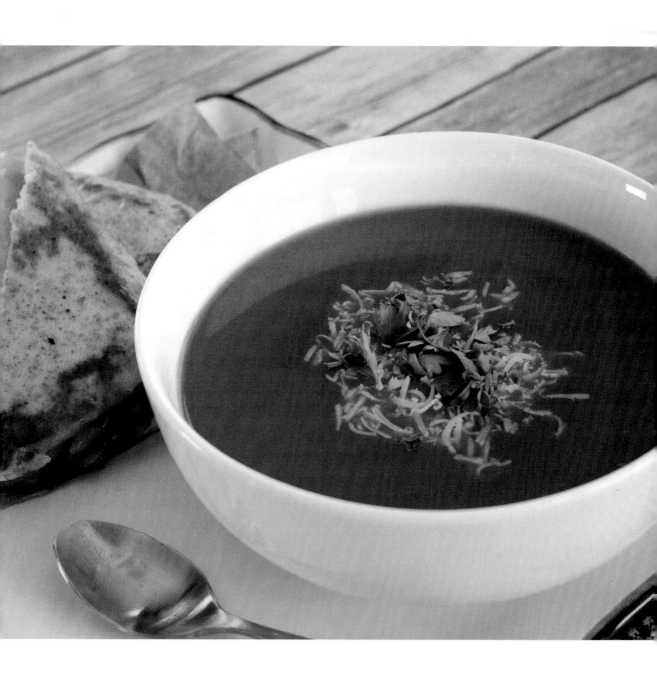

cream of sweet stuff soup

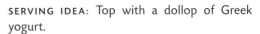

1 medium sweet potato, peeled and
   diced small

4 baby carrots, or ½ large carrot,
   diced small

3 frozen whole okra

1 cup chicken broth or bone stock
   (pages 495–496)

¾ cup unsweetened almond or
   cashew milk

1 teaspoon coconut oil

¼ teaspoon Super Sweet Blend

⅛ teaspoon ground cinnamon

3 generous pinches Mineral Salt

1½ scoops Integral Collagen (optional)

Think an E soup couldn't possibly be creamy? Wipe away that notion with this easy recipe. This bowl of golden goodness tastes like fall but can be enjoyed all year. It is chock-full of beta-carotene from the sweet potato and carrots, and has just enough fat to help your body absorb all the vitamins and minerals. One teaspoon of fat is all it takes to get wonderful creaminess when okra tag-teams in an E recipe.

1. Put all the ingredients except the collagen in a small saucepan. Cover and turn the heat to high, bringing the mixture to a quick boil. Lower the heat and simmer the veggies until tender (takes just a few minutes).

2. Transfer the mixture to a blender and add the collagen (if using). Make sure the lid is secure, and blend well for a few seconds. Turn the blender off and vent the hot air, then continue to blend until completely smooth.

3. Return the puree to the saucepan and simmer for a couple more minutes. Taste and adjust the seasonings to "own it."

SERVING IDEA: Top with a dollop of Greek yogurt.

NOTE: The collagen in this recipe gives you around 15 grams of protein, which is suitable for a lunch. If you want to stick with an NSI, substitute some diced cooked chicken breast.

**NSI (IF USING CHICKEN INSTEAD OF COLLAGEN)
DF (WITHOUT THE YOGURT TOPPING)**

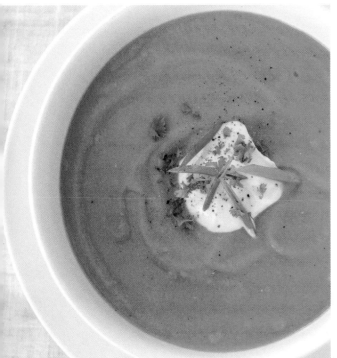

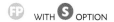
3 to 4 ounces browned ground lean meat of any kind (Serene uses venison or grass-fed beef)

Cumin, hot sauce, Mineral Salt, nutritional yeast, onion powder, and garlic powder, for seasoning

1½ cups hot (not quite boiling) water

1 teaspoon miso

1 teaspoon coconut oil

1 scoop Integral Collagen

2 to 3 pinches Mineral Salt

1 teaspoon nutritional yeast

⅛ teaspoon garlic powder

¼ teaspoon onion powder

Cayenne and/or black pepper to taste

1 cup very thinly sliced green cabbage, or 1 cup Troodles (page 222), or 1 single-serve package Not Naughty Noodles

1 teaspoon dried parsley

Nourish both your body and your mind with this deeply soothing soup. The ingredients in this recipe fortify your liver, which is so important to maintain while your body is in weight-loss mode. Allergen-free and purist Mamas will love this soup for its superfood qualities and for the magic of collagen and coconut oil creaming this up without the need for any dairy. But don't overlook this recipe if you are a Drive Thru Sue—this is about as easy as it gets. If you do not like venison or cannot afford grass-fed beef, don't shy away from making this, either. Use any ol' ground meat you have, like turkey, because the other ingredients in this soup still push it into superstar healthy mode.

Miso is a traditional Asian fermented food with an incredible savory taste and is packed with nutrients. You can find it easily at any health food store, online, or at international grocery stores. It comes in a range of strengths, from mild light to strong dark red. Even though miso is made from soybeans, don't confuse it with unfermented or unsprouted soy, which we are not too keen on.

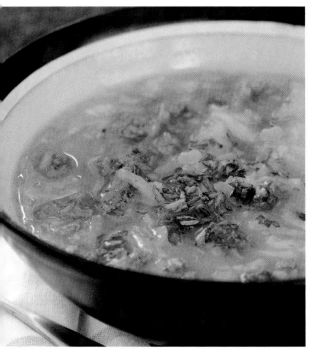

1. If you do not already have cooked ground meat ready, brown ground meat of choice and set aside (brown enough so you can use leftovers for other quick meals). Spice it with a few dashes of the following spices: cumin, hot sauce, Mineral Salt, nutritional yeast, and onion and garlic powders.

2. Pour the hot water into a blender. Add the miso, coconut oil, collagen, and all the seasonings except the parsley. Blend until it's a creamy puree.

3. Transfer the puree to a small saucepan. Add the cabbage (or noodles) and meat, and bring the soup to a simmer over medium-low heat. Add the parsley and serve.

NOTE: You can make this an **S** by adding a swirl of cream, using more beef without worrying if it's lean, and optional grated cheese.

DF (WITHOUT THE CREAM OR CHEESE TOPPING)

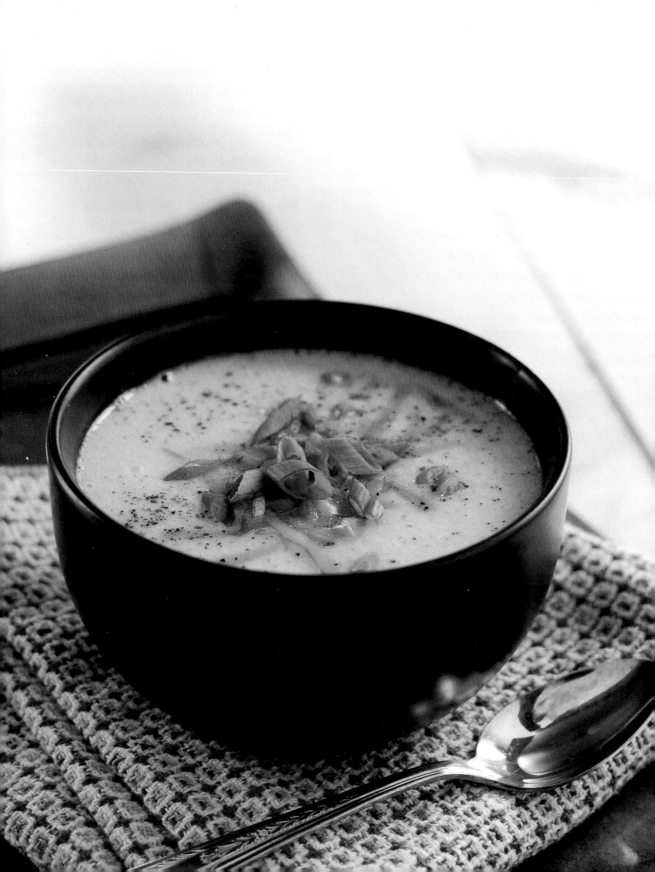

loaded fotato soup

SINGLE SERVE

8 ounces frozen cauliflower
(half a 16-ounce bag)

2 cups chicken broth or bone stock
(pages 495–496)

1 (.75-ounce) Light Laughing Cow
cheese wedge (for dairy-free option,
use 1 to 2 tablespoons Laughin'
Mama Cheese, page 484)

4 generous pinches Mineral Salt

⅛ teaspoon black pepper

¼ teaspoon onion powder

⅛ teaspoon garlic powder

Cayenne pepper to taste

1 to 2 squirts Bragg liquid aminos
(optional)

2 teaspoons nutritional yeast (optional)

Gluccie, or xanthan gum if you don't
have Gluccie

2 teaspoons turkey bacon bits

This quick soup from our first book became a favorite among the Trim Healthy Mama community because it is so creamy, dreamy yet it is a weight-kicking Fuel Pull. This blended veggie soup can be adapted for many nonstarchy veggies. Try it with yellow squash, zucchini, or broccoli. Top it with some grated cheese, if you'd prefer to put this in an S setting.

1. Put the cauliflower and broth in a saucepan, cover, and bring to a quick boil. Simmer until the cauliflower is tender (takes just a few minutes).

2. Transfer the cauliflower and about 1 cup broth to a blender. Secure the lid and blend well for a few seconds. Turn the blender off and vent the hot air, then continue to blend again until a smooth puree.

3. Pour the puree back into the saucepan, then add the cheese wedge and whisk until the cheese melts. Add the seasonings, liquid aminos, and nutritional yeast (if using).

4. Thicken the soup to desired consistency by sprinkling in the Gluccie from a salt shaker little by little while whisking briskly. Stop sprinkling a little before desired thickness is achieved. This soup should be a thick consistency to resemble a potato-based soup, but your soup will continue to thicken a little more after you stop sprinkling.

5. Taste and adjust the seasonings to "own it."

NOTE: You can up the protein content by adding some leftover chicken breast or stirring in a scoop of Integral Collagen and you'll still remain in **FP** mode. Or enjoy some Superfood Chocolate Chews (page 383) or a Praline Protein Bar (page 391) for dessert; however, that will take you into **S** mode.

NSI (IF USING XANTHAN INSTEAD OF GLUCCIE AND OMITTING THE NUTRITIONAL YEAST) DF (IF USING 1 TO 2 TABLESPOONS LAUGHIN' MAMA CHEESE, PAGE 484)

zesty sweetie soup

SINGLE SERVE

1 medium sweet potato, peeled and
diced small

1½ cups water

1 scoop Integral Collagen

1 teaspoon extra-virgin coconut oil, or
1 to 2 teaspoons MCT oil

6 pinches Mineral Salt (or 3 pinches
salt and 1 teaspoon light miso)

½ teaspoon ground cumin

1 teaspoon apple cider vinegar

1 teaspoon hot sauce of choice

⅛ teaspoon each garlic and onion
powder

Black pepper to taste

Cayenne pepper to taste

2 teaspoons nutritional yeast

¼ cup diced canned or ripe tomatoes

2 to 4 ounces foil-packed salmon, or
¼ to ½ cup diced cooked chicken
breast (optional)

Sweet potato is the star again in this soup, but this time the flavors are zesty and perhaps a little bit naughty, instead of sweet and mild as in the Cream of Sweet Stuff Soup (page 114).

1. Place the sweet potato in a small saucepan with the water, cover, and bring to a quick boil over high heat. Reduce the heat and simmer until tender.

2. Transfer the sweet potato and some cooking water to a blender. Add all the remaining ingredients except the tomatoes and salmon or chicken (if using). Blend to a smooth puree, venting the hot air periodically for safety. Pour the puree back into the saucepan, add the tomatoes and the salmon or chicken, and simmer for another minute or two.

3. Taste and adjust the seasonings to "own it."

SERVING IDEA: Garnish with parsley flakes and a sprinkling of grated pecorino cheese.

NOTE: If you don't have any cooked meat or salmon handy, just leave it out. You can always add 2 teaspoons Just Gelatin during the blending to up the protein content.

DF

cheesy dream soup

SINGLE SERVE

2 cups hot (not quite boiling) water

1 scoop Integral Collagen

1 teaspoon Just Gelatin

1 teaspoon coconut oil, butter, MCT oil, or tahini (sesame butter)

2 tablespoons grated pecorino romano or finely grated Parmesan cheese, or ½ inch cube any sharp aged cheese, the sharper the better (dairy-free people can use 2 tablespoons Hello Cheese, page 487)

1 tablespoon nutritional yeast

6 to 7 generous pinches Mineral Salt

1½ teaspoons miso or soy sauce

⅛ teaspoon garlic powder

1 wedge raw onion (roughly ⅛ of a small onion)

⅛ teaspoon black pepper

Cayenne pepper (to taste—we like more, and more, and maybe a tad more)

¼ to ¾ teaspoon Gluccie, for thickening

½ teaspoon apple cider vinegar or lemon juice (optional)

¼ teaspoon Liquid Smoke (optional)

1 doonk each of turmeric and paprika (optional)

SERENE CHATS: *This is a favorite of my oldest son, Arden. Of course, being an older teenager and now standing at six-foot-five, he burns fuel like a race car with a gas leak so he dunks a pile of my buttered Artisan Sourdough toast (page 206) in it . . . by pile, I mean a mountain.*

1. Place all the ingredients in a blender (use only ¼ teaspoon Gluccie) and process for a couple minutes. Transfer the puree to a small saucepan and bring to a simmer over medium-low heat. The soup will begin to thicken slightly. If it's not thickening enough for you, add a bit more Gluccie and whisk like crazy.

2. Simmer the soup for another 1 to 2 minutes, then taste and adjust the seasonings to "own it."

NOTE: We're slightly over **FP** fat grams here with the cheese and oil, but not by much. It is okay for a Fuel Pull to go over slightly sometimes if the meal is not paired with "push the limit" carbs. Hey, feel free to up the oil and the cheese and make this a full-blown **S**, if you want.

DF (IF USING HELLO CHEESE INSTEAD, PAGE 487)

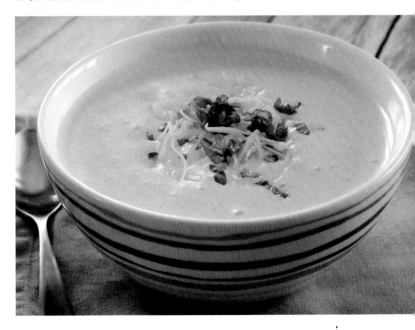

tuscan tomato soup

SINGLE SERVE

1¾ cups hot (not quite boiling) water

2½ tablespoons tomato paste

1 scoop Integral Collagen

2 teaspoons Just Gelatin

1 teaspoon coconut oil, or 1 to
   2 teaspoons MCT oil (see Note)

6 generous pinches Mineral Salt

2 teaspoons balsamic vinegar

4 shakes of Italian seasoning

3 frozen whole okra pods

¼ teaspoon onion powder

⅛ teaspoon garlic powder

Black and cayenne pepper to taste

A wonderful tomato soup for our dairy-free peeps, but it's also a nice alternative to the Just Like Campbell's Tomato Soup (page 112) even if you aren't dairy-free. One cannot get enough tomato soup in one's life, can one?

1. Pour the hot water into a blender. Add all the remaining ingredients and blend well until smooth.

2. Transfer the puree to a small saucepan. Bring to a simmer over medium-low heat, then taste and adjust the seasonings to "own it."

SERVING IDEA: Garnish with 1 tablespoon grated pecorino romano cheese to stay in **FP** mode or go heavier with other cheese of your choice to head into **S** mode.

NOTE: See page 44 of *Trim Healthy Mama Plan* for why 2 teaspoons of MCT oil can sometimes be used in a **FP** or **E** setting.

DF (IF USING HELLO CHEESE, PAGE 487, INSTEAD OF THE PECORINO)

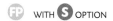
1½ cups hot (not quite boiling) water

⅔ cup frozen chopped spinach, or ⅔ cup tightly packed chopped fresh spinach

4 frozen whole okra pods

1 scoop Integral Collagen

1 teaspoon Just Gelatin

1 teaspoon coconut oil or butter, or 1 to 2 teaspoons MCT oil (or more, for **S** version)

6 generous pinches Mineral Salt

⅛ teaspoon black pepper

⅛ teaspoon cayenne pepper, or to taste

2 teaspoons nutritional yeast

1 teaspoon apple cider vinegar or vinegar of choice

1 tablespoon finely grated Parmesan or pecorino cheese

1 teaspoon light miso or soy sauce

⅛ teaspoon garlic powder

⅛ teaspoon onion powder

SERENE CHATS: *This is the single version of the family soup that I call Popeye's Power Soup (page 104). When I am not pulling my hair out at our nighttime dinner table, wiping up spilled water, and squelching squabbles, I love to savor this soup at lunch, for its sophistication. When my toddler is sleeping, I enjoy it slowly, taking a deep breath, a welcome break from the hectic day. It's a great way to savor a moment's peace.*

1. Place all the ingredients except half the spinach in a blender and puree until smooth.

2. Transfer the puree to a small saucepan and add the remaining spinach. Bring to a quick boil over high heat, then reduce the heat to low and simmer for a few minutes, until the spinach is no longer chewy but falls apart in your mouth. Taste and adjust the seasonings to "own it."

NOTE: Add some optional diced cooked chicken for more protein. The soup already has around 13 grams of protein, so it is not necessary if your other meals and snacks in the day provide ample amounts.

DF (IF USING 1 TABLESPOON HELLO CHEESE, PAGE 487, INSTEAD OF THE PARMESAN)

The following four soups all call for a single-serve package of Not Naughty Noodles as an ingredient, available from www.trimhealthymama.com. See page 27 on what to look for in store-bought versions.

thai on the fly soup

SINGLE SERVE

1½ cups chicken broth or bone stock (pages 495–496)

1 teaspoon red curry paste

½ to 1 teaspoon toasted sesame oil

1 squirt Bragg liquid aminos or soy sauce

3 pinches Mineral Salt

¼ to ½ teaspoon Super Sweet Blend, or ½ doonk Pure Stevia Extract

Cayenne pepper to taste

1 tablespoon nutritional yeast

1 single-serve package Not Naughty Noodles, rinsed, drained, and snipped smaller

3 to 4 ounces diced cooked chicken breast or quick pouch salmon

1 diced green onion (white and green parts)

It doesn't get easier than this soup—but oh my, the flavor!

1. Put all the ingredients except the noodles, chicken or salmon, and green onion in a blender and puree for a few seconds (this helps the sesame oil not to separate). Transfer the puree to a small saucepan. Add the noodles, chicken, and green onion, and bring to a simmer over medium-low heat. Taste and adjust the seasonings to "own it."

SERVING IDEA: Top with diced fresh cilantro, if desired.

NOTE: If desired, stir in 1 scoop Integral Collagen after placing soup in a bowl.

NSI (IF USING STORE-BOUGHT KONJAC NOODLES AND USING YOUR FAVORITE HANDY ON-PLAN SWEETENER) DF

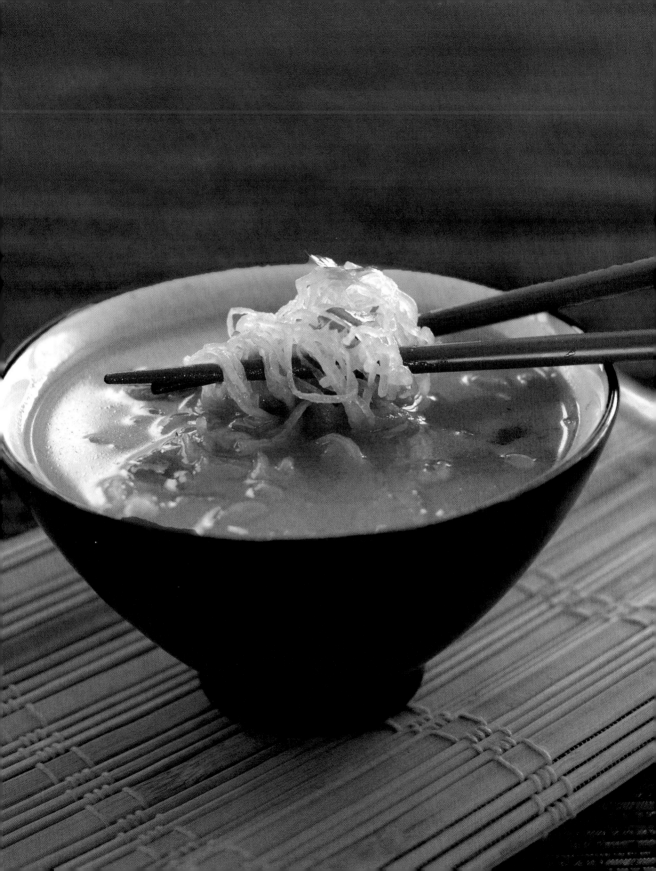

hot pot soup

(S)

SINGLE SERVE

1½ cups chicken broth or bone stock
  (pages 495–496)
3 to 4 generous pinches Mineral Salt
1 tablespoon nutritional yeast
¼ teaspoon onion powder
⅛ teaspoon garlic powder
Cayenne pepper to taste
1 single-serve package Not Naughty
  Noodles, rinsed, drained, and
  snipped smaller
2 tablespoons heavy cream
3 to 6 ounces cooked meat (any kind,
  seasoned; about ¾ cup)
1 to 2 squirts Bragg liquid aminos
  (optional)

The broth in this soup is rich and creamy, and offers a good dose of S fuel satisfaction. This soup is ready in less than 5 minutes.

1. Put the broth and seasonings in a small saucepan over medium-low heat and bring to a simmer. Add the noodles along with the cream and meat and liquid aminos (if using). Simmer for 1 minute, then taste and adjust the seasonings to "own it."

NSI (IF USING STORE-BOUGHT KONJAC NOODLES INSTEAD)

asian gold soup

(S)

SINGLE SERVE

¾ cup chicken broth or bone broth
  (pages 495–496)
¾ cup light canned coconut milk, or
  3 tablespoons full-fat coconut milk
  (plus ½ cup more chicken broth)
½ teaspoon curry powder
¼ teaspoon turmeric
3 to 4 generous pinches Mineral Salt
2 teaspoons lime juice (fresh or bottled
  from concentrate is fine)
½ teaspoon fish sauce
Cayenne pepper to taste
1 squirt Bragg liquid aminos
1 single-serve package Not Naughty
  Noodles, rinsed, drained, and
  snipped smaller
3 to 6 ounces canned salmon

Turmeric and curry powder bring healing treasures to your body, while the spiced coconut flavor makes your taste buds say, "Yes, please!"

1. Place the broth and coconut milk in a small saucepan and add the seasonings. Stir to combine over medium-high heat. Add the noodles and salmon, trying to include some skin and bones (if you are not afraid of bones, don't skip them; they are easily chewable and will give you much needed glycine—just ignore this suggestion about bones and skin if we are freaking you out and use pouch salmon). Simmer the soup for a couple minutes, then serve.

NOTE: The canned salmon is a wonderful quick option for this soup and works perfectly with the flavors going on. You can use leftover canned salmon to make Salmon Mousse (page 465) with the rest; the mousse is a fantastic snack with cucumber slices. If you HATE salmon . . . okay, diced cooked chicken is a fine option. We didn't list it in the ingredients this time because we're really trying to force you to *eat you some salmon!!!*

NSI (IF USING STORE-BOUGHT KONJAC NOODLES)   DF

1 tablespoon Trim Bouillon Mix
   (page 491)
1 cup water
1 single-serve package Not Naughty
   Noodles, drained, rinsed, and
   snipped smaller
1 scoop Integral Collagen or Just
   Gelatin (or both for more protein)

Make a batch of Trim Bouillon Mix (page 491) and keep it handy. With that sitting in your cupboard, this soup can become your no-brainer, go-to, ultra-speedy, make-life-easy snack or the main part of a meal. There's nothing but noodles, flavor, and health-promoting goodness. It has protein in the form of collagen and/or gelatin, but you can skip the collagen/gelatin if you want this to be a side dish with a sandwich that contains another source of protein. Or put some chicken in it in place of the collagen/gelatin. But if you can afford to keep one or both of these rich glycine sources of protein around, that is the quickest route to getting 'er done.

1. Place all the ingredients in a small saucepan over medium-low heat. Stir, then simmer until heated though. Taste and adjust the seasonings, then serve.

NOTE: The gelatin in the soup will gel if it gets cold, but will stay liquid while hot.

NSI (IF USING STORE-BOUGHT KONJAC NOODLES AND IF LEAVING OUT THE COLLAGEN AND GELATIN) DF

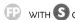 **FP** WITH **S** OPTION

1½ cups Purist Bone Stock (page 495)

1 teaspoon extra-virgin coconut oil

3 pinches Mineral Salt, or 1 teaspoon light miso

1 teaspoon nutritional yeast

Pinch of cayenne pepper

½ teaspoon dried parsley

SERENE CHATS: *This soup broth sounds so simple, but the stock almost literally "creams up" into "mother's milk" and makes the world seem a better place. This recipe doesn't float Pearl's boat, but it is one of my favorite treats as a comfort snack. I put it in an insulated coffee mug and sip my cares away all afternoon. Or, it is great as part of a larger meal. It soothes me like nothing else, bar God, of course—and a giant hug from hubby.*

You can add a swirl of raw pastured raw cream to the blender as an optional S twist, taking an already creamy toddy into the next dimension of amazingness. Along with the creamy mouth feel, there is health science behind this drink. It is naturally rich in glycine, which is an anti-spasmodic, anti-excitatory amino acid that relaxes the nerves. Drink up, my Purist Pals. Goodness awaits you.

1. Heat the stock in a small saucepan over medium-high heat. Place the hot stock in a blender and add the remaining ingredients. With the lid on securely, blend until creamy and frothy.

SERVING IDEA: Enjoy this soup in a cup that holds the heat so the delicious broth stays warm until the last sip.

NSI (IF LEAVING OUT NUTRITIONAL YEAST) DF

1 scoop Integral Collagen

1 teaspoon extra-virgin coconut oil

1 teaspoon light miso, or 3 pinches Mineral Salt

1 teaspoon nutritional yeast

Pinch of cayenne pepper

½ teaspoon dried parsley

SERENE CHATS: *I always throw a couple of these zippies into my purse if I have to be away from home for a day, or especially if I have to go out of town for a couple of days. Obviously, we purists can't carry big stockpots around with us, so this portable version of my Purist Primer (opposite) uses Integral Collagen for a protein- and nutrient-rich tide-me-over for when I am somewhere devoid of healthy options. It brings a little bit of the comfort of home to me when I am out and about. If you catch me at an airport or on a plane, I might just have this yummy concoction in my insulated coffee mug (and if I look happy and contented, now you'll know why). This is an especially wonderful treat during the fall and winter, although I drink it year-round.*

1. Place all the ingredients in a small zippy plastic bag.

SERVING IDEA: Carry the bag in your purse when traveling. When ready to enjoy, rip or snip a hole in the bottom corner and squeeze out into a stainless steel coffee mug with a good lid. Fill with hot water from any nearby café or gas station carafe. Stir with a coffee stirrer until completely dissolved and place on your lid. Give a gentle but purposeful swirl a couple of times to help combine the coconut oil with the rest of the ingredients. Sip and enjoy this warming healing elixir wherever you are and take your health with you on the go.

NOTE: **from Serene** This can also be made at home in your blender, and I often have it after dinner when I get the munchies but have no fresh stock on hand. If you are in a hotel and don't mind carrying one of those smallish hand-held immersion blender wands, then you can whip it quickly and it becomes a creamy soup instead of a broth-y clear liquid. Or, even niftier, if you have one of those battery-operated little coffee frothing wands that fit in your purse, then you can go for the creamy option anytime, anywhere.

DF

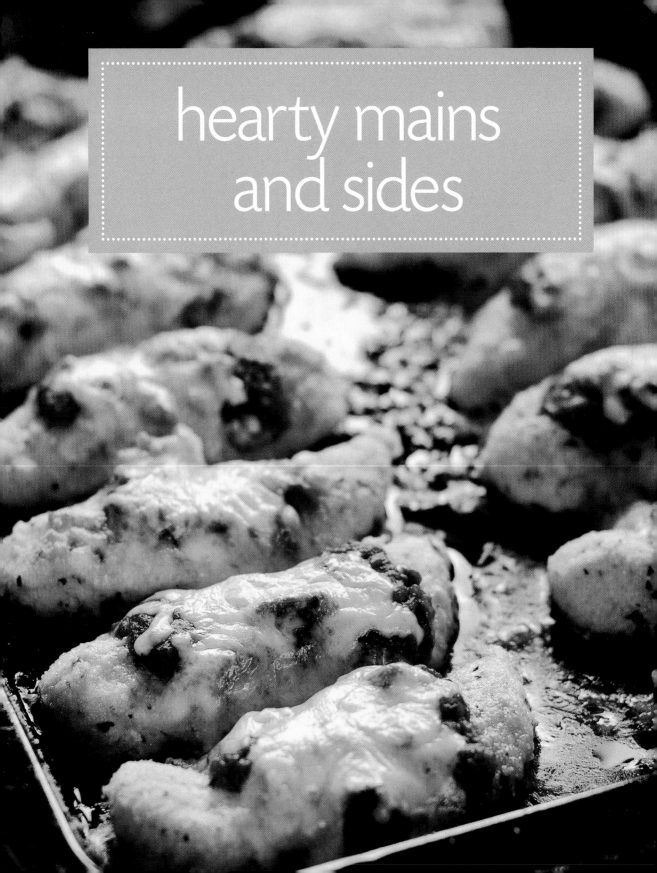

hearty mains
and sides

● = S ● = E ● = FP   MORE THAN ONE DOT INDICATES OPTIONS

SIDES

● = S   ● = E   ● = FP   MORE THAN ONE DOT INDICATES OPTIONS

OVEN DISHES

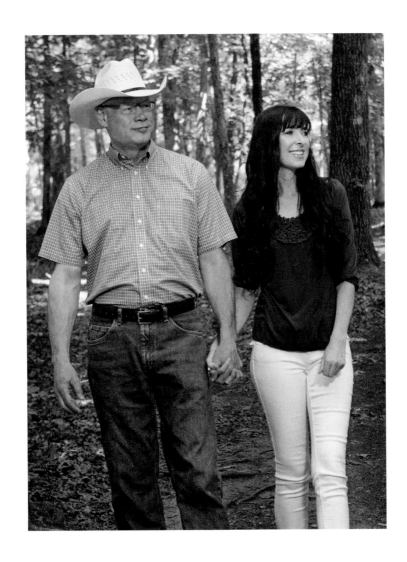

cornbread crusted mexican pie Ⓢ

FOR THE FILLING

2 pounds thawed ground meat of any
  kind (beef and venison work great)

2 (10-ounce) cans Rotel-style tomatoes
  and chilies (drain 1 of the cans)

3 large eggs, whisked well or beaten in
  a food processor

2 cups grated cheese of choice (or for
  dairy-free, 2 cups grated Hello
  Cheese, page 487)

2 teaspoons chili powder

2 teaspoons ground cumin

1½ teaspoons Mineral Salt

1 teaspoon onion powder

1 teaspooon paprika

FOR THE CORNBREAD TOPPING

¾ cup egg whites (carton is easier,
  but you can use fresh)

¾ cup Trim Healthy Mama Baking
  Blend

¼ cup water

2 tablespoons butter or coconut oil

½ teaspoon Super Sweet Blend
  (¾ teaspoon if you like a sweeter
  cornbread)

⅓ teaspoon Mineral Salt

¼ teaspoon paprika

Scant ¼ teaspoon turmeric

1½ teaspoons aluminum-free baking
  powder

2 tablespoons frozen corn kernels

Coconut oil cooking spray

Nothing else to say but *make this*! Yes, we're yelling through a megaphone here. We predict this will become a family favorite in your home as it is in ours. Children go nuts over this pie. If they cannot tolerate a lot of spice, though, choose mild canned tomatoes with chilies rather than the hotter version. Want to bring your man onboard the THM train? Serve him this with a smile and see what happens.

1. Preheat the oven to 350°F.

2. Make the filling. Brown the meat in a large skillet over medium-high heat. If the meat is not grass-fed beef, drain off most of the fat.

3. Add the tomatoes and chilies, eggs, half the cheese, and the seasonings and combine well. Pour into a 9 × 13-inch baking dish, spreading out the filling evenly. Top with the remaining cheese.

4. Make the cornbread topping. Put all the topping ingredients into a food processor and process until well combined. Spread the batter gently and evenly over the filling (topping does not have to go to the very edges of the dish). Spray the topping with the coconut oil.

5. Bake the pie for 35 minutes. Broil the top for another 3 to 5 minutes. Watch carefully so the cornbread crust does not burn but gets a nice golden brown.

SERVING IDEAS: Enjoy with a big side salad, which may be enough, but a side of green beans or buttered broccoli is always a winner with this meal.

NOTE: The small amount of corn here should not interfere with your **S** fuel.

DF (IF USING HELLO CHEESE, PAGE 487)

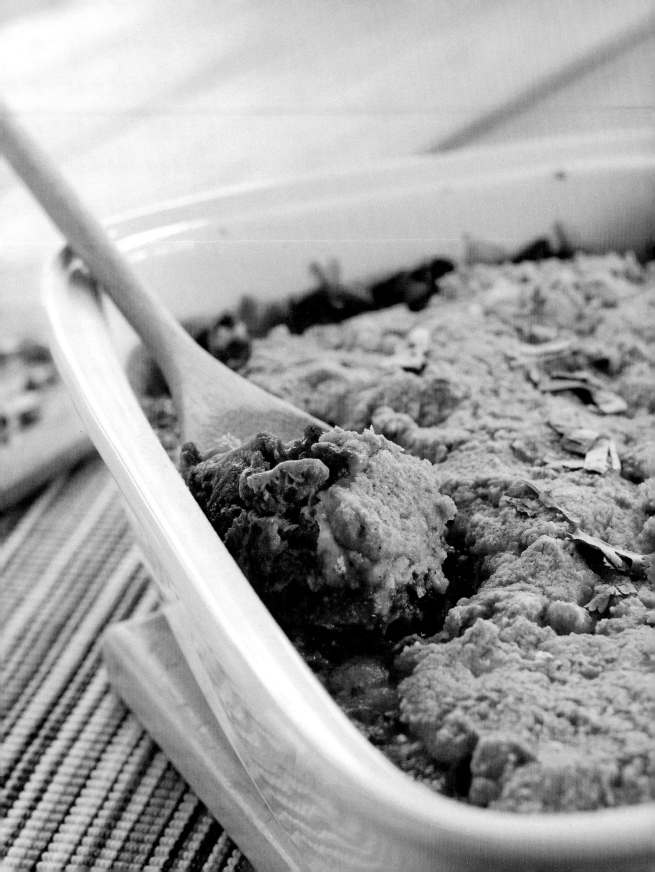

wise shepherd's pie

FAMILY SERVE – FEEDS 6 TO 8 (HALVE INGREDIENTS IF YOUR FAMILY IS SMALLER)

4 celery stalks, diced

1 large carrot, diced

1 large onion, chopped

2 garlic cloves, minced, or ½ to ¾ teaspoon garlic powder

2 tablespoons butter

2 pounds thawed ground beef or venison (or ground lamb, if you are lucky)

¾ cup beef broth (chicken broth works, too)

½ (6-ounce) can tomato paste

1 tablespoon Worcestershire sauce

1½ teaspoons Mineral Salt, or to taste

1 teaspoon onion powder

1 teaspoon black pepper

¼ teaspoon cayenne pepper (optional)

½ teaspoon crumbled dried rosemary

2 teaspoons dried parsley

1 cup frozen peas, or 1 (15-ounce) can green beans, drained and chopped smaller

1 batch Mashed Fotatoes (page 219), bacon bits and green onions omitted)

We grew up in New Zealand, which is a land of over 40 million sheep and less than 5 million people, so you can bet a big shepherd's pie was frequently on our dinner table. We come from a long line of sheep keepers, and our grandfather was listed in the *Guinness Book of World Records* for having the fastest time shearing a sheep (couldn't help boasting for a minute). Our childhood shepherd's pie was made with ground lamb; it was the ultimate comfort food dished out by our mother and the aroma of the lamb, seasoned with rosemary, filled our home. Lamb is so expensive here in the United States, so we use beef or venison to make this dish. We love shepherd's pie made this wise way, which uses cauliflower for the mashed topping, instead of potatoes, to keep blood sugars stable. Give this a try!

1. Preheat the oven to 350°F.

2. In a large skillet, sauté the celery, carrot, onion, and garlic in the butter over medium-high heat until the vegetables are starting to wilt and soften, about 3 minutes. Add the ground meat and brown it, stirring it into the veggies until cooked through. (If the meat isn't all that lean, cook it first, drain off the fat, then add the vegetables.)

3. Add the broth, tomato paste, Worcestershire sauce, and seasonings. Stir well, then remove the skillet from the heat and add the peas or green beans.

4. Pour the meat and veggie mix into a 9 × 13-inch baking dish. Spread the mashed cauliflower on top of the meat and spread out to cover well. Use your fork to trace long, vertical lines over the top. Bake for 30 minutes, then broil for a few minutes, until the top is golden brown (watch that it doesn't burn).

NOTE: If certain members of your family are not too keen on Mashed Fotatoes, make up just half the recipe and split the filling into two smaller baking dishes. Top one dish with Mashed Fotatoes and the other with mashed potatoes. That's an extra step that may keep the peace in some homes, and peace is a wonderful thing!

NSI

troodle casserole

⑤

2 pounds thawed ground meat (beef, venison, or turkey all work well)

3 to 4 garlic cloves, minced

2 (14-ounce) jars sugar-free pizza sauce or spaghetti sauce (see Note), or 3½ cups homemade sauce

⅓ teaspoon Mineral Salt

⅓ teaspoon black pepper

¼ teaspoon cayenne pepper

1 to 2 doonks Pure Stevia Extract

½ cup finely grated Parmesan cheese (green can kind is fine)

5 medium zucchini, made into Troodles (page 222)

8 ounces part-skim mozzarella cheese, grated

Turkey pepperoni slices

Sliced olives

This is a great dinner in summer, when gardens are abundant with zucchini—or enjoy it any time of the year by using store-bought zucchini.

1. Preheat the oven to 350°F.

2. Brown the meat and garlic in a large skillet over high heat. (If the meat releases a lot of fat, brown it alone and drain off the fat, then sauté the garlic with the meat for a couple minutes.) Add the sauce and seasonings, as well as the Parmesan, and simmer, stirring, until heated through.

3. Put the cooked Troodles in a colander and press down to eliminate excess water. Arrange the Troodles in a 9 × 13-inch baking dish and pour on and stir in the meat sauce. Sprinkle with the grated mozzarella, then arrange the pepperoni slices and olives on top. Bake for 25 to 30 minutes or until bubbly.

SERVING IDEAS: Enjoy with a very large side salad with an olive oil–based vinaigrette and Swiss Garlic Bread (page 196) on the side, if desired.

NOTE: Walmart's Great Value Pizza Sauce has only 3 net carbs.

NSI

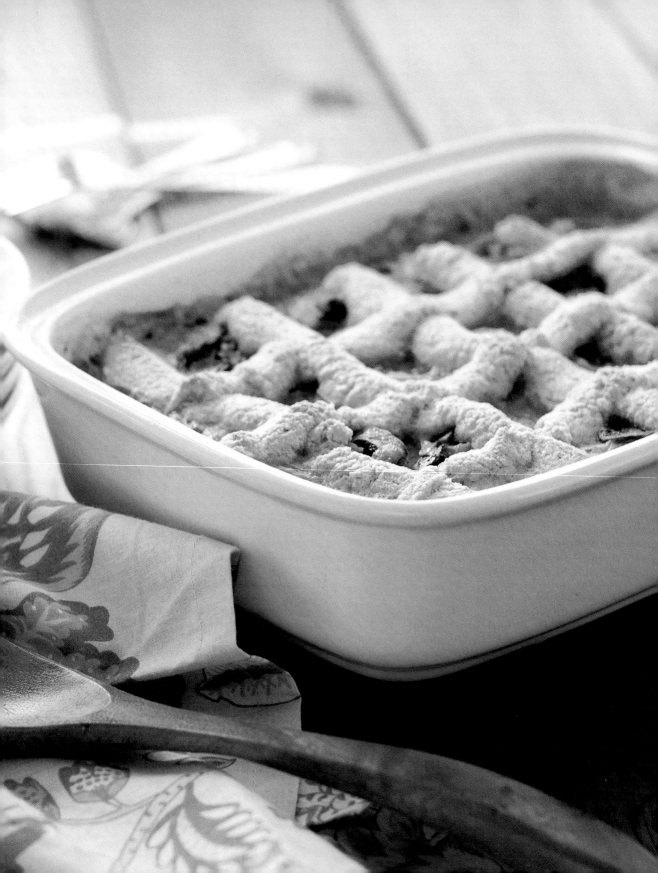

chicken pot pie

(S)

FOR THE FILLING

1 medium onion, diced

3 celery stalks, thinly sliced

1 large carrot, thinly sliced

8 ounces button mushrooms, thinly sliced

1 tablespoon butter

1¾ cups chicken broth

1 tablespoon Trim Bouillon Mix (page 491)

1½ cups unsweetened almond or cashew milk

1 teaspoon Mineral Salt

¾ teaspooon black pepper

1½ teaspoons dried thyme

1 teaspoon Gluccie

¼ cup heavy cream

1½ pounds (2 to 3 cups) diced cooked chicken (Drive Thru Sue's can even use canned chicken)

1 cup frozen peas

FOR THE CRUST

¾ cup egg whites (carton is easier, but fresh is fine)

¾ cup Trim Healthy Mama Baking Blend

4 tablespoons water

3 tablespoons butter or coconut oil

4 pinches Super Sweet Blend

4 pinches Mineral Salt

1½ teaspoons aluminum-free baking powder

Coconut oil cooking spray

Craving some comfort food? Here you go.

1. Preheat the oven to 350°F.

2. Make the filling. In a large skillet, sauté the onion, celery, carrot, and mushrooms in the butter with ¼ cup broth and the bouillon mix until wilted and tender. Add the remaining 1½ cups broth, the almond milk, salt, pepper, and thyme to the skillet and bring to a simmer. Push the veggies to the side and slowly add the Gluccie from a spice shaker, whisking like crazy. Allow to simmer for a few minutes and thicken a bit, then add the cream and stir. Remove from the heat.

3. Spread the chicken in a 9 × 13-inch baking dish along with the peas. Add the sautéed veggies and sauce over the top.

4. Make the crust. Put all the ingredients in a food processor and process until well combined.

5. Spread the batter gently over the top of the pie, using the back of a spoon so it is even thickness (does not have to go to the very edges of the dish), or put the batter in a zippy bag, snip one corner, and pipe over the top in a pattern of your choice.

6. Spray the top of the pie with coconut oil, then bake for 35 minutes or until bubbly. Broil the top for another 3 to 5 minutes, watching carefully so the crust does not burn but gets a nice golden brown.

loaded spaghetti squash casserole

1 large spaghetti squash

2 cups grated cheddar cheese

1½ to 2 pounds (3 cups) diced cooked chicken or cooked lean ground meat

6 tablespoons (¾ stick) butter

½ cup heavy cream

1 cup sour cream, or ⅓ less fat cream cheese, or Greek yogurt

¼ cup bacon pieces or chopped turkey bacon

Mineral Salt and black pepper to taste

Ooey, gooey, cheesy goodness! Spaghetti squash has never been so yummy! You can make this casserole a full meal by including diced cooked chicken or ground beef (or venison), or omit the meat and enjoy this as a side. Jennifer Griffin is a wonderful creator of Trim Healthy Mama recipes, and we give her the credit for this hit recipe in the THM community. Check out more of her recipes at www.ahomewithapurpose.com.

1. Preheat the oven to 350°F.

2. Cook the squash until tender, then scoop out the "spaghetti" using a fork. (You can cook the squash in a crockpot all day; or slice it in half and bake face down on a coconut oil–sprayed baking pan at 350°F for 45 minutes; or cook the two halves for 4 to 5 minutes in a pressure cooker.) Keep the oven set to 350°F.

3. In a large bowl, mix the squash with 1 cup of the cheddar cheese and the remaining ingredients. Mix well and place in a 9 × 13-inch baking dish. Top with the remaining cheddar cheese and bake for 30 minutes or until bubbly.

NSI

zucchini canoes

 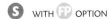
FAMILY SERVE – FEEDS 6 TO 8 (HALVE INGREDIENTS IF YOUR FAMILY IS SMALLER)

4 to 6 medium to large zucchini

Coconut oil cooking spray

1 pound (1½ to 2 cups) diced cooked chicken breast, or browned ground meat, or diced sprouted tofu, seasoned with salt and black pepper

2 to 3 ripe medium tomatoes, chopped

8 ounces cheddar cheese or part-skim mozzarella cheese, grated (for dairy-free, use grated Hello Cheese, page 487)

4 green onions, white and green parts finely diced

¼ cup bacon bits (turkey or otherwise)

Black olives, for garnish (optional)

Zucchini is on sale? Or perhaps your garden is abundant with them? This is a fun family dinner to help you use up all those healthy zucchini.

1. Preheat the oven to 400°F.

2. Cut the zucchini lengthwise and scoop out the seedy middle. Spray a large cooking sheet with coconut oil spray and arrange the zucchini halves on it. Bake for 10 minutes, or until somewhat softened. Keep the oven at 400°F.

3. In a medium bowl, combine the chicken and tomatoes. Stuff the zucchini centers with the mixture, then top with sprinkles of grated cheese, green onion, olives (if using), and bacon bits. Bake for another 10 to 15 minutes.

NOTE: If you use chicken breast and grated Hello Cheese (page 487), you can consider your dish **FP.**

NSI DF (IF USING HELLO CHEESE, PAGE 487)

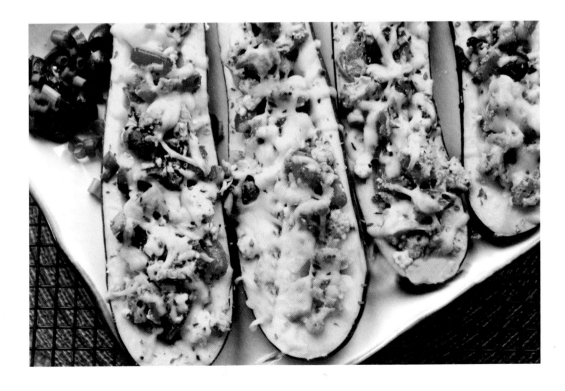

lazy lasagna

2 pounds thawed ground meat (beef and venison work well)

2 (12-ounce) jars no-sugar-added pizza or spaghetti sauce (see Note)

1½ tablespoons dried oregano

½ teaspoon Mineral Salt

1 teaspoon onion powder

1 teaspoon garlic powder

⅛ teaspoon cayenne pepper

1 to 2 doonks Pure Stevia Extract (optional)

2 (10-ounce) packages frozen chopped spinach, thawed

1 (8-ounce) package ⅓ less fat cream cheese

1 (14-ounce) container 1% cottage cheese

2 large eggs

8 ounces part-skim mozzarella cheese, grated

¼ cup finely grated Parmesan cheese (for sprinkling over top; green can kind is fine)

PEARL CHATS: I've made plenty of zucchini and eggplant lasagnas in the last few years that fit S mode, but they call for cutting the veggies into thin layers as faux noodles, and sometimes also require pre-cooking the veggies. I'm so over that. These days my life is way too busy for those extra steps; I need ultra-easy meals, so I thought about spinach. It's super cheap when you buy it in frozen bricks, it doesn't require cutting—hmmm—couldn't that work as a lasagna noodle layer? My children are not the hugest spinach fans, but they scarf this down and tell me it is the best lasagna ever! This is my go-to lasagna now; I've ditched all the others.

1. Preheat the oven to 350°F.

2. Brown the meat in a large skillet over high heat, then drain off any excess fat if necessary. Add the sauce and seasonings, and simmer over low heat for several minutes.

3. Put the spinach in a colander and squeeze and push to get all the liquid out.

4. Put the cream cheese, cottage cheese, and eggs in a food processor and process until smooth.

5. Layer half the meat sauce in the bottom of a 9 × 13-inch baking dish. Top with half the cheese mixture, then layer on half the spinach. Follow with half the grated mozzarella. Repeat the layers, ending with the mozzarella. Top with a good sprinkling of Parmesan cheese. Bake for 40 minutes or until bubbly.

NOTE: Walmart's Great Value Pizza Sauce has only 3 net carbs.

NSI (IF USING YOUR HANDY ON-PLAN SWEETENER)

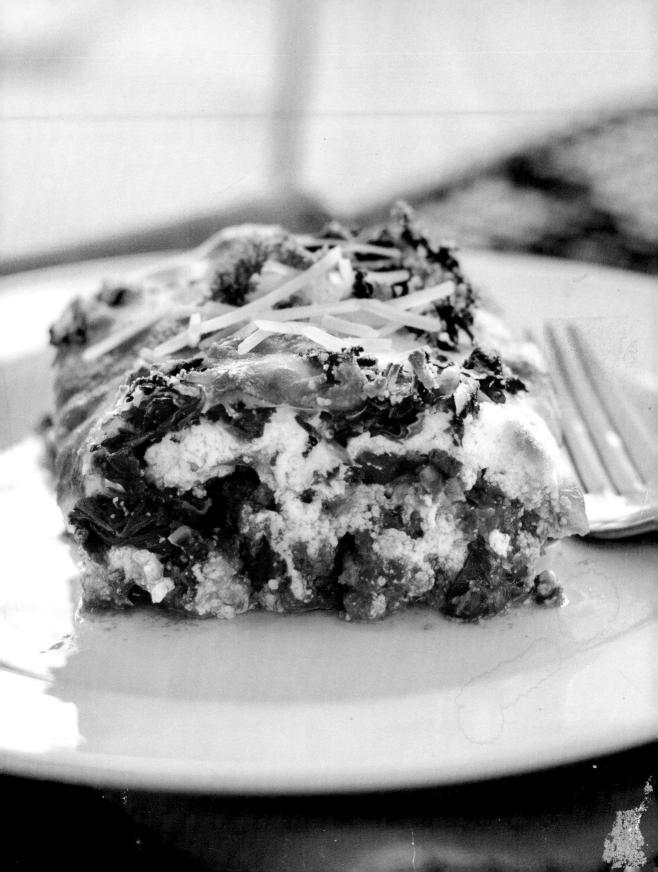

nacho stuffed peppers

FAMILY SERVE – FEEDS 6 TO 8 (HALVE INGREDIENTS IF YOUR FAMILY IS SMALLER)

1½ pounds small bell peppers (the small colorful ones you can buy in zip-top baggies)

1 pound thawed ground beef or venison

½ medium onion, finely diced

1½ tablespoons "Macho" Nacho Seasoning (page 492)

8 ounces cheddar cheese, grated (for dairy-free, use Hello Cheese, page 487)

1 to 2 green onions, white and green parts diced (optional)

Pitted black olives, diced (optional)

Pickled jalapeño peppers, diced, to taste (optional)

1. Preheat the oven to 350°F.

2. Slice the peppers in half and scoop out any seeds or ridges so the peppers become little boats; also slice off the stem ends.

3. Brown the meat with the onion in a large skillet over high heat. Add the seasoning and stir well.

4. Stuff the pepper boats with the meat and onion, then top with the grated cheese and green onions, olives, and jalapeños (if using). Bake for 15 to 20 minutes. Broil at the end for just a few minutes for crispier tops, but keep a watch out that they don't burn.

SERVING IDEAS: Enjoy with a large, crisp side salad.

NSI DF (IF USING GRATED HELLO CHEESE, PAGE 487)

creamy pearlchilada bake

(S)

FAMILY SERVE – FEEDS 6 TO 8 (HALVE INGREDIENTS IF YOUR FAMILY IS SMALLER)

FOR THE ENCHILADAS

1½ pounds (2 to 3 cups) shredded
   cooked chicken (or 2 [12-ounce]
   cans chicken breast, drained; diced
   sprouted tofu also works for
   vegetarians)
1 (12-ounce) jar salsa of choice
1 teaspoon chili powder
1 teaspoon ground cumin
½ teaspoon Mineral Salt
½ teaspoon onion powder
½ teaspoon garlic powder (optional)
1 family-serve batch Wonder Wraps
   (page 204)
8 ounces cheddar or pepper jack
   cheese, grated
Coconut oil cooking spray

FOR THE CREAM SAUCE

1 (12- to 14-ounce) container
   1% cottage cheese
1 cup sour cream
½ cup chicken broth
½ teaspoon Mineral Salt
¼ teaspoon black pepper

FOR THE TOPPING

4 ounces cheese of your choice,
   grated
Mexican hot sauce, such as Valentina
Chopped green onions (white and
   green parts)
Chopped pitted olives

PEARL CHATS: Serene named this dish for me. She told me I cannot call these enchiladas, as they simply are not enchiladas! Her husband, Sam, is from New Mexico, so "apparently" she now knows all about enchiladas. She was quite bossy about it, and told me this *shall* be their name. Okay, okay, so maybe this dish is not truly authentic, but my family thinks it is truly yummy. It came about because I was in the mood for enchiladas but had no tortillas or enchilada sauce. I created this out of what I had on hand, and it turned into something I make often now.

You can use store-bought low-carb tortillas, if you prefer (I do that occasionally), but Wonder Wraps are a no-Frankenfood way to eat these. They work really well and are much healthier. I find myself stepping toward Serene's purist ways every now and then. It's a good idea to make the Wonder Wraps ahead of time, whenever you have a spare 15 to 20 minutes—or if you have a spare teenager wandering around your home, then put him or her to work. Wonder Wrapping is fun and quite therapeutic. The wraps keep well in the refrigerator, and if they are sitting pretty in the fridge all ready to go, this recipe is a snap to put together.

1. Preheat the oven to 350°F.
2. Make the enchiladas. Put the chicken in a medium bowl with the salsa and seasonings. Combine well.
3. Fill each wrap with some of the chicken mixture and some grated cheese. Roll each wrap closed (they do not need to be sealed at the top and bottom). Coat a 9 × 13-inch baking dish with coconut oil cooking spray. Squeeze all the wraps into the baking dish so they fit tightly next to each other.
4. Make the sauce. Put all the sauce ingredients in a blender and puree. Pour over the wraps in the dish.
5. Add the topping. Top with grated cheese, swirl several squirts of hot sauce over the top, then garnish with the green onions and olives.
6. Bake for 30 to 35 minutes, or until bubbly.

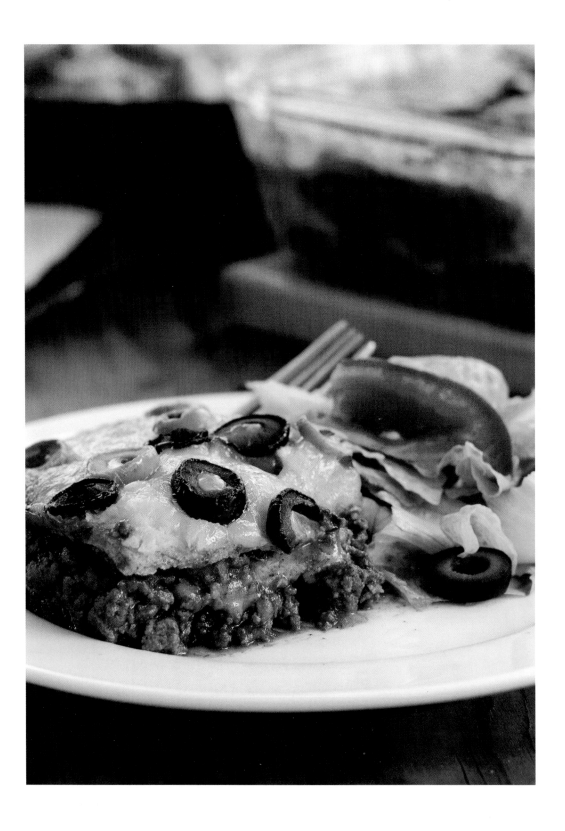

enchilada wonder casserole

FAMILY SERVE – FEEDS 6 TO 8 (HALVE INGREDIENTS IF YOUR FAMILY IS SMALLER)

3 pounds thawed ground beef, venison, or turkey (or use shredded cooked chicken)

FOR THE ENCHILADA GRAVY

3 tablespoons MCT oil or cooking coconut oil (you don't want coconut flavor)

½ teaspoon Gluccie

¼ cup chili powder

2 cups chicken broth

10 ounces tomato paste

1 teaspoon dried oregano

1 teaspoon ground cumin

½ teaspoon Mineral Salt

2 pickled jalapeño peppers, minced, or 1 fresh jalapeño, minced with 1 tablespoon apple cider vinegar and a pinch of salt (optional; for more heat)

Coconut oil cooking spray

1 family-serve batch Wonder Wraps (page 204)

8 ounces sharp cheddar, grated, or 8 ounces grated Hello Cheese (page 487)

1 (15-ounce) can pitted black or green olives, drained and sliced

SERENE CHATS: *You bet I'm not allowing Pearl to use the official* enchilada *word in her title. My husband's family is serious about their enchiladas, and the casserole form is always an important dish at birthdays or on special occasions on that side of our family. The tradition and love for this dish was passed on from my husband to our children, so I've had to put a lot of thought into how to "trimhealthymamafy" the authentic flavors so that it could still pass muster in our home. Pearl threw together a bunch of stuff she saw in her fridge on a whim—what???!!! I had to think and experiment and tweak until I got it perfect. That's why I get to use the word* enchilada *and she doesn't—'nuff said. This simple recipe is both Drive Thru Sue friendly and purist/allergen-free friendly, depending on what cheese you use. Drive Thru Sue's can use 8 ounces of grated sharp cheddar, while those who can't or prefer not to use pasteurized cheese, can use Hello Cheese (page 487). My family can barely tell the difference between the two versions.*

1. Preheat the oven to 350°F.
2. Brown the ground meat and drain excess fat.
3. Meanwhile, put all enchilada gravy ingredients in the blender and blend well.
4. Add the enchilada gravy to the browned meat.
5. Spray a 9 × 13-inch baking dish with coconut oil cooking spray and start your layering. Begin with a gravy meat layer using half the meat mixture, then a layer of Wonder Wraps, slightly overlapping. Sprinkle half the grated cheese on the wraps, then repeat with the remaining meat mixture. Add a second layer of Wonder Wraps, then the remaining cheese. Finish with the garnish of sliced olives on top of the cheese.
6. Bake for 30 minutes.

DF (IF USING GRATED HELLO CHEESE, PAGE 487)

2½ pounds thawed ultra-lean (at least 96%) ground turkey or venison (or use regular ground turkey and rinse well under hot water after browning)

FOR THE ENCHILADA GRAVY

1½ tablespoons MCT oil or cooking coconut oil (you don't want coconut flavor)

½ teaspoon Gluccie

¼ cup chili powder

2 cups chicken broth

10 ounces tomato paste

1 teaspoon dried oregano

1 teaspoon ground cumin

½ teaspoon Mineral Salt

2 pickled jalapeño peppers, minced; or 1 fresh jalapeño, minced with 1 tablespoon apple cider vinegar and a pinch of salt (optional; for more heat)

I batch Laughin' Mama Cheese (page 484)

1 cup carton egg whites or 8 large egg whites

½ teaspoon Mineral Salt

½ teaspoon cumin

Coconut oil cooking spray

1 family-serve batch Wonder Wraps (page 204)

2 (15-ounce) cans diced tomatoes, drained, or same amount of fresh (squeeze out juice)

2 (4-ounce) cans diced green chilies

SERENE CHATS: *This is a tweak on the Enchilada Wonder Casserole (page 145). Despite this being a Fuel Pull, it's hearty good eats! In fact, it might just become your favorite way of eating enchiladas, and will allow you more of that fuel juggle we keep urging you to keep in your life.*

1. Preheat the oven to 350°F.

2. Brown the ground meat and rinse away excess fat.

3. Meanwhile, put all the enchilada gravy ingredients in a blender and blend well.

4. Add the enchilada gravy to the browned meat.

5. In the blender, blend the Laughin' Mama Cheese with the egg whites, extra salt, and extra cumin.

6. Spray a 9 × 13-inch baking dish with coconut oil cooking spray. Start your layering, beginning with half of the gravy-meat mixture, then a layer of Wonder Wraps, slightly overlapping. Drizzle half the cheese mixture over the top, then sprinkle half the tomatoes over the cheese. Repeat the layers—meat/gravy, Wonder Wraps, cheese/egg white mix, diced toms—then top with a finale of diced green chilies.

7. Bake for 30 minutes, uncovered, then cover with aluminum foil (or another tray as a lid) and bake an additional 20 minutes. When done, let set for 15 to 20 minutes before serving.

NOTE: Usually we suggest a 3 to 4 ounce meat limit for **FP** meals. Once ground beef is browned, it loses weight. So even if just slightly over **FP** amounts here, it still can fit **FP** mode.

DF

fakertot casserole

FAMILY SERVE – FEEDS 6 TO 8 (HALVE INGREDIENTS IF YOUR FAMILY IS SMALLER)

1½ to 2 pounds thawed ground beef

1½ teaspoons Mineral Salt

1 teaspoon black pepper

⅓ cup diced onion

½ cup heavy cream

4 ounces cream cheese

4 tablespoons (½ stick) butter

1½ cups beef broth

½ teaspoon garlic powder

½ cup finely diced button mushrooms

½ teaspoon Gluccie

2 (16-ounce) bags frozen cauliflower florets

2 cups grated cheddar cheese

This recipe from Amanda Coers was a runaway hit in the THM community because—who doesn't like tatertots? And in casserole form, well, that just makes everything better. Check out her other Trim Healthy Mama recipes at www.thecoersfamily.com.

1. Preheat the oven to 400°F.

2. Cook the ground beef in a large skillet until browned, then drain off excess fat. Add salt, pepper, and the onion, and cook for a few more minutes, stirring it into the meat.

3. Place the cream, cream cheese, butter, broth, garlic powder, and salt and pepper to taste in a medium saucepan. Cook over medium heat, whisking occasionally, then turn down the heat and let simmer while you stir in the mushrooms.

4. Slowly add the Gluccie to the sauce and whisk well to avoid lumps. Simmer the sauce for 3 to 5 minutes more, stirring, then remove from heat.

5. Layer the cauliflower in a 9 × 13-inch baking dish. Spread the meat mixture on top, then pour the sauce over the entire dish. Top with the shredded cheese. Cover the dish with aluminum foil and bake for 25 to 30 minutes. Remove foil and continue to bake for another 10 minutes to brown the top.

NSI (IF USING XANTHAN INSTEAD OF GLUCCIE TO THICKEN THE SAUCE)

wonder-wrap–ful lasagna

Ⓢ

FAMILY SERVE – FEEDS 6 TO 8 (HALVE INGREDIENTS IF YOUR FAMILY IS SMALLER)

2 to 3 pounds thawed ground beef,
   venison, or turkey

1 (6-ounce) can tomato paste

1 (8-ounce) can tomato sauce

¾ teaspoon Mineral Salt

1 to 2 teaspoons Italian seasoning mix

Black pepper and cayenne pepper
   to taste

Onion and garlic powder to taste

1 (14-ounce) container 1 or 2% cottage
   cheese or part-skim ricotta
   (dairy-free peeps can sub
   1½ batches Laughin' Mama Cheese,
   page 484)

2 large eggs plus 4 egg whites

Coconut oil cooking spray

1 family-serve batch Wonder Wraps
   (page 204)

12 ounces part-skim mozzarella
   cheese, grated (for dairy-free, use
   12 ounces grated Hello Cheese,
   page 487)

SERENE CHATS: *Here's another casserole using Wonder Wraps. Now that I always have Hello Cheese (page 487) handy, I can enjoy making casseroles a whole lot more frequently—and that's making my husband an even happier man. I tolerate dairy well, but foods dense in calories, like hard, full-fat pasteurized cheese, are personally not the way I, as a purist, like to get my fat. I prefer avocados, walnuts, raw cheese, coconut, MCT, and red palm oil. It's not that I stay completely away from pasteurized hard cheeses, but they're not so high on my list of "good guys." You can stay with regular hard cheese—Pearl does. All of our Trim Healthy Mama journeys look unique, and that's perfectly okay. But lately, I sub grated Hello Cheese for all the fatty cheese called for in most casseroles; my children don't even seem to notice I've switched. I have found a great cultured 1% cottage cheese that I am in love with, called Nancy's (Daisy's is great, too), with no fillers, so I'm fine using cottage cheese.*

1. Preheat the oven to 350°F.

2. Brown the meat in a large skillet over high heat, then drain off any excess fat. Add the tomato paste, tomato sauce (holding back 2 tablespoons), and the seasonings. Stir to combine.

3. In a bowl, combine the cottage cheese and eggs and egg whites.

4. Spray a 9 × 13-inch baking pan with coconut oil cooking spray. Spread the remaining 2 tablespoons tomato sauce on the bottom of the pan. If making a three-layer lasagna, use one-third of the Wonder Wraps to cover the bottom of the pan, then one-third of the cottage cheese mixture, one-third of the meat, and one-third of the grated mozzarella; repeat twice. If doing a two-layer lasagna, use half of the items and repeat once.

5. Bake for 35 minutes, or until bubbly.

DF (IF USING HELLO CHEESE, PAGE 487, AND LAUGHIN' MAMA
CHEESE, PAGE 484, INSTEAD OF THE COTTAGE CHEESE AND
MOZZARELLA)

cheeseburger pie

S

2 to 2 ½ pounds ground beef or venison

3 teaspoons onion powder

1½ teaspoons Mineral Salt

½ teaspoon black pepper

12 ounces cheese of your choice, grated

2 large eggs

½ cup mayonnaise

½ cup heavy cream

PEARL CHATS: This decadent dish wins over reluctant husbands by the thousands! Any way you like your cheeseburger you can apply to this pie. You could include a layer of finely diced sautéed onions, dill pickles, jalapeños, or even a layer of tomatoes to the basic recipe below. Our children love to top this pie with a little mustard and a lot of ketchup. Serve it with a large side salad and you've got dinner! (By the way, Drive Thru Sue's could get away with using a packet of onion soup mix instead of the seasonings here.)

1. Preheat the oven to 350°F.
2. Brown the meat in a large skillet over high heat, then drain off excess fat. Add the onion powder, salt, and pepper and mix well.
3. Spread the meat mixture in a 9 × 13-inch baking dish and mix in half the grated cheese.
4. In a bowl, combine the eggs, mayonnaise, and cream. Pour over the meat, then top with the remaining grated cheese. Bake for 35 minutes, or until bubbly.

NOTE: Greek yogurt can be subbed for mayonnaise.

NSI

spinach and sausage quiche ⓢ

FOR THE CRUST

1 cup Trim Healthy Mama Baking Blend

5 tablespoons cold butter

2 large egg yolks (save the whites for the filling)

1 tablespoon cold water

FOR THE FILLING

10 large eggs plus 2 egg whites

4 to 6 cooked chicken sausage links, thinly sliced

1 (10-ounce) package frozen chopped spinach, thawed and squeezed of excess water

2 cups grated cheese of your choice

½ teaspoon Mineral Salt

½ teaspoon black pepper

Dried basil to taste (optional)

Sliced fresh mushrooms, ripe tomatoes, and pitted olives (optional)

This quiche has a wonderfully rich crust, but you can skip the crust if you want to make things easier on yourself or use a quick Simple Simon Pie Crust (page 324), omitting the sweetener, as it requires no pre-baking. Another option for a simple crust is to combine 1 cup almond flour with 1 egg white and bake for 10 minutes to crisp it before filling.

1. Preheat the oven to 350°F.

2. Make the crust. Place the Baking Blend and butter in a food processor and process until well combined, like coarse meal. Add the egg yolks and pulse to mix well. Add the tablespoon cold water and pulse again. You should be able to press the mixture together and have it stick; if it doesn't, add a little more cold water.

3. Gather the mixture into a ball and flatten the ball. Put the flattened ball between 2 sheets of parchment and roll out to a large circle if you are using a pie plate or a large rectangle if using a 9 × 13-inch baking pan. Remove the top parchment and use the rolling pin to invert the crust into the baking dish. If the crust breaks apart, gently press it back together and press into the pan. Bake the crust for 10 minutes. Let cool briefly to set. Keep the oven at 350°F.

4. Make the filling. In a bowl, whisk together the eggs, egg whites, sausage slices, spinach, grated cheese, seasonings, and optional ingredients like mushrooms, tomato, and olives. Pour into the crust and bake for about 45 minutes, or until the filling is set.

NSI (IF GOING CRUSTLESS OR MAKING ALMOND FLOUR CRUST)

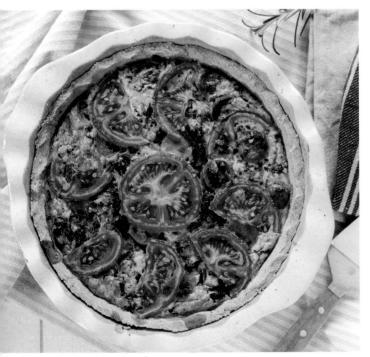

fussless fuel pull quiche

2½ cups egg whites (carton is easier, but fresh is fine)

1 (10-ounce) bag chopped spinach, thawed and squeezed of excess water

1 (15-ounce) can petite tomatoes, drained

9 ounces natural lean deli meat, diced (such as turkey)

5 tablespoons finely grated Parmesan cheese (for dairy-free, use grated lighter version of Hello Cheese, page 487)

3 tablespoons nutritional yeast

½ teaspoon Mineral Salt

½ teaspoon black pepper

½ teaspoon red pepper flakes

1 teaspoon onion powder

½ teaspoon garlic powder

1 teaspoon Italian seasoning mix

2 tablespoons Whole-Husk Psyllium Flakes

Sometimes you just need easy, and you also need to lighten up your meals occasionally if you have been stuck in heavy mode. This is light, but still delightfully yummy.

1. Preheat the oven to 350°F.
2. Combine all the ingredients in a bowl. Pour into a 9 × 13-inch baking dish and bake for 30 to 35 minutes, or until bubbly.

DF (IF USING GRATED HELLO CHEESE, PAGE 487, INSTEAD)

tuscan sausage and egg bake

(S)

FOR THE BREAD CUBES

1 cup Trim Healthy Mama Baking Blend

4 small pinches Super Sweet Blend

4 pinches Mineral Salt

2 teaspoons aluminum-free baking powder

4 tablespoons water

1 cup plus 2 tablespoons liquid egg whites (carton or fresh, but carton is easier)

FOR THE CASSEROLE

2 tablespoons ghee (clarified butter) or butter (if using ghee, add ¼ teaspoon Mineral Salt)

½ teaspoon dried basil, plus 1½ teaspoons for garnishing

½ teaspoon ground cumin

½ teaspoon paprika

¼ teaspoon garlic powder

Coconut oil cooking spray

1 fresh jalapeño pepper, diced

1 large onion, diced

2 (15-ounce) cans diced tomatoes, with juice

⅓ cup pitted green olives, diced

4 to 5 cooked turkey, beef, pork, or chicken sausage links, sliced

1 cup grated pecorino romano or sharp cheddar (for dairy-free, use Hello Cheese, page 487)

⅓ cup frozen diced okra

2 tablespoons tomato paste

1½ cups chicken broth

1 teaspoon Mineral Salt

¼ teaspoon Gluccie

8 large eggs

¼ cup diced pitted green olives, for garnishing

Cracked black pepper to taste, for garnishing

1 tablespoon balsamic vinegar, for drizzling on top

What's not to love about this hearty combination of hunks of bread, sausage, cheese, and golden poached eggs, all mixed up and in perfect harmony with a Tuscan tomato sauce? Even though we're talking eggs here, this is a dinner in our homes, and it's also a hit at brunches and potlucks. It looks like a lot of ingredients, but most of them are spices. The first time around this preparation might seem a tad daunting, but after you've tried it once, you'll find it's quite easy.

1. Preheat the oven to 350°F.

2. Make the breads. Whisk together the Baking Blend, Super Sweet, salt, baking powder, water, and egg whites in a mixing bowl or process in a food processor.

3. Lightly coat an 8-cup muffin tin with coconut oil cooking spray. Divide the batter among the muffin cup holes. Bake for 15 minutes. Remove from the oven and let cool a little. Cut into cubes. Keep the oven set at 350°F.

4. Make the casserole. Fry the bread cubes in a large skillet with the ghee or butter, basil, cumin, paprika, and garlic powder.

5. Lightly spray a 9 × 13-inch baking dish with the cooking spray. Transfer the seasoned bread cubes to the baking dish.

6. Sauté the jalapeño and onion in the same skillet with some of the tomato juice until soft, about 3 minutes. Add to the baking dish and toss with the bread. Add the olives, sausage, tomatoes, and grated cheese, and stir to blend.

7. In a blender, combine the okra, tomato paste, broth, salt, and Gluccie until smooth. Pour over the mixture in the baking dish. Gently stir the "innards" of the casserole to mix things up a bit.

8. Create 4 evenly spaced cavities in 2 rows, making 8 "nests" for your eggs. Gently crack an egg into each cavity. Sprinkle the top of the casserole with the green olives, basil, and cracked black peppercorns, then drizzle on the vinegar.

9. Cover the casserole with foil and bake for 30 minutes. Remove the cover and bake approximately 5 minutes more if you want slightly runny poached eggs (keep an eye on the yolks; you might need more or less time depending on your oven) or 15 to 20 minutes more for solid yolks.

DF (IF USING HELLO CHEESE, PAGE 487, INSTEAD OF THE PECORINO)

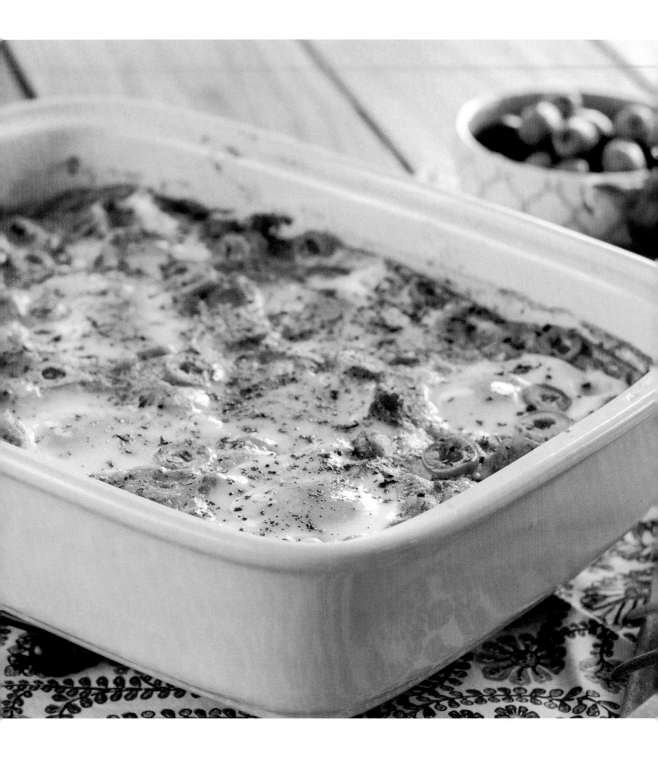

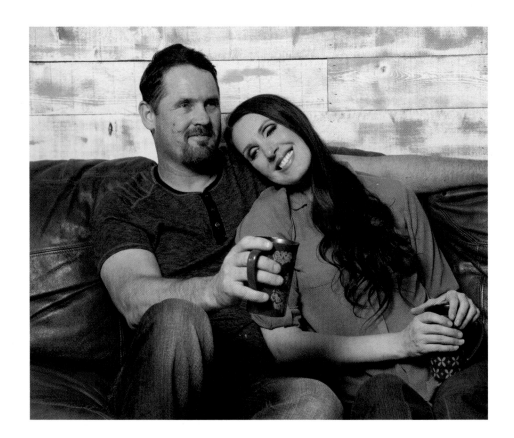

mini meat loaves

FAMILY SERVE – MAKES 16 MINI MEAT LOAVES AND FEEDS 6 TO 8
(HALVE INGREDIENTS IF YOUR FAMILY IS SMALLER)

3 pounds thawed ultra-lean ground turkey (96 to 99%)

1 cup egg whites (from carton or use fresh egg whites)

½ cup 0% Greek yogurt

½ cup soaked and cooked quinoa

2 medium onions, finely diced

2 ripe tomatoes, diced small

4 celery stalks, thinly sliced

2 tablespoons diced pickled jalapeño pepper

1½ teaspoons Mineral Salt

½ teaspoon black pepper

1 teaspoon onion powder

½ teaspoon garlic powder

Few dashes of hot sauce of your choice

Coconut oil cooking spray

1 (6-ounce) can of garlic and herb style tomato paste

Don't forget about your Fuel Pull meals! Your body needs a lighter meal every now and then, and you can make one deliciously with this recipe.

1. Preheat the oven to 350°F.

2. Put the ground turkey in a large bowl with the egg whites, yogurt, and quinoa. Mix well.

3. In a medium skillet, sauté the onions, tomatoes, and celery until tender, then add to the bowl. Stir in the jalapeño and seasonings; add the hot sauce, and mix very well.

4. Lightly spray two 8-cup muffin tins with coconut oil cooking spray. Fill the holes with the meat mixture. Spread some of the seasoned tomato paste on the tops and bake for 35 to 45 minutes or until cooked through.

NSI

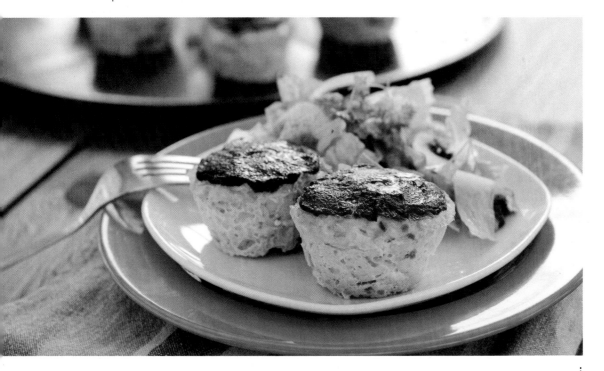

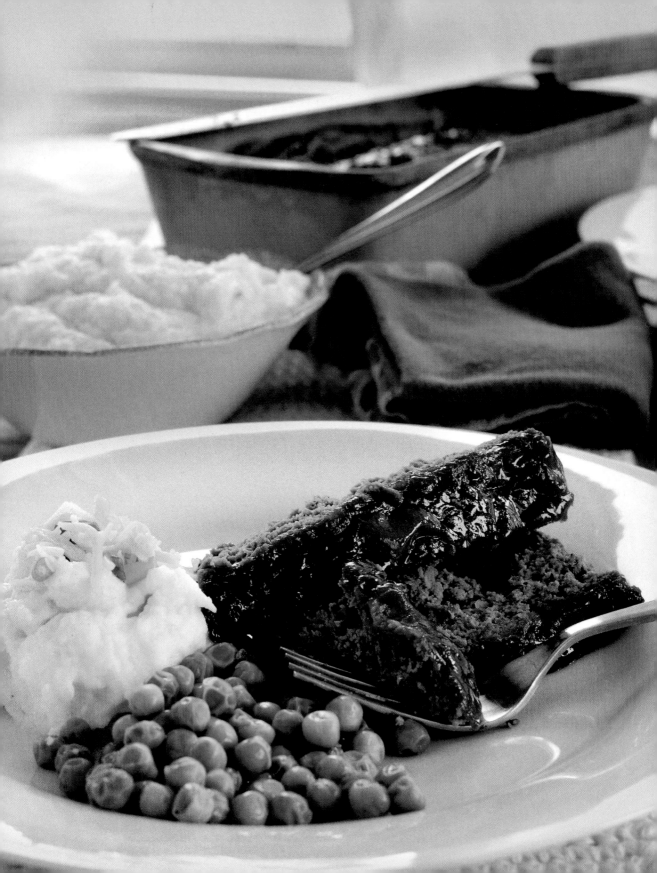

mama's famous meatloaf

⑤

FAMILY SERVE – FEEDS 6 TO 8 (HALVE INGREDIENTS IF YOUR FAMILY IS SMALLER)

FOR THE LOAF

½ large onion

3 pounds thawed ground beef (or venison or turkey)

3 large eggs

2 teaspoons onion powder

3 teaspoons dried minced onion

2 teaspoons garlic powder

2½ teaspoons Mineral Salt

¾ teaspoon black pepper

3 tablespoons prepared yellow mustard

6 tablespoons Trim Healthy Ketchup (page 482) or store bought sugar-free

3 tablespoons Trim Healthy Mama Baking Blend

FOR THE TOPPING

⅓ cup Trim Healthy Ketchup (page 482) or store bought

2 tablespoons prepared yellow mustard

2 to 3 tablespoons Gentle Sweet, or 1 tablespoon Super Sweet Blend

Here's a traditional meatloaf just like your mama or grand-mama used to make. The processed onion keeps the loaf incredibly moist, but little children who are picky about onions won't even know they're in there.

1. Preheat the oven to 350°F.

2. Make the loaf. Put the onion half in a food processor with 1 heaping cup of the ground meat. Process until the onion is completely broken down and absorbed by the meat (you may have to stop processing and scrape down sides with a spatula, then start again a couple times).

3. Put the meat-onion mix in a large bowl and combine with the remaining meat, the eggs, the seasonings, mustard, ketchup, and Baking Blend. Put in a 9 × 13-inch baking dish. Bake for 45 minutes.

4. Make the topping. Mix the ketchup, mustard, and Gentle Sweet, and spread on top of the loaf. Bake for 10 minutes more. Broil for the last few minutes for a browned and bubbly topping.

DF

pearl's easy meatloaf

S

3 pounds thawed ground beef or
  venison

1½ cups salsa of choice

½ cup sour cream

3 large eggs, lightly beaten

2 packets taco seasoning (see Note)

⅓ cup ground Joseph's pitas (store
  bought)

PEARL CHATS: Here's meatloaf with a Mexican twist. This gets devoured in my home, and if you do happen to have leftovers, it is great as an S sandwich the next day.

1. Preheat the oven to 350°F.

2. In a bowl, combine the meat with the salsa, sour cream, eggs, and taco seasoning. Stir in the salt and bread crumbs.

3. Mix well, then place in a 9 × 13-inch baking dish and bake for 1 hour.

NOTE: Wick Fowler's taco seasoning does not have sugar or other junk. Or, to make your own taco seasoning, combine 2 teaspoons ground cumin, 1½ teaspoons paprika, 3 teaspoons chili powder, 2 teaspoons onion powder, 1 teaspoon garlic powder, and 2½ teaspoons Mineral Salt. This will replace the 2 packets taco seasoning.

NSI

sausage balls

- 2 pounds of your favorite thawed ground sausage (we use inexpensive turkey or venison, but you can use pork)
- ½ cup Trim Healthy Mama Baking Blend or a combination of almond flour and oat fiber or coconut flour
- ½ medium onion (very finely diced), or ¼ cup dried minced onion mixed with ¼ cup water
- 1 large egg
- 8 ounces extra-sharp cheddar cheese, grated (if using fatty sausage), or 12 ounces cheese (if using lean sausage)
- 1½ teaspoons Mineral Salt
- 1 teaspoon onion and/or garlic powder
- 1 teaspoon ground sage
- 1 teaspoon black pepper
- ¼ to ½ teaspoon cayenne pepper (you won't need this if you choose to use hot sausage)

These flavorful balls are great either hot or cold. Enjoy them as part of a quick grab-and-go out-of-the-fridge breakfast or snack, or enjoy them hot as the main protein portion of your dinner. They're a hit at parties, too!

1. Preheat the oven to 375°F.
2. Mix all the ingredients in a large bowl. The fastest results will be with your hands. Squeeze the mixture into balls with those same sticky hands. Place the balls on 2 parchment-lined 9 × 13-inch baking sheets.
3. Bake for 20 minutes. Some of the cheese will melt out during the baking, but that's okay—it makes them even yummier. Use a spoon to push the melted cheese back toward each ball (you don't have to get fussy about it—you just don't want to waste any cheese). Return the balls to the oven and broil the top of the balls for 3 to 5 more minutes, watching carefully so they don't burn.

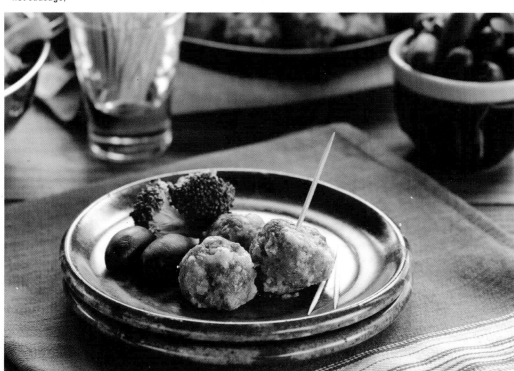

bone-in roast beef

S

2 (3- to 4-pound) thawed bone-in beef roasts

3 teaspoons Mineral Salt

Onion powder and/or garlic powder, dried rosemary, black pepper, and cayenne pepper, to sprinkle on roasts

PEARL CHATS: I love that bone-in roasts provide glycine, a sadly missing amino acid in our modern world. But as healthy as this is, that is not the main reason I make this dish. It is for the sheer love of it. The roasting meat makes my house smell amazing and my family cannot get enough of it. I prepare two roasts at the same time, each 3 to 4 pounds. I cook them long and slow, which makes the meat incredibly succulent, then I crisp it at the end. I try to keep some leftovers for the next day (which means hiding it from my teenage boys). I also make an S sandwich with slices of it for my husband and use other pieces to top a quick lunch salad for myself.

1. Preheat the oven to 225°F.
2. Put each roast in a 9 × 13-inch baking pan. Sprinkle 1½ teaspoons salt on each, then sprinkle liberally with the other seasonings (except for the cayenne pepper if you have little ones who are sensitive to spice). Pour about 1 cup of water around each roast. Cover each roast with aluminum foil and bake for 3½ hours (for example, put your roasts in the oven around 2 p.m. if you want to eat by 6).
3. Remove the foil, then turn the temp up to 400°F and roast for another 20 minutes. Ladle some of the meat juices on top of the roasts, then broil the top of the meat for five minutes before taking out of the oven (watch that top of meat does not burn).

NSI DF

chicken parmy

FAMILY SERVE – FEEDS 6 TO 8 (HALVE INGREDIENTS IF YOUR FAMILY IS SMALLER)

¾ cup Trim Healthy Mama Baking Blend or ground Joseph's pitas (store bought)

¾ cup finely grated Parmesan cheese

2 tablespoons Italian seasoning

2 teaspoons dried parsley

¼ teaspoon Mineral Salt

½ teaspoon black pepper

2 teaspoons garlic powder

Coconut oil cooking spray

2½ pounds thawed boneless, skinless chicken breasts or tenderloins

4 tablespoons (½ stick) butter, melted

1½ cups no-added-sugar pizza or spaghetti sauce (see Note)

1½ cups grated part-skim mozzarella cheese

If you like things easy and tasty, this will rock your dinner world.

1. Preheat the oven to 425°F.

2. In a bowl, whisk together the Baking Blend with the Parmesan cheese and the seasonings. Spread the breading mix on a large dinner plate.

3. Lightly coat a large baking sheet with coconut oil cooking spray.

4. Dip each chicken breast into the melted butter, then into the breading and pat to coat well on both sides. Place the chicken pieces on the baking sheet and sprinkle any leftover breading mix evenly over the tops of the chicken.

5. Bake for 20 minutes (or 15 minutes for tenderloins). Take the chicken out of the oven, top each breast with 2 tablespoons sauce, and sprinkle with a little of the mozzarella. Put back in the oven and bake for another 5 to 10 minutes, or until the cheese is melted and the sauce is bubbling.

SERVING IDEAS: Serve with a side salad and Green Fries (page 218) or Roasted Asparagus (see page 227), or enjoy over Troodles (page 222).

NOTE: Great Value Pizza Sauce from Walmart has just 3 carbs. Purists can make their own sauce from equal parts tomato paste (BPA-free cans) and water, with salt and oregano to taste and an optional doonk of Pure Stevia Extract.

NSI (IF USING GROUND-UP JOSEPH'S PITAS FOR THE CRUMB MIXTURE)

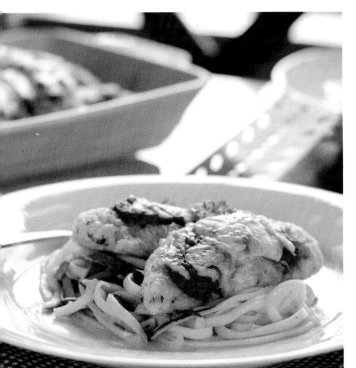

bangin' ranch drums

(S)

FAMILY SERVE – FEEDS 6 TO 8 (HALVE INGREDIENTS IF YOUR FAMILY IS SMALLER)

½ cup mayonnaise (Body-Burn Mayonnaise, page 470, or store bought)

½ cup plain 0% Greek yogurt

2 teaspoons garlic powder, or 3 garlic cloves, minced

1 tablespoon dried minced onion

2½ teaspoons Mineral Salt

1½ teaspoons black pepper

1 tablespoon dried parsley

6 pounds thawed chicken drumsticks

If any of your family members are skeptical about the Trim Healthy Mama way of life, then bake these for dinner and watch them all come around. Who can resist crispy, juicy chicken on the bone, baked with the flavors of ranch seasoning?

1. Preheat the oven to 375°F.

2. Mix the mayonnaise and yogurt in a bowl. Add the seasonings and mix well.

3. Put the chicken drumsticks in 2 large shallow, well-greased baking pans. Put half of the mayonnaise mix in each pan and, using your hands, coat the chicken well with the dressing.

4. Bake, uncovered, for 45 to 50 minutes.

SERVING IDEA: Serve with Rohnda's Ranch Dressing (page 471) as an additional dipping sauce for the chicken, if desired.

NSI

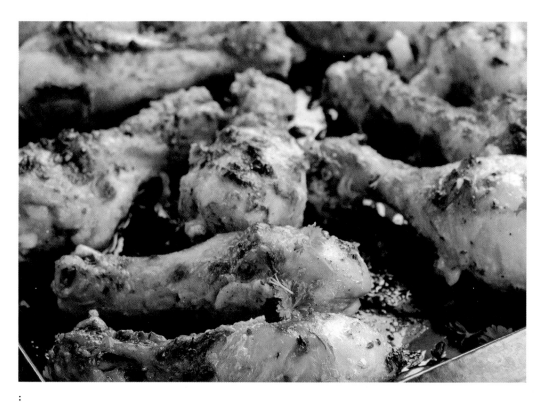

crispy lickin' chicken

S

6 to 8 pounds frozen chicken leg quarters (thigh and drumstick, usually sold in 4-pound bags)

2 teaspoons MSG-free Creole seasoning

2 teaspoons Mineral Salt

1 teaspoon black pepper

¾ teaspoon garlic powder

3 tablespoons nutritional yeast

3 tablespoons hot sauce of your choice

3 tablespoons finely grated Parmesan cheese (green can kind is fine)

2 tablespoons Liquid Smoke

3 teaspoons paprika

2 teaspoons onion powder

This bone-in, skin-on recipe is super high in the amino acid glycine, which your body needs. Boy, oh boy, what a yummy way this is to get your glycine! If you opened this book and did what we call the "flick trick" to any random page, and this is the first recipe you see, you might think, "Ho hum, a crispy chicken recipe. Looks nice." You wouldn't realize our fervent desire for you to eat more glycine-rich foods. That subject is discussed in full in *Trim Healthy Mama Plan,* so consider this a shameless plug to get you to read that.

This chicken is super crispy, with the perfect amount of finger-lickin' greasiness, but it's also a little reminiscent of jerky in its chewiness. Don't be put off by the time it takes to bake. It isn't laborious—you don't even have to thaw the chicken. It starts frozen, so we suggest you begin cooking by mid-afternoon. The only work you do is a bit of sprinkling on of spices, a little bit of basting, and then generating some patience while you smell the delicious aroma wafting from your oven.

Unless you have a small family and want to halve this recipe, make the full amount. It's extra delicious cold as leftovers. Just chill it, uncovered, in the fridge. There's something about that delicious savory chewiness that is so satisfying to gnaw on when the munchies hit.

1. Preheat the oven to 350°F.

2. Place the frozen chicken quarters on 2 large baking pans. Sprinkle the Creole seasoning on the chicken and bake for 1 hour. Baste the chicken with the juices that pool in the bottoms of the pans every so often—about four times during the first hour.

3. Remove the pans and drain off the juice (you can save this yummy juice to make a gravy, if desired). Sprinkle the chicken with all the remaining seasonings and cheese, making sure to distribute them evenly. Return the pans to the oven, lower the heat to 200°F, and continue to roast the chicken for a few more hours. Delish!

NSI

peanut popper chicken ⓢ

3 pounds thawed boneless chicken thighs or breasts, cut into bite-size pieces
1 cup Pressed Peanut Flour
3 tablespoons chunky natural-style sugar-free peanut butter (optional)
½ cup water
1¼ to 1½ teaspoons Mineral Salt
¾ teaspoon black pepper
¼ to ½ teaspoon cayenne pepper
½ teaspoon onion powder
2 tablespoons butter or coconut oil

1. Preheat the oven to 425°F.
2. Put the chicken pieces in a large bowl, add the peanut flour, peanut butter (if using), water, salt, pepper, cayenne, and onion powder, and combine to coat well.
3. Melt the butter, then pour into a 9 × 13-inch baking pan. Place the seasoned chicken on top, spreading it out to leave room between the pieces. Bake for 15 minutes.
4. Run the pan under the broiler for 5 to 10 minutes, or until the tops of the chicken pieces are golden brown and get ultra-crispy. Watch closely after 5 minutes, so they don't burn.

DF (IF USING COCONUT OIL INSTEAD OF BUTTER)

spicy chicken wings ⓢ

6 pounds thawed chicken wing segments
Mineral Salt to taste
½ cup (1 stick) butter, melted
1 (12-ounce) bottle Frank's hot sauce or your favorite (with 0 carbs)
Cayenne pepper to taste

1. Preheat the oven to 425°F.
2. Place the chicken wings in two or three 9 × 13-inch baking pans. Sprinkle lightly with salt.
3. Pour the melted butter into a bowl and add the hot sauce. Mix well. (If you want more heat, add several shakes of cayenne pepper to the butter/sauce mix.)
4. Pour the sauce over the chicken and bake for 1 hour. Broil the tops of the wings until crispy at the ends.

NSI

papster thighs

(S)

FAMILY SERVE – FEEDS 6 TO 8 (HALVE INGREDIENTS IF YOUR FAMILY IS SMALLER)

6 to 8 pounds thawed bone-in chicken thighs (or about 2 small thighs for each person; larger thighs should be enough for 1 person)

Mineral Salt, black pepper, cayenne pepper, garlic or onion powder, and paprika (smoked or regular), for sprinkling

We love paprika, and since we can't help giving our beloved foods nicknames, this spice is affectionately referred to as "The Papster" in our homes. It is the perfect spice to offset these chicken thighs, which fall apart because they are so tender yet they are also crispy on top.

1. Preheat the oven to 225°F.

2. Place the thighs skin side up in 2 or 3 large baking pans. Sprinkle the tops of the chicken generously with the seasonings. Cover the pans with foil and bake long and slow, for 3 hours.

3. Remove the foil, turn the oven up to 425°F, and crisp the chicken for the last 20 minutes. (If the tops of the chicken are not quite crispy enough, at the end you can broil for just a few minutes, but watch closely so they don't burn.)

NSI DF

---

creamy herb chicken

(S) WITH OPTION

FAMILY SERVE – FEEDS 6 TO 8 (HALVE INGREDIENTS IF YOUR FAMILY IS SMALLER)

Coconut oil cooking spray

2½ pounds thawed boneless, skinless chicken breasts

1 cup plain 0% Greek yogurt

½ cup mayonnaise

1 cup finely grated Parmesan cheese, plus additional for topping (green can kind is fine or use freshly grated)

3 tablespoons dried parsley

2 tablespoons dried oregano

¾ teaspoon Mineral Salt

¾ teaspoon black pepper

1 teaspoon garlic powder

1. Preheat the oven to 425°F.

2. Spray a large 9 × 13-inch shallow baking pan with coconut oil cooking spray. Arrange the chicken breasts in the pan.

3. Mix all other ingredients and generously spread on the chicken. Sprinkle a little more Parmesan on top of each piece. Bake for 25 minutes, or until the tops of the chicken are golden brown and the meat is cooked through.

SERVING IDEAS: This is perfect with Troodles (page 222) or Not Naughty Noodles, or simply with a side salad.

NOTE: If desiring this to be in **FP** mode, omit the mayonnaise and increase the yogurt by another ½ cup; also, reduce the Parmesan cheese to ½ cup.

NSI

sweet potato bar

6 to 8 medium sweet potatoes

2½ pounds thawed boneless, skinless chicken breasts

Mineral Salt, black pepper, chili powder, ground cumin, and garlic powder, for sprinkling on the chicken

Coconut oil cooking spray

FIXIN' IDEAS

Plain 0% Greek yogurt (for dairy-free, use Laughin' Mama Cheese, page 484)

Diced cucumber

Ripe tomatoes

Sweet onions

Salsa of choice

Shredded lettuce

Your oven is going to do double duty here, cooking both your protein and your healthy carb at the same time. So, load those sweet potatoes high with all the good fixings! Your children may want some butter on their potatoes, as growing children do well with Crossovers, but if you're still in weight-loss mode, we doubt you'll miss the butter if you pile on all the E-friendly toppings. Remember, though, that a Crossover is not a cheat. We all can enjoy them from time to time, and some of us need more of them than others. You will likely have leftovers of this chicken, but that is great for other meals.

1. Preheat the oven to 375°F.

2. Put the sweet potatoes directly on the middle rack of the oven, off to one side.

3. Put the chicken on a large dinner plate and generously season with the spices.

4. Lightly coat a large shallow baking pan with coconut oil cooking spray and arrange the chicken in the pan. Bake next to the sweet potatoes for 35 minutes, or until cooked through. Take the chicken out and allow to cool while the potatoes continue baking.

5. Cut the chicken into small pieces and put into a bowl.

SERVING IDEA: Arrange the fixin' ideas in separate bowls. When the potatoes are done (about 45 minutes), split them open, creating room for the fixins. Pile the potatoes high with your choice of goodies; you can even drizzle on 1 teaspoon coconut oil or butter for your **E** fat quota.

NSI DF (IF USING LAUGHIN' MAMA CHEESE, PAGE 484)

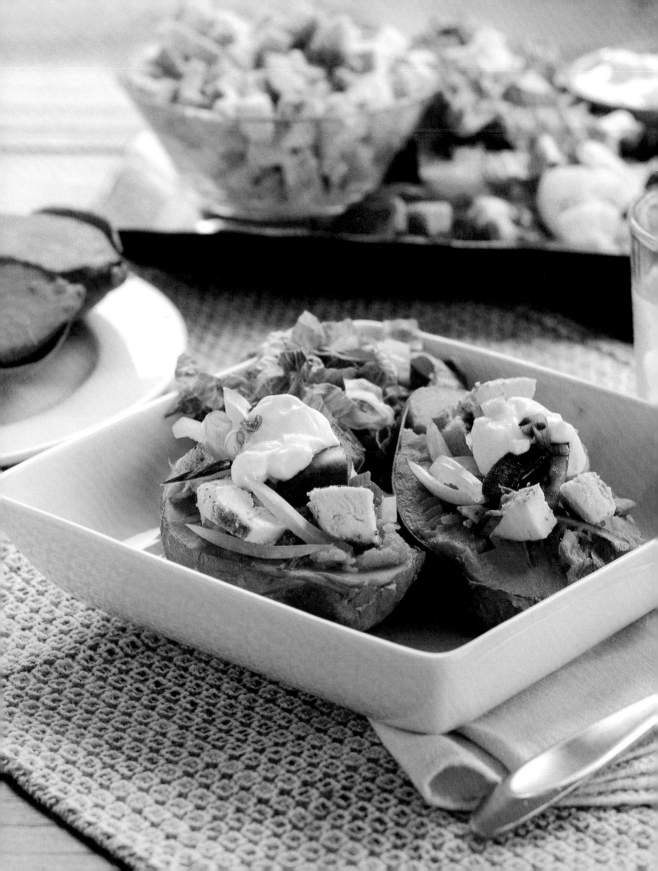

super prepared roasted chicken

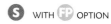

FAMILY SERVE – FEEDS 6 TO 8 WITH LEFTOVERS FOR THE REST OF THE WEEK OR TO FREEZE (HALVE IF YOUR FAMILY IS SMALLER)

3 whole thawed chickens

3 teaspoons Mineral Salt

3 teaspoons black pepper

3 teaspoons dried sage

3 teaspoons paprika

Being "super prepared" means thinking far enough ahead that you not only prepare enough for one meal but also have plenty left over for storing in zippy bags that can be used for future quickie meals. If you have a small family, or if you are single, you might see the ingredient list here and think, "Why the heck would I roast three chickens at once?" Trust us. This is going to help you stay on plan and make your life so much easier. You'll use one or two chickens (depending on the size of your family) for a dinner. The third will be for other meals in the week. Divide the light meat from the dark, if you want. The white breast meat can work well for E and FP, but you can use any of it for S. If you don't think you'll use all the chicken in the week, freeze single-serve portions in zippies so they can easily be thawed for quick soups and salads.

The added bonus here is that you will have all the bones you need ready for an awesome stock! Now that's thinking ahead. (See pages 495–496 to learn how to make stock with the bones.)

1. Preheat the oven to 450°F.

2. Remove any gizzards or necks from the chickens and save for stock—or just throw away. Place the chickens next to one another in a very large roasting pan, or split them between 2 pans. Rub 1 teaspoon of the seasonings on each bird.

3. Roast for 15 minutes, then reduce the temperature to 350°F, and roast for 2 hours more. You can lower the temperature to 300°F and cook for 3 hours, or cook them long and slow at 250°F for 5 hours—your choice. Occasionally during the roasting, dip a ladle into the pan juices and baste the tops and sides of the birds. You may need to add a little water to the pans toward the end of a long and slow roast. Or, alternatively, for the long and slow-roast version, add a cup of chicken broth or dry red wine, and cover to roast.

NOTE: You can go beyond these simple spices and add more pizzazz with some cayenne pepper, Cajun or Creole seasoning, nutritional yeast, Dijon mustard, and so on. Use your imagination and personal flair.

NSI DF

EXTRA SKILLET STUFF

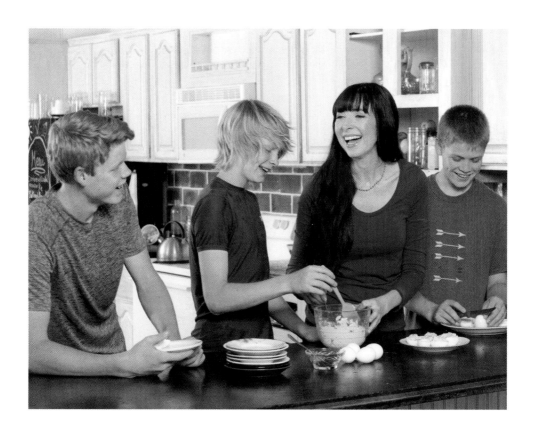

wonder fish tacos

PEARL CHATS: Every year our two families (along with our sister Vange, her husband, and ten children) all caravan down from the Tennessee woods to Florida for a camping trip at the beach. It is chaos—fun, wild, and crazy—but we wouldn't have it any other way. Well, I shouldn't lie . . . they camp, I don't. I can't summon any love for sandy tents (that always get flooded from storms), mosquitoes, middle-of-the-night walks to the bathrooms. Nah, Serene can have it. Our children join their cousins in tents while my husband and I rent a condo next to the campground and secretly laugh at what everyone else has to go through. But I digress; this chat is not about the camping. It is about the fish tacos on a roadside stand in Florida that changed my world.

Coming from Down Under, the pairing of fish and tacos was never part of our early culinary experience. I was 40 before I first tasted them, but one bite and I was a goner! That roadside stand used fresh ocean-caught fish, but I've still been able to have similar, delicious success at home using inexpensive frozen tilapia and incorporating other fresh flavors and ingredients, like cabbage, cilantro, and lime juice.

Following are two equally delicious versions of fish tacos, one for E and one for S. My husband usually enjoys S meals more than E for dinner (I'm always sure to feed him plenty of E breakfasts), but he gets filled up on these E-style tacos and does not miss the fats he ordinarily craves in the evening. So while both versions are good, do give the E version a try first. I have a sneaking suspicion you need to get more E meals into your life.

It's a good idea to make your Wonder Wraps earlier in the day or week. Wonder Wraps keep well in the fridge, so if you have an afternoon or evening free, spend some time Wonder Wrappin' (or get a spare teenager to do it). The other option is to only use Wonder Wraps yourself. Those family members who don't need to watch their weight can use regular whole-grain soft or crunchy tacos. While these are called Wonder Fish Tacos, if a Drive Thru Sue used a store-bought low-carb tortilla (or two small ones) instead, then I'm sure not going to yell at her—but let's not tell Serene.

FAMILY SERVE – FEEDS 6 TO 8 (HALVE INGREDIENTS IF YOUR FAMILY IS SMALLER)

Juice of 2 limes

½ head green cabbage, cored and finely chopped, or 1 (8-ounce) bag coleslaw mix

2 pounds thawed tilapia fillets (or use any white fish available to you)

Mineral Salt, black pepper, and chili powder, for sprinkling on fish

Coconut oil cooking spray

4 teaspoons butter or coconut oil

2¼ cups cooked black beans, drained, or 1½ (15-ounce) cans black beans, rinsed and drained (the leftover half can is the exact amount of beans to use in Bean Boss Soup, page 109, later in your week)

1½ cups 0% plain Greek yogurt

1½ cups cooked brown rice

1½ teaspoons ground cumin

½ bunch fresh cilantro, chopped

1 family-serve batch Wonder Wraps (page 204)

1 medium onion, thinly sliced

Hot sauce of choice (optional)

1. Squeeze the lime juice over the cabbage and set aside.

2. Season the fish with a light sprinkle of salt, pepper, and chili powder.

3. Place a large skillet over medium-high heat, coat lightly with coconut oil spray, then add 2 teaspoons of the butter. Put half the fish fillets in the skillet and sauté for 2 to 3 minutes on each side, or until flaky (doesn't matter if the fish falls apart). Remove the fillets and set aside, then add the remaining butter and repeat with the remaining fish fillets.

4. Put the beans, yogurt, rice, and cumin in a medium saucepan and warm over medium heat until hot. Add the cilantro and give a light sprinkle of salt and pepper.

5. If desired, heat the Wonder Wraps lightly in the oven for a minute or two, or microwave for a few seconds. Stuff the wraps in any order with the fish pieces, beans and rice mixture, cabbage, and onion. Sprinkle with hot sauce (if using).

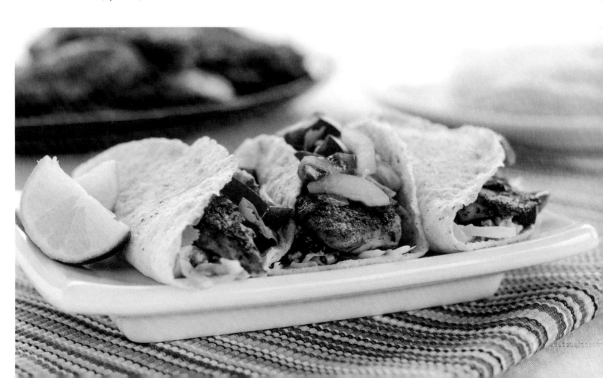

WONDER FISH TACOS

1 bunch fresh cilantro

8 ounces sour cream

Juice of 1 or 2 limes

2 pounds thawed tilapia fillets (or use any white fish available to you)

Mineral Salt, black pepper, and chili powder, for sprinkling on fish

4 tablespoons (½ stick) butter or coconut oil

1 family-serve batch Wonder Wraps (page 204)

½ green cabbage, cored and finely chopped, or 1 (8-ounce) bag coleslaw mix

2 or 3 avocados, pitted, peeled, and cut into thin slices

Hot sauce of choice (optional)

1. Put the cilantro in a food processor and process until fine but not pureed. Transfer to a bowl and mix with the sour cream, then add the lime juice and set aside.

2. Sauté the fish in a large skillet as directed for the **E** version (on page 171), but using 2 tablespoons butter for each batch.

3. Stuff the wraps with the fish, cabbage, and avocado slices, then top with the sour cream mixture, followed by a drizzle of hot sauce (if using).

chicken-fried tofu

FAMILY SERVE – FEEDS 6 TO 8 (HALVE INGREDIENTS IF YOUR FAMILY IS SMALLER)

2 (15-ounce) blocks firm sprouted tofu

4 tablespoons Trim Bouillon Mix
(page 491)

4 tablespoons Trim Healthy Mama
Baking Blend (you can use ground
Joseph's pita crumbs if you don't
have any Baking Blend)

4 tablespoons coconut oil or butter

Your children are going to gobble this up! If you want a break from meat, you won't lose any taste with this tofu. Sprouted tofu is much higher in protein than regular, the sprouting process making it easily digested and offering more vitamins and minerals. This is a cinch to make!

1. Pour the water out of the tofu packet (does not matter if a little stays), and cut the tofu into ⅓-inch slices (you can do this right inside the packet). Combine the bouillon mix and Baking Blend on a large dinner plate, then coat both sides of each piece of tofu.

2. Melt 2 tablespoons coconut oil or butter in a skillet set over medium-high heat. Put half the tofu in the skillet and brown for a couple minutes on each side. Repeat with the remaining coconut oil or butter and tofu.

SERVING IDEAS: Delicious served with a side veggie of choice and a salad.

DF

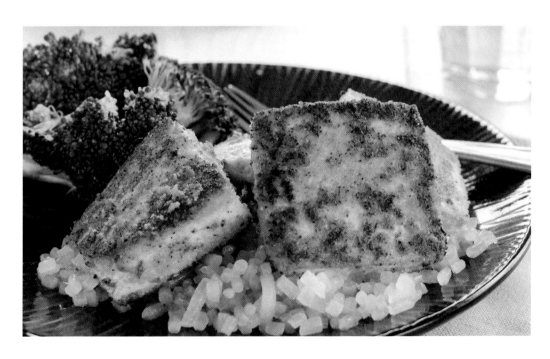

salisbury steak

(S)

FOR THE PATTIES

2½ pounds ground beef

2 large eggs

2 tablespoons Trim Healthy Mama Baking Blend

¼ teaspoon black pepper

1 teaspoon Mineral Salt

1 teaspoon onion powder

1 teaspoon garlic powder

1 tablespoon Worcestershire sauce

2 tablespoons coconut oil or butter

FOR THE GRAVY

1 large or 2 small onions, thinly sliced

1½ cups beef broth

1 teaspoon Mineral Salt

8 to 10 ounces button mushrooms, sliced

2 tablespoons Trim Healthy Mama Baking Blend

¾ to 1 teaspoon Gluccie

Here's hearty "man food" that we women love, too! Sometimes this is known as hamburger steak, but either way it is going to be a winner in your home. The recipe makes 8 to 10 substantial patties.

1. Make the patties. In a large bowl, combine the ground beef, eggs, Baking Blend, pepper, salt, onion powder, garlic powder, and Worcestershire sauce. Form into 8 to 10 balls and then flatten into patties.

2. Heat half the oil in a large skillet over medium heat. Fry half the patties until nicely browned, about 4 minutes per side. Remove to a plate and keep warm. Add the remaining oil to the skillet and fry the other patties. Set aside with the rest of the patties.

3. Make the gravy. Add the sliced onions to the skillet with a splash of beef broth and the salt. Cook for 8 to 10 minutes, stirring to loosen any bits of meat and drippings from the pan. Add the mushrooms and sauté a few minutes more.

4. Sprinkle the Baking Blend over the mixture in the skillet and toss to blend well. Gradually mix in the remaining beef broth. Simmer over medium-low heat, and whisk vigorously while sprinkling in up to 1 teaspoon Gluccie, until the gravy starts to thicken.

5. Turn the heat to low, return the patties to the skillet, cover, and simmer for another 15 minutes without stirring too much, as you don't want to break up the patties.

DF (IF USING COCONUT OIL IN PLACE OF BUTTER)

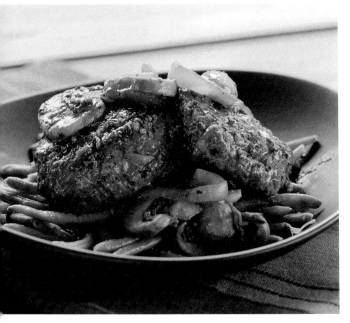

potsticker patties

1 medium to large zucchini, chopped into 4 large pieces

1 (8-ounce) package button mushrooms

1 medium onion, cut into 2 or 3 large pieces

1 large egg

1¾ teaspoons MSG-free Creole seasoning (Tony Chachere's is good)

⅓ cup old-fashioned oats, ground, or 3 tablespoons Trim Healthy Mama Baking Blend

1 pound thawed ground turkey

Coconut oil and/or butter, for cooking

PEARL CHATS: I was trying to come up with a name for these patties that would reflect how budget friendly they are. The hidden veggies stretch 1 pound of inexpensive ground turkey into enough to feed 6 to 8 hungry people. You're going to double the number of burgers that 1 pound usually makes by adding onion, mushrooms, and zucchini. Picky children won't know the difference because the immune-supporting veggies are all processed smooth. I tested these on a pack of about 10 cousins coming in and out of my home, and they quickly scarfed them down and declared that they tasted just like potstickers—so that name stuck and the budget-saving title got buried.

Warning: Try to avoid your children seeing the meat and veggie mixture before it is cooked. It is honestly ugly and scary looking. But amazingly, once cooked, these patties transform into much prettier creations that do not give children nightmares.

1. Put the zucchini, mushrooms, and onion in a food processor and process on high until pureed (you may have to stop the food processor and scrape it down a couple of times). Add the egg, Creole seasoning, and oats or Baking Blend and process again for another 30 seconds.

2. Place the puree in a large bowl and add the ground turkey. Combine well with a fork. Form the mixture into patties.

3. Heat the coconut oil in a large skillet over medium-high heat. Sauté the patties until crisp and cooked through, turning once.

NOTE: The small amount of ground oats used here is spread through the whole mixture, so it is not problematic enough to interfere with **S** mode.

NSI (IF USING GROUND OATS) DF

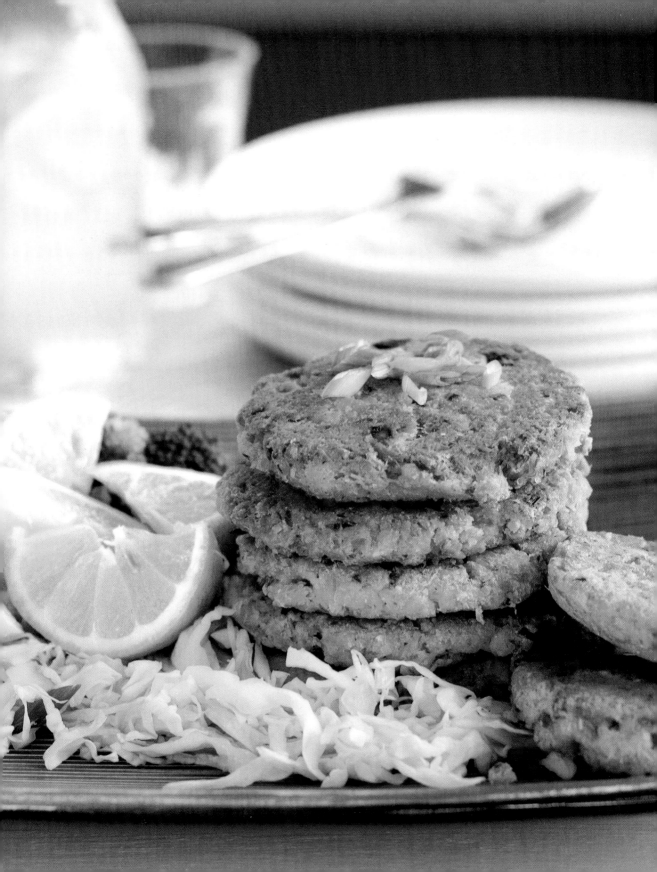

super salmon patties

(S)

FAMILY SERVE – FEEDS 6 TO 8 (HALVE INGREDIENTS IF YOUR FAMILY IS SMALLER)

2 to 3 (15-ounce) cans wild pink
  salmon (use 3 cans only if you have
  huge eaters)
2 to 3 large eggs (1 for each can of
  salmon)
2 to 3 tablespoons Trim Healthy Mama
  Baking Blend, or ⅓ cup ground
  Joseph's pitas (store bought), or
  ⅓ cup old-fashioned rolled oats
  ground into flour
¼ to ⅓ cup finely diced onion (optional)
2 tablespoons minced pickled
  jalapeños (optional)
Light sprinkle of MSG-free seasoning
  salt
Coconut oil, for frying

PEARL CHATS: Talk about healthy and yummy! This recipe is easy and budget friendly. My children nicknamed these "Crabby Patties," after that crazy Sponge Bob cartoon character who obsesses over crabby patties. However, these are made from salmon, not crab. They're great for the whole family and are a perfect way to take in those important omega-3 fatty acids, especially by picky children who ordinarily may not want to eat salmon. Salmon is our highest food source of dimethylaminoethanol (DMAE), which is essential for brain health and is found to be effective for conditions like lack of concentration and ADD. It lifts and firms the skin, so that's good for us Mamas, too. Salmon is one of the best sources of macro-trace minerals such as iodine and zinc, and it also provides an abundance of our fat-soluble vitamins A and D.

1. Drain the cans of salmon and put the fish into a large bowl. Mash the fish with a fork; any little bones are soft so they will easily mash in. These bones are full of calcium and glycine, so it's best to leave them in. Add the eggs and Baking Blend, and stir well. Add the onion and jalapeño (if using), and add a very light sprinkle of seasoning.

2. Heat the coconut oil in a large skillet over medium-high heat. Sauté the patties until heated through and lightly browned on both sides, turning once.

NSI (IF USING GROUND OATS OR GROUND JOSEPH'S PITAS INSTEAD OF BAKING BLEND) DF

jalapeño onion burgers

FAMILY SERVE – FEEDS 6 TO 8 PEOPLE (HALVE INGREDIENTS IF YOUR FAMILY IS SMALLER)

3 pounds thawed ground beef

2 teaspoons ground cumin

2 teaspoons chili powder

2 teaspoons Mineral Salt

1 teaspoon black pepper

2 to 4 tablespoons minced pickled jalapeños

¼ large onion, finely diced

1 large egg

Butter or coconut oil, for cooking (if using lean beef)

Succulent, moist burgers with oodles of flavor! Enjoy these wrapped in large lettuce leaves or between slices of Swiss Bread (page 196), or in a Joseph's pita (store bought). But these burgers don't even need casings. They're delicious on a plate, loaded with sautéed onions, mushrooms, a slice of cheese, mayo, and ketchup—all eaten with a fork.

1. Combine all the ingredients except the oil in a large bowl. Form into patties.

2. Put a large skillet over medium heat and brown the patties on both sides until cooked through (use butter or coconut oil only if your ground meat is lean). Or, grill the burgers on an inside or outside grill.

NSI DF (IF NOT TOPPING THE BURGER WITH CHEESE)

fried breaded fish

FAMILY SERVE – FEEDS 6 TO 8 PEOPLE (HALVE INGREDIENTS IF YOUR FAMILY IS SMALLER)

1 cup Trim Healthy Mama Baking Blend, or ⅔ cup ground Joseph's pitas (store bought) and ⅓ cup old-fashioned rolled oats ground into flour

1½ teaspoons Mineral Salt

1½ teaspoons black pepper

1½ teaspoons onion powder

2 pounds thawed white fish fillets, such as tilapia

Coconut oil and butter, for frying

Flaky white fish fillets with a crisp breading. Mmmmm—a hit with children and even more amazing with Trim Healthy Ketchup (page 482).

1. Combine the Baking Blend, salt, pepper, and onion powder on a large dinner plate. Rinse the fish fillets so they are damp, not dry. Place each fillet onto the breading mix to coat well, then turn over and coat the other side; the flour will stick because of the moisture.

2. Heat an equal amount of coconut oil and butter in a large skillet set over medium-high heat. Fry 3 to 4 fillets at a time, turning once, about 3 minutes per side.

NSI (IF USING GROUND OATS AND JOSEPH'S PITAS) DF (IF USING COCONUT OIL TO FRY)

FAMILY SALADS

These salads stand proudly alone as entire meals. They have ample protein, and you can really go to town with hearty portions. Nothing else will be needed in your meal unless you want to serve your children some whole-grain bread and butter on the side for extra carbs. If you're the type who needs bread with your salad, Swiss Bread (page 196) will always come to your rescue, or pile on those Blendtons (page 476).

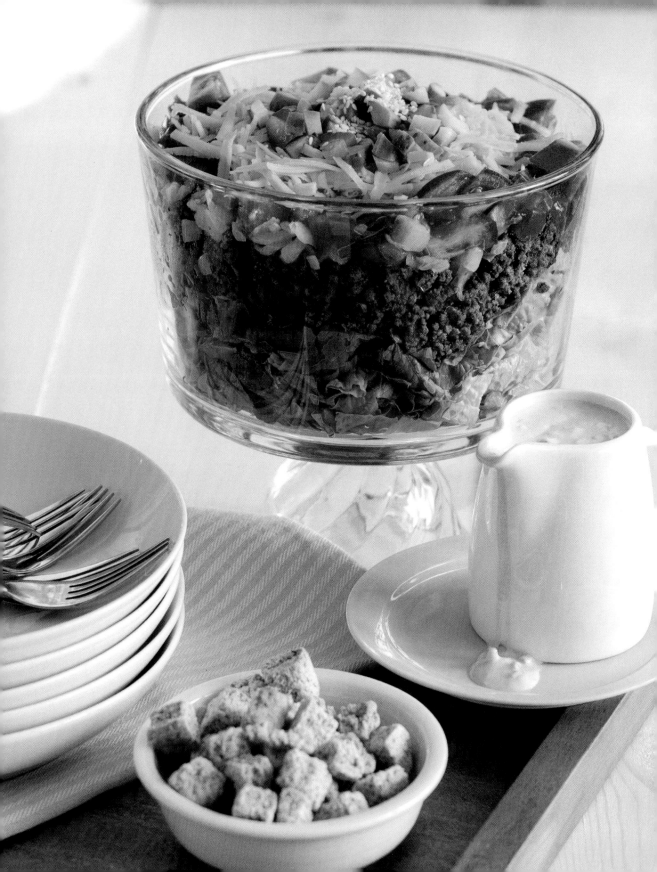

trim mac salad

2 to 2½ pounds thawed ground beef

½ cup water, beef broth, or bone stock (pages 495–496)

1½ tablespoons Worcestershire sauce

2 teaspoons paprika

1 teaspoon Mineral Salt

1 teaspoon black pepper

1 large onion, finely diced

1 tablespoon butter

3 or 4 large heads crisp romaine lettuce, shredded or roughly chopped

3 or 4 ripe tomatoes, roughly chopped

8 ounces cheddar cheese, grated or finely shredded

3 or 4 dill pickles, chopped, or ⅓ cup dill relish

Thousand Island Dressing (page 472)

¼ to ⅓ cup sesame seeds

All the flavor of the most famous burger in the world, without the weight problems that can come with it. It's all about that special sauce, right? That's a cinch when you use our Thousand Island Dressing (page 472). Now the whole family can sit down to enjoy the taste of fast food for dinner and you don't have to fret about the health consequences. Do you have children who don't want to eat salad? What a great way for them to learn how to get addicted to salad when there's yumminess like this.

For the sake of ease, we brown the ground beef rather than make patties. It's just quicker, yet still tastes great in the salad. If you prefer to use beef patties for a more authentic burger experience, go ahead. You'll want to cut the burgers into bite-size pieces once they are cooked.

1. Brown the meat in a large skillet over medium-high heat, about 10 minutes, then pour off any excess fat. Add the water, Worcestershire sauce, paprika, salt, and pepper.

2. In a separate smaller skillet, sauté the onion in the butter until translucent.

3. Assemble individual salad bowls by layering first the lettuce, then the meat, then the onion, then the tomatoes, cheese, and pickles, and then the Thousand Island Dressing. Top with the sesame seeds and Blendtons (page 476), if desired. (Or just layer in one big bowl and let people serve themselves.)

NSI

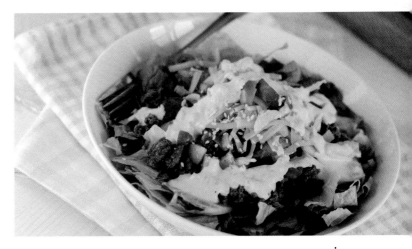

zesty southwestern chop up (S)

3 or 4 heads crisp romaine lettuce, chopped

4 to 6 cups diced cooked chicken, sprinkled to taste with Mineral Salt, black pepper, and ground cumin

2 large orange or red bell peppers, cored, seeded, and chopped

2 cups cherry tomatoes, chopped

8 green onions, white and green parts finely diced

2 avocados, pitted, peeled, and chopped into small cubes

1 (15-ounce) can of black beans, rinsed and drained, or 1½ cups cooked black beans, drained

1 batch Zesty Avo Cream Dressing (page 471)

This salad is rich in the good fats that avocados provide, not only in the salad itself but also in the dressing. Eat up!

1. Place all the ingredients except the dressing in a large bowl (or bowls, if you want to make up individual bowls for each person). Toss with the dressing and serve!

NOTE: The amount of beans in this recipe should not interfere too much with the **S** fuel, as they come in at ¼ cup or less per serving.

NSI DF (IF USING THE DOUBLE AVOCADO OPTION FOR THE DRESSING IN PLACE OF THE YOGURT)

grand greek salad

(S)

FOR THE CHICKEN MARINADE

3 tablespoons extra-virgin olive oil

1½ teaspoons dried oregano

½ teaspoon Mineral Salt

½ teaspoon black pepper

Juice of 1 lemon

2½ pounds thawed chicken breasts or tenderloins, cut into small pieces

Coconut oil cooking spray

FOR THE SALAD

3 or 4 crisp heads romaine lettuce, chopped

2 medium cucumbers, peeled and chopped

2 large ripe tomatoes, chopped

½ purple onion, thinly sliced

½ to ¾ cup Kalamata or other pitted black olives

6 ounces feta cheese, crumbled

Grand Greek Dressing (page 475), or Drive Thru Sue's can use store-bought Caesar dressing slightly thinned with water

This salad is grand because it's both full of flavor and full of oomph. You sure don't have to leave the table hungry. Swiss Garlic Bread (page 196) is a perfect accompaniment to this meal.

1. Marinate the chicken. Combine the olive oil, oregano, salt and pepper, and lemon juice in a glass or ceramic bowl and add the chicken. Cover and put in the fridge to marinate for 30 minutes (or you can put it in earlier in the day for a longer marinade).

2. While the chicken is marinating, prepare the salad. Put the lettuce in a large bowl or into individual bowls. Top with the cucumbers, tomatoes, onion, olives, feta cheese, and dressing. (Put the onion in a bowl on the side if you have children who are not keen on them.)

3. Coat a large skillet with coconut oil cooking spray and heat over medium-high heat. Add the chicken and brown on all sides. Cook until done through and crisp, about 10 minutes.

4. Top salads with the chicken pieces or place it in a side bowl so each member of the family can take what he or she wants.

NSI

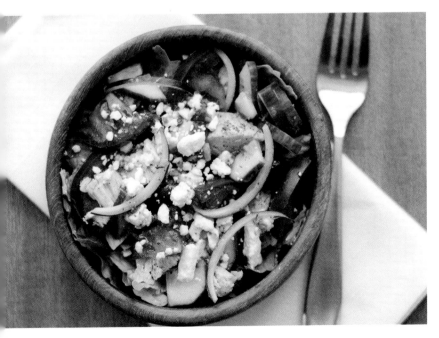

taco salad

2 to 2 ½ pounds thawed ground meat of choice

½ teaspoon garlic powder

2 tablespoons chili powder

2 teaspoons ground cumin

2½ teaspoons paprika

1¾ teaspoons Mineral Salt

¼ teaspoon black pepper

¼ teaspoon cayenne pepper (pull back if your little ones cannot handle heat)

1½ teaspoons onion powder

½ cup water

3 or 4 crisp hearts of romaine lettuce

2 or 3 ripe tomatoes, diced (optional)

½ medium onion, diced (optional)

1 or 2 (15-ounce) cans mild chili beans (for the Crossover people in the family), rinsed and drained, or 1½ to 3 cups cooked beans, drained

8 ounces or more cheddar cheese, grated

Salsa of choice

Sour cream

Blendtons (page 476) or Joseph's Crackers (page 453) or crumbled Mad Melbas (page 456)

Chopped pitted black olives

This is an easy "fall back on" meal that always makes our families happy. We use ground venison for the meat (which goes great with the taco seasonings), but use any ground meat of your choice. Our children pile beans on their salads, which is a cheap tummy filler and turns their meal into a healthy Crossover (not saying they don't have a few corn chips on top, too). We skip the beans if we desire a pure S meal or just sprinkle a very small handful (less than ¼ cup) over our salads.

1. Brown the meat in a large skillet over medium-high heat, about 10 minutes or until cooked through. If necessary, drain off excess fat. Add the seasonings and water, and simmer over low heat for a few more minutes.

2. Assemble the salads, starting with the lettuce and adding the tomatoes and onion (if using), followed by the ground meat, beans, and grated cheese. Top with dashes of salsa, dollops of sour cream, the Blendtons, and the olives.

NSI

3 or 4 heads crisp romaine (or if your budget is super tight, iceberg)

2 tablespoons extra-virgin olive oil

Juice of 1 lemon

3 to 4 doonks Pure Stevia Extract

Mineral Salt, black pepper, and chili powder, to sprinkle

4 (5-ounce) cans tuna packed in water, drained

1½ to 2 cups 1% cottage cheese

3 cups cooked brown rice

1 cup mango chunks, frozen or fresh (or other fruit except berries, as you need more **E** fuel here)

Blendtons (page 476) or 2 Wasa crackers, crumbled (optional)

Red pepper flakes (optional)

Tuna and rice are some of the cheapest real foods you can buy. We have to say "real" because it's true that you can buy a bunch of white carbs like ramen noodles, chips, or white bread on sale and get a cart full of so-called food for very little money. But in reality you have not bought any real food; you have simply bought yourself a blood sugar spike. This salad uses real food, is real yummy, and is also really cheap! Can't beat that.

1. Rip the romaine into small pieces and place in a large bowl. Pour the olive oil onto the lettuce and massage it in with your hands (this softens the leaves and makes all the greens feel like they have a fattier mouth feel, even though we're in **E** mode). Add the lemon juice, then the stevia, and sprinkle on the seasonings. Toss them with the lettuce.

2. Add the tuna, cottage cheese, and brown rice. Put the mango chunks in a food processor and pulse several times until they are broken down into smaller pieces (but have not turned into mango mush). Add to the salad.

3. Toss the salad well, then sprinkle on the Blendtons and an optional sprinkle of some red pepper flakes (if using).

NSI (IF YOU SUBSTITUTE YOUR FAVORITE ON-PLAN SWEETENER FOR THE STEVIA AND USE WASA CRACKERS IN PLACE OF THE BLENDTONS)

QUICK SINGLE SALADS

This idea of making salad your full meal a few times a week is an awesome habit to get into. Lunch is the perfect occasion to get your salad on! You'll receive plenty of protein, and since leafy greens are such great fillers, you can eat as much as you want of them. Don't put a measly amount of salad on your plate. Load up! Top with delicious, life-giving dressings and watch your health flourish and your weight head down in the right direction.

salads in a jar

These salads can be your rescue if you have limited time during the day to make lunch or if you work outside the home. You make them up ahead of time (usually on a Sunday afternoon), and your salad will stay crisp and fresh for the week. Find some wide-mouth quart jars with lids. They can fit a lot of salad, and you won't come away hungry. Or, if your appetite is not that hearty, you can pack a lot tightly into a pint jar. Pour the salad onto a plate when it is time to eat.

Following are four versions of Salad in a Jar: E, Heavy S, Deep S, and FP. You can learn more about the differences between Heavy S and Deep S in the "Just the Numbers" chapter of *Trim Healthy Mama Plan*. These are just skeleton suggestions for you to get going with your own creative ideas. Throw more or less of your preferred nonstarchy veggies into these salads. (We did not include onion, but you certainly can—just keep it away from the Deep S recipe.) Use different fruits or grains for E, if you prefer.

Of course, you do not have to make these in a jar. Take the ingredient ideas from each type of salad and make up an E, FP, or Heavy or Deep S salad straight on a plate if you're in your own kitchen at meal time and would rather not prep ahead. The main thing is this: don't get stuck eating the same type of salad every day. Keep juggling those fuels for a revved metabolism. We know the Heavy S option with ranch dressing and grated cheese is conventional and convenient; enjoy that from time to time, but don't neglect the others.

NOTE: It's important to follow the order of directions, rather than just throwing the salad stuff in a jar. These salads work best when the dressing goes in first and the lettuce goes in last.

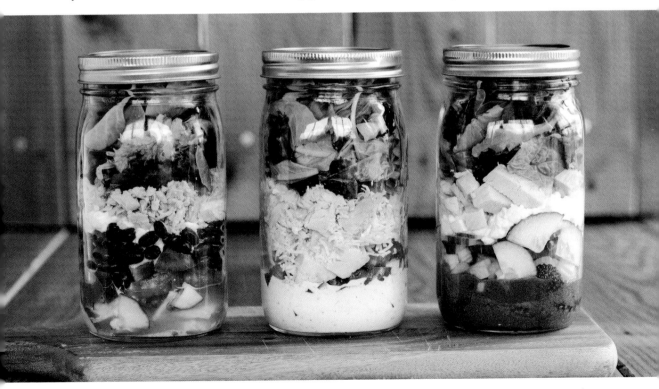

SINGLE SERVE

1 teaspoon MCT or olive oil

3 tablespoons vinegar of choice
   (balsamic tastes great but turns
   veggies brown—if you don't care
   about that, go for it; if you don't like
   brown veggies, try apple cider, or
   white wine vinegars)

1½ doonks Pure Stevia Extract, or your
   favorite stevia blend to taste

Mineral Salt and black pepper to taste

⅓ cup diced cucumber, or more as
   desired

⅓ cup diced ripe tomato, or more as
   desired

½ cup cooked black beans and ½ large
   apple, diced and sprinkled with
   lemon juice to retain color; or ½ cup
   rice or quinoa and ⅓ cup frozen or
   fresh mango pieces, diced

⅓ cup 1% cottage cheese (for dairy-
   free, omit this)

3 to 6 ounces diced cooked chicken
   breast or canned tuna

Enough ripped or chopped lettuce to
   fill to top of jar

1. Put the oil, vinegar, and stevia into the bottom of the jar.
   Add a sprinkle or two of salt and pepper, then stir.

2. Add the cucumber and tomato, followed by your choice of
   beans + fruit or grain + fruit. Follow with the cottage cheese
   and chicken or tuna.

3. Top with the lettuce all the way to the top of the jar. Screw
   the lid on tightly and refrigerate.

NOTE: If you'd rather not use the vinaigrette here, substitute
a store-bought light dressing. Bolthouse Farms has some nice
yogurt-based lean dressings. Try to use one with less than 3 to 5
grams of fat. You can also use Slim Belly Vinaigrette (page 474).

NSI (IF YOU SUBSTITUTE YOUR FAVORITE ON-PLAN SWEETENER FOR
PURE STEVIA EXTRACT) DF (IF YOU LEAVE OUT THE COTTAGE CHEESE)

SALAD IN A JAR (FP)

SINGLE SERVE

3 tablespoons Slim Belly Vinaigrette
   (page 474)

5 fresh or frozen strawberries, hulled
   and sliced

1 large celery stalk, thinly sliced

½ cup peeled and diced cucumber

⅓ to ½ cup 1% cottage cheese (for
   dairy-free, omit this)

3 to 4 ounces diced cooked chicken or
   canned tuna

Enough ripped or chopped lettuce to
   fill to top of jar

1. Put the dressing in the bottom of the jar.

2. Add the strawberries, followed by the celery and cucumber,
   followed by the cottage cheese and chicken or tuna.

3. Top with enough lettuce to reach all the way to the top of
   the jar. Screw the lid on tightly and refrigerate.

NSI DF (IF COTTAGE CHEESE IS OMITTED; YOU CAN USE SOME
GRATED HELLO CHEESE, PAGE 487)

DEEP S SALAD IN A JAR

SINGLE SERVE

3 tablespoons Tangy and Sweet
  Vinaigrette (page 472); or 2 to
  3 tablespoons olive oil or MCT oil and
  1 to 2 tablespoons vinegar of choice
Mineral Salt and black pepper to taste
½ cup peeled and diced cucumber
¼ to ⅓ cup thinly sliced celery or
  green bell pepper (optional)
4 to 6 ounces diced cooked meat or
  fish of choice (use more if desired)
1 tablespoon grated Parmesan cheese
  (optional; green can kind is fine; this
  gives a bit more flavor to the salad
  and really is just a garnish amount)
Enough ripped or chopped lettuce to
  fill to top of jar

1. Put the dressing in the bottom of the jar. Sprinkle in the salt and pepper.

2. Add the cucumber and celery or green pepper (if using), followed by the meat of choice and the grated Parmesan.

3. Top with lettuce all the way to the top of the jar. Screw the lid on tightly and refrigerate.

NSI DF (IF LEAVING OUT PARMESAN CHEESE)

HEAVY S SALAD IN A JAR

SINGLE SERVE

Any S Dressing (pages 470–475)
⅓ cup diced cucumber, or more as
  desired
⅓ cup diced ripe tomato, or more as
  desired
½ avocado, pitted, peeled, and sliced,
  doused with lemon juice to retain
  color; or a handful of nuts (optional)
¼ cup grated cheese of your choice
  (optional)
3 to 6 ounces diced cooked chicken,
  beef, fish, or sprouted tofu
Enough ripped or chopped lettuce to
  fill to top of jar

Use any of the S dressings on pages 470–475 or your favorite plan-approved store-bought dressing with 2 grams or less of carbs. Try thinning store-bought dressings like ranch, blue cheese, and Caesar so they go further and don't pour needless soybean oil calories down your throat.

1. Pour into the jar the amount of dressing you desire (or think is sensible).

2. Add the cucumber and tomato, followed by the avocado or nuts (if using). Add the cheese (if using), followed by the meat of choice.

3. Top with the lettuce all the way to the top of the jar. Screw the lid on tightly and refrigerate.

NSI DF (WITHOUT THE GRATED CHEESE, OR SUBSTITUTE GRATED HELLO CHEESE, PAGE 487)

waldorf cottage cheese salad ⓔ

2 teaspoons finely chopped nuts

Cayenne pepper and Bragg liquid aminos or Mineral Salt, for dusting (see Note)

1 medium apple

1 tablespoon lemon juice

2 celery stalks, thinly sliced

1 cup 1% cottage cheese

Red pepper flakes (optional)

Here's a wonderfully filling way to get more E lunches in your life. The sweetness of the apple mixed with the spiciness of the nuts makes for a delicious meal. Since we're in E mode here, don't use too many nuts. Chop them very small, and put lots of spice on them so you get oodles of flavor for just a small amount.

1. Mix the nuts with a little cayenne pepper and season with a small squirt of the liquid aminos or a sprinkle of salt. Toss in a small dry skillet over medium heat until brown and crispy, about 2 minutes (watch that nuts don't start to smoke and burn). Set aside.

2. Dice the apple, put in large ceramic cereal bowl, and toss with the lemon juice. Add the celery and cottage cheese, and mix well.

3. Top with the spicy nuts; if desired, sprinkle with red pepper flakes.

NOTE: You could also use store-bought spicy nuts, like Blue Diamond Bold Habenero BBQ.

NSI

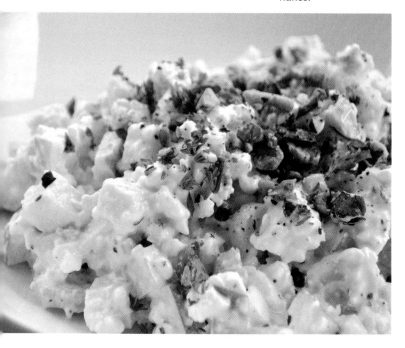

three-minute sensational salad

(S)

SINGLE SERVE

Couple of very large handfuls baby field greens or enough to fill a large dinner plate

1 (4- to 6-ounce) packet of tuna

2 teaspoons MCT oil or extra-virgin olive oil

1 to 2 teaspoons toasted sesame oil

1 teaspoon tahini (sesame paste)

Balsamic vinegar to taste

2 tablespoons grated light sheep's-milk cheese, like pecorino romano, or Parmesan (green can kind is fine; for dairy-free, use grated Hello Cheese, page 487)

Small sprinkle of toasted sesame seeds or chopped walnuts

Mineral Salt, black pepper, and cayenne pepper, for seasoning

Handful of Blendtons (page 476; optional)

This is a regular when we write together at each other's houses. It's super quick and tasty; there is no need to make up any dressing beforehand, since it goes right on the plate. This takes us 3 to 5 minutes to prepare, we get nicely filled up, then we're back to more Trim Healthy Mama "bidness," sipping a Collagen Tea (page 436).

1. Put the greens on a large dinner plate. Add the tuna, then drizzle on the oils, tahini, and vinegar.

2. Toss, then add the cheese, sesame seeds, and seasonings. Sprinkle the Blendtons on top (if using).

NSI DF (WITHOUT THE CHEESE, OR SUBSTITUTE HELLO CHEESE, PAGE 487)

lime lover's tofu toss

(S)

SINGLE SERVE (1 LARGE SINGLE LUNCH OR DINNER SERVING OR 2 SIDE SERVINGS)

5 to 6 ounces sprouted tofu

2 tablespoons lime juice

1 tablespoon MCT oil or extra-virgin olive oil

6 pinches Mineral Salt

¼ teaspoon onion powder and/or 2 teaspoons finely diced green onion

⅛ teaspoon garlic powder

1 tablespoon nutritional yeast

⅛ teaspoon black pepper

¼ packed cup finely diced fresh cilantro

1 large celery stalk, finely diced

1 small handful chopped toasted walnuts

1. Smash the tofu with a fork and combine in a large bowl with the remaining ingredients. Toss well.

NOTE: See our thoughts about tofu on page 194.

NSI (IF USING OLIVE OIL INSTEAD OF MCT OIL AND LEAVING OUT NUTRITIONAL YEAST) DF

superfood-loaded salad

SINGLE SERVE

Leafy greens

4 to 8 ounces tuna, salmon, grilled chicken, turkey chunks, steak strips, or use boiled eggs, fried eggs, cubed or crumbled sprouted tofu—your choice

2 tablespoons superfood oils (extra-virgin olive oil, MCT oil, and toasted sesame oil are good choices)

1 tablespoon balsamic vinegar, or to taste

2 tablespoons Superfood Salad Sprinkles (page 493)

OPTIONAL TOPPINGS

Small sprinkling of walnuts or other favorite nuts

½ avocado, peeled, pitted, and cubed

Sprinkling of grated Hello Cheese (page 487) or light raw sheep's-milk cheese like pecorino romano, or feta

Olives or capers to taste

Blendtons (page 476)

½ medium carrot, grated or diced, or ripe tomato, sliced; or other favorite veggie

SERENE CHATS: *This is a huge salad that has nothing in common with dry, boring rabbit food. It makes you want to eat more salad, not because you have to but because you crave it!*

We don't go around belittling iceberg lettuce, and even enjoy it ourselves from time to time; but no iceberg is allowed in this salad. It's all about optimum nutrition. We are not sticklers for everything organic either, but try to at least stick to organic with your salad greens for this recipe. Fill your bowl with greens—they are the feature here. Pile them high, as they will wilt under the dressing and reduce in volume. For this, you'll need a much larger container than a cereal bowl, sistah! Baby green mixes are delicious and so is just plain ol' full-grown crispy romaine.

This is not the salad for large amounts of regular pasteurized cow's-milk cheeses or—shock and horror!—don't let me see you pouring store-bought ranch over it. Save those for your Heavy S salads and for when I'm not looking. Right now, I'm looking and this salad goes with the Superfood Salad Sprinkles recipe (page 493). Your dressing and toppings must be optimally superfood-ish, so while I'll let a little grated cheddar slip in, I'd prefer it if you used the other toppings in the ingredients. Pearl talks a good Drive Thru Sue gab, but don't be fooled—she eats lots of superfood salads without store-bought ranch and you can, too!

I might be a weirdo, but I enjoy eating this salad with my favorite pair of chopsticks. It makes me relax and take the time to chew my greens up properly and not just shovel in and inhale. I also have a favorite beautiful bowl and—watch out, world—if I can't find it when it's time for my superfood salad, especially if it's been hijacked by a six-year-old boy and found in the sand pit with three dead worms and a dehydrated mud pie in it.

1. Fill a large salad bowl enthusiastically with the greens. Top with the meat, poultry, eggs, or fish of choice.

2. Drizzle on the oil and vinegar, then dust the salad with the sprinkles. Toss well (see Note).

3. Choose from among the toppings and enjoy.

NOTE: The toss step is the key to this superfood salad. Combined with the moistness of the oil, the savory mix coats each leaf and gives a flavor burst and heartier feel with each bite.

NSI DF (WITHOUT THE CHEESE OPTIONS)

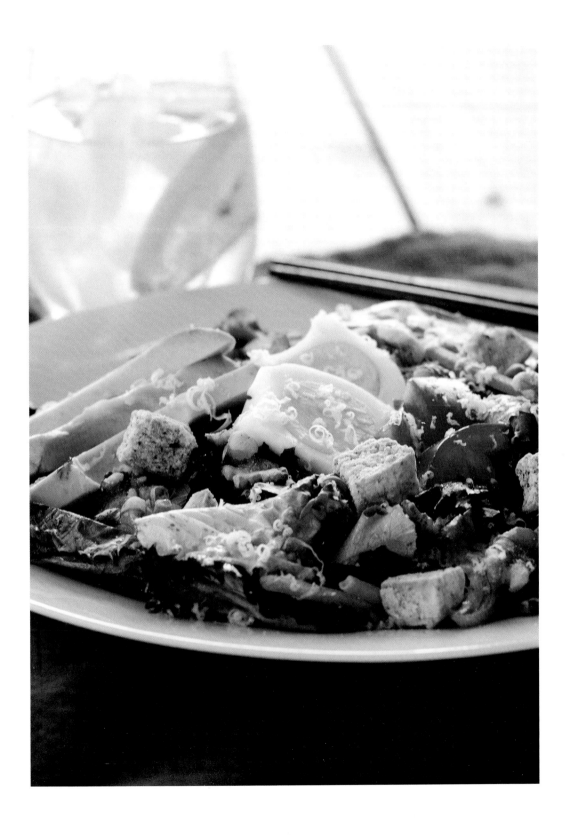

asian sesame tofu toss

S

SINGLE SERVE (1 LARGE SINGLE LUNCH OR DINNER SERVING OR 2 SIDE SERVINGS)

5 to 6 ounces sprouted tofu

1 large celery stalk, finely diced

2 teaspoons toasted sesame oil

2 teaspoons MCT oil or extra-virgin olive oil

2 teaspoons rice vinegar

2 teaspoons nutritional yeast

1 teaspoon soy sauce

1½ teaspoons toasted sesame seeds

¼ teaspoon onion powder and/or 2 teaspoons minced green onion

⅛ teaspoon garlic powder

⅛ teaspoon black pepper

⅛ teaspoon ground cumin (optional)

¼ teaspoon Liquid Smoke (optional)

3 pinches Mineral Salt (optional)

We know the whole scoop about soy and all its problems, and we agree with all that when it comes to overdoing regular unfermented or unsprouted soy. But properly cultured soy used in smaller amounts as part of a balanced diet (as in the cultures where it hails from) can be a healthful food and not the villain we are told to steer clear of. (We do not recommend uncultured or unsprouted soy products.)

After years of abstaining from tofu when we stopped our vegetarian ways, we decided it was time to take a more balanced approach. Sprouted tofu has brought this yummy comfort food back to our tables. Tofu may not be for everyone, and you sure don't have to eat it on plan—but wow, this is good! We enjoy this salad in lettuce cups or just as is, with a small smoothie, shake, or frap on the side.

1. Smash the tofu with a fork and combine in a large bowl with the remaining ingredients. Toss well. Taste, and if it needs a bit more salt, add the pinches of salt.

NSI (IF USING OLIVE OIL INSTEAD OF MCT AND OMITTING NUTRITIONAL YEAST) DF

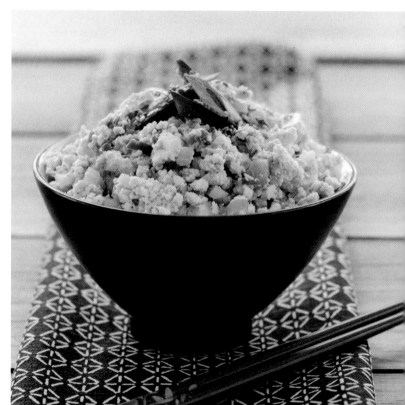

BREADS AND PIZZA CRUSTS

Why would we be so cruel as to take bread and pizza from your life? Enjoy!

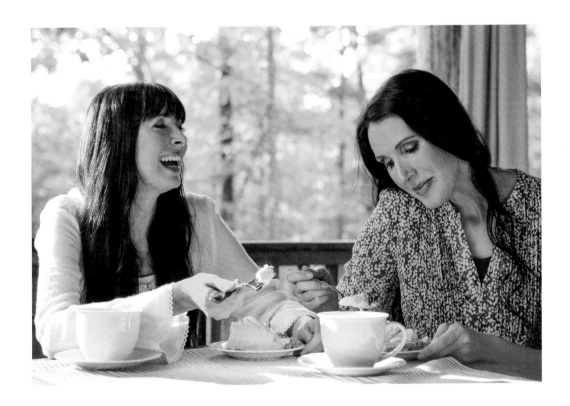

swiss bread

SINGLE SERVE (MAKES 2 ROUNDS OR ONE LARGE PIECE OF BREAD, DEPENDING ON THE SHAPE OF THE PAN)

¼ cup Trim Healthy Mama Baking Blend

2 large egg whites

1 tablespoon water

1 small pinch Mineral Salt

2 pinches Super Sweet Blend

½ teaspoon aluminum-free baking powder

Coconut oil cooking spray

We call this Swiss Bread because, like Switzerland, it doesn't take sides. It can be your go-to bread replacement for any meal. You can eat it with either S or E meals, or keep it in Fuel Pull mode. It makes a wonderfully ooey-gooey grilled cheese or a great side to soup or stew, especially when topped with a bit of buttah for S. Enjoy it as an FP sandwich with lean fillings, but have fruit on the side for an E option. The ideas for flavors are limitless. Add rosemary, garlic or onion powder, jalapeño, or cheese (the cheese would make it an S)—whatever flavors you can dream up!

1. Preheat the oven to 350°F.

2. Mix all the food ingredients in a medium bowl. Coat 2 of the holes in an 8-cup muffin tin with coconut oil spray or coat a bread-shaped small baking pan. Fill the other holes in the muffin tin with water (this gives a nice steaming effect and helps improve the texture of the bread). If using a small baking pan, put an oven-safe bowl with water in the oven. Fill the 2 holes with the bread mix or put into the small pan.

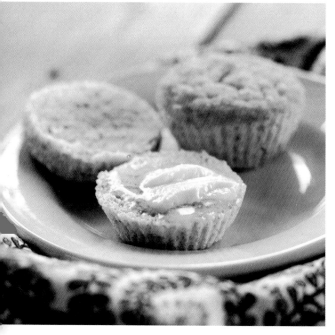

3. Bake for 13 to 15 minutes; do not overbake. Allow the bread to sit for a few minutes before removing from the muffin tin or cutting open. Alternatively, put the bread mix in a microwave-safe container (bread-shaped Pyrex works best) and nuke for 1 minute.

NOTE: Feel free to quadruple this recipe, which then fills all 8 holes of the muffin tin and will give you 8 bread rolls when made in the oven.

VARIATION: For Swiss Garlic Bread, melt 2 teaspoons butter (or coconut oil) and mix with 1 minced garlic clove or a sprinkle of garlic powder in a skillet, slice Swiss bread (or roll shapes) in halves and brown in the garlic butter. Alternatively, smear the slices with butter and minced garlic or garlic powder, and put under the broiler for a couple minutes, watching carefully that they do not burn.

DF

cheddar herb biscuits

SINGLE SERVE (MAKES 2 SMALL BISCUITS)

1 large egg, lightly beaten

¼ cup Trim Healthy Mama Baking Blend

Pinch of Mineral Salt

¼ teaspooon each garlic powder, onion powder, and dried dill (or other dried herb)

½ teaspoon aluminum-free baking powder

1 tablespoon grated cheddar cheese

½ tablespoon cold butter, cut into small pieces

Coconut oil cooking spray

Jessica Myers (our Trim Healthy Mama social group manager) immediately began creating up a storm of recipes as soon as she tried our Trim Healthy Mama Baking Blend. Her husband now prefers these to regular biscuits!

1. Preheat the oven to 350°F.

2. Mix the egg, Baking Blend, salt, seasonings, and baking powder in a medium bowl, until a soft dough forms (it will be sticky). Gently fold in the cheese and butter.

3. Coat 2 holes of an 8-cup muffin tin with coconut oil spray. Divide the dough into 2 balls and drop them into the 2 holes. Bake for 15 minutes.

swiss loaf

6 large egg whites

1 cup water

1 tablespoon apple cider vinegar

1½ cups Trim Healthy Mama Baking Blend

3½ tablespoons Whole-Husk Psyllium Flakes

Scant ¼ teaspoon Mineral Salt

½ teaspoon Super Sweet Blend

1½ teaspoons aluminum-free baking powder

1½ teaspoons baking soda

Coconut oil cooking spray

PEARL CHATS: Of all our goals for this book, our numero uno was to come up with an FP loaf of bread that you can cut, slather butter on, and not turn into a Crossover in the process. Fats with bread are what we all long for, right? Our lofty goal was to create a protein-based loaf that wasn't dry or too heavy and eggy. One that you can put under fried eggs for S or use to make a sandwich and still have room for fruit on the side for E.

The single Swiss Bread (page 196) wasn't hard to get right, but the Swiss Loaf gave us more trouble. There were many failures along the way—flat loaves, squishy loaves, yucky loaves, dry loaves, eggy loaves. But we got closer and closer, and when the final loaf came out of the oven, we cut into it and knew the goal was achieved. Our children and husbands love this. No, it's not your high, fluffy loaf of bread from the store, but it's pretty darn good—and so good for you!

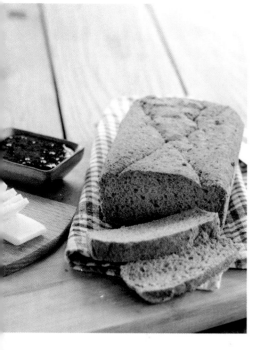

1. Preheat the oven to 400°F.

2. Place the egg whites in a food processor, add the water and vinegar, and process for 15 seconds. Add the other food ingredients, pulse to combine for a few seconds, scrape down the sides of the processor bowl with a spatula, then pulse again for 10 seconds. Allow the mixture to sit for 3 or 4 minutes.

3. Lightly spray a 4½ × 8½-inch loaf pan with coconut oil spray (pan size is important; too big a pan and your loaf will be flat). Pour the dough into the pan, then smooth the top gently with your spatula. Cut a large X in the top, then gently widen it so the top cracks evenly. Put the bread on the middle rack of the oven, then immediately turn the oven temperature down to 375°F. After 20 minutes, cover the top of the loaf with foil and continue baking for another 40 minutes for a full hour total.

4. Remove the loaf from the oven and let cool briefly, then remove from the pan and allow to cool on a wire rack or on the top of the loaf pan for a couple hours. Protein-rich breads are much better after having sat out for a while. If you cut into it too soon, it will appear too moist. The texture will be even better the next day, after drying out a little.

NOTE: You can freeze extra bread in baggies, separating the pieces with wax paper or coffee filters.

DF

trim corn bread

1 cup Trim Healthy Mama Baking
Blend

2 large eggs plus ½ cup egg whites
(carton or fresh)

¼ cup water

4 tablespoons coconut oil or butter

½ teaspoon Super Sweet Blend
(optional)

⅓ teaspoon Mineral Salt

⅛ teaspoon turmeric

⅓ teaspoon paprika

3 tablespoons frozen corn kernels

2 teaspoons aluminum-free baking
powder

1. Preheat the oven to 425°F.

2. Put the Baking Blend, eggs and egg whites, water, 3 table-spoons coconut oil, Super Sweet Blend (if using), salt, turmeric, and paprika in a food processor. Add the corn, and process for several seconds. Turn off, scrape down the bowl sides with a spatula, and process again. Add the baking powder and process one more time for a few seconds.

3. Melt the remaining 1 tablespoon coconut oil in an 8-inch square baking pan in the hot oven. Take the pan out, swish around the fat to cover the bottom and sides, then pour the batter into the pan. Alternatively, pour the batter into the holes of a greased 8-cup muffin tin.

4. Bake for 20 minutes.

NOTE: The corn kernels in this recipe are a small amount and should not cause a fuel clash, but you can leave out if desired.

DF (IF USING COCONUT OIL RATHER THAN BUTTER)

soft sprouted bread

2 cups warm water (105°F)

1 tablespoon honey (this is needed to activate the yeast)

1 tablespoon active dry yeast

3½ to 4 cups sprouted bread flour (kamut, spelt, or whole wheat; see Note)

1 tablespoon butter or ghee (clarified butter)

1 teaspoon Mineral Salt

Coconut oil cooking spray

If you don't want to shell out the dollars that stores charge for sprouted bread, make your own at home for less expense. This bread is absolutely soft and lovely (a nicer texture than the store-bought versions, we think), perfect for an E style sandwich, or under an egg-white scramble, or when smeared with a good amount of butter as a Crossover for your children, or when you reach or are close to your goal weight.

1. Put the warm water in a small bowl, stir in the honey, and let it dissolve. Add the yeast and give it a gentle stir. Allow to sit for about 10 minutes, or until the yeast has frothed and bubbled on top of the water.

2. Place 3 cups of the flour in a large bowl, or in the bowl of a stand mixer, or in a food processor. Pour in the yeast mixture and salt and stir until well combined. It will still be quite sticky. Start kneading, adding more flour 1 tablespoon at a time, until the dough is smooth and elastic, not sticky, but still moist and pliable. In a food processor, this takes from 1 to 5 minutes. In a stand mixer with a dough hook, it takes 8 to 12 minutes. By hand, it takes 20 to 30 minutes.

3. Once the dough is kneaded, divide it into 2 portions, or into your desired shapes. Lightly spray two 4½ × 8½-inch loaf pans with coconut oil and place dough in them. Cover and allow to rise for about 1 hour, or until doubled in size. Score if desired.

4. Preheat the oven to 350°F.

5. Bake the loaves for 35 to 40 minutes. If the tops of the loaves are getting too browned, cover them loosely with foil for the last 10 minutes. Allow the loaves to rest for at least 10 minutes before removing from the pans and slicing.

VARIATION: For rolls instead of loaves, roll the dough into balls, score across the top, allow to rise, and bake them on a greased shallow baking sheet for 20 minutes.

NOTE: Kamut and spelt will not rise quite as high as whole wheat, but the flavor is great and they have less gluten for those who are sensitive.

NSI DF (GHEE [CLARIFIED BUTTER] IS OFTEN TOLERATED AS A DAIRY-FREE OPTION)

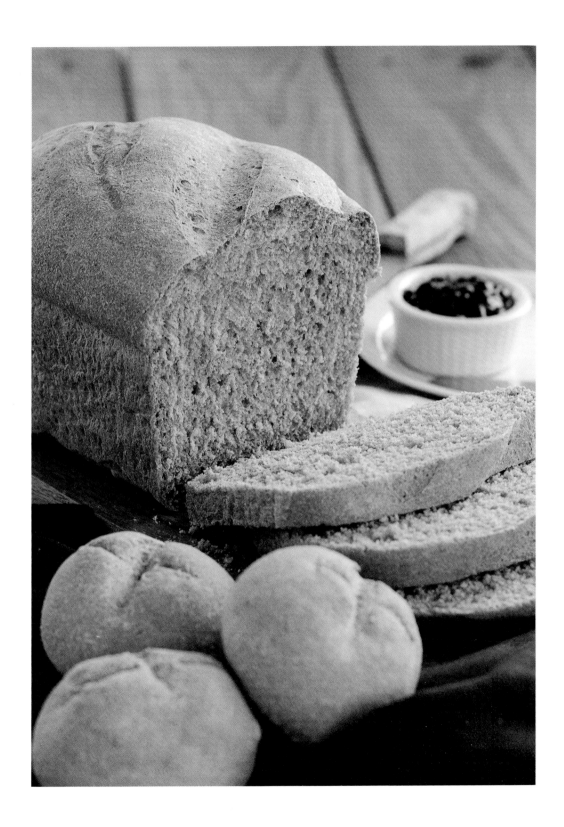

southwestern pan bread

MULTIPLE SERVE

(3 official **E** servings or up to ⅓ of the batch for each serving. That means you'll cut the pan bread into 6 super-large pieces of bread and use 2 pieces for a really big, filling **E** sandwich. Or, you can cut the bread into 8 or 10 slices, which will give you 4 to 5 servings for more medium-size sandwiches, but be sure to have some fruit on the side for extra needed **E** fuel if making a smaller sandwich.)

1 cup old-fashioned rolled oats, ground into flour in a blender

1 cup low-fat cottage cheese

1 cup egg whites (carton or fresh, but carton is easier)

2 teaspoons aluminum-free baking powder

2 pinches Mineral Salt

Scant ¼ teaspoon ground cumin

Scant ¼ teaspoon onion powder

⅛ teaspoon garlic powder (optional)

2 tablespoons salsa of choice

Coconut oil cooking spray

Here's a budget-friendly way to make a great E sandwich if you don't want to buy sprouted bread, or make the more involved Soft Sprouted Bread (page 200) or Artisan Sourdough Bread (page 206). No special ingredients or kitchen skills needed here. This is so simple you might chuckle out loud at the ease. Make a batch at the beginning of the week, put the slices in zippies, and you'll have sandwich bread in the fridge for some well-needed E fuel whenever you need it.

The Southwestern flavors are mild here, so they only enhance most E sandwiches you may want to make with lean deli meat or chicken breast. This pan bread also works great as a breakfast-type sandwich with crispy egg whites and Laughing Cow cheese. If you don't want the hint of Southwest, omit all the seasonings except the salt.

1. Preheat the oven to 350°F.

2. Combine the ground oats in a blender with the cottage cheese, egg whites, baking powder, and seasonings. Stir in the salsa.

3. Coat a 9 × 13-inch shallow baking pan with coconut oil cooking spray or line the pan with parchment. Pour the batter into the pan so it covers the entire space. Bake for 20 minutes. After the first 5 to 8 minutes, prick the bread with a fork to release any air bubbles.

4. Let cool briefly, then cut into desired pieces.

NSI

bread in a mug

SINGLE SERVE

¼ cup egg whites (carton or fresh)
2 tablespoons golden flax meal and
   2 tablespoons almond flour, or
   4 tablespoons golden flax meal
1 teaspoon coconut oil or butter
2 teaspoons water
Pinch of Mineral Salt
Seasonings of your choice
½ teaspoon aluminum-free baking
   powder
Coconut oil cooking spray

You can find golden flax meal and almond flour at most grocery stores, but if not, brown flax meal should work just fine. This bread is great for a quick S sandwich.

1. Mix well all the ingredients except cooking spray directly in a mug or in a small bowl.
2. Drive Thru Sue's can microwave in a mug or bread-shaped Pyrex dish for 1 minute to 1 minute 20 seconds. Or bake in a small greased Pyrex dish in the oven at 350°F for 15 minutes.

NSI DF

golden flat bread

FAMILY SERVE – MAKES 10 TO 12 SLICES

2 cups golden flax meal
¾ teaspoon Mineral Salt
¾ teaspoon Super Sweet Blend
¼ cup coconut oil
1 cup egg whites (carton or fresh)
½ cup water
1 tablespoon aluminum-free baking
   powder
Dried rosemary (optional)
Finely grated Parmesan cheese
   (optional), for sprinkling over top

Once again, no special ingredients are required for this recipe, which is a boon for our budget-friendly Mamas. The bread is a hearty focaccia type that you can dip, top, and dunk with. It's great as a side to an S or Fuel Pull soup. And it's delicious with the rosemary and Parmesan cheese sprinkled over top.

1. Preheat the oven to 350°F.
2. Put the flax meal, salt, Super Sweet Blend, coconut oil, egg whites, and water in a food processor and process until smooth. Add the baking powder and process again for just a few seconds, or mix in a bowl by hand. Allow the batter to sit for about 5 minutes to thicken.
3. Line a 9 × 15-inch baking sheet with parchment. Pour on the batter and spread thinly to the edges with moistened fingers. If desired, sprinkle the top with the rosemary and Parmesan. Bake for 20 minutes.
4. Let cool briefly, then cut into 10 to 12 pieces, or tear off hunks as desired.

NSI DF

wonder wraps

makes 2 to 3 small to medium wraps (if this is not enough for those with heartier appetites, you can up the single serve to
1 tablespoon psyllium with ½ cup egg whites and still easily be in FP mode)

2 teaspoons Whole-Husk Psyllium
    Flakes
⅓ cup egg whites (carton or fresh)
2 small pinches Mineral Salt
1 pinch each garlic and onion powder
1 teaspoon nutritional yeast (optional)
Dash of hot sauce of choice
Coconut oil cooking spray

These wraps can revolutionize your food world. They're a great choice for purists who don't want to use any Frankenfood, or low-carb wraps from the store, but they're easy enough for any Drive Thru Sue to master.

It's a great idea to make the family-size batch every week, and keep them in your fridge (put teenagers or older children to work—we have teens who are better than we are at this now). Wonder Wraps make fast, no-think lunches for home or work, and they are sturdy enough to hold up well when stuffed with meats and veggies. For instance, it might be as simple and quick as stuffing the wraps with diced avocado and tomato. Or, you can create wonderful whole meals like Wonder Fish Tacos (pages 171–172), Enchilada Wonder Casserole (page 145), or Wonder-Wrap-Ful Lasagna (page 148).

Don't abandon this if you (or your teen) mess up a little on your first attempt—practice makes perfect. The key is to spread them out as thin as you can on your griddle, using the back of your spoon. Don't keep them thick, or they'll be like rubber wraps, and nobody wants that. Watch the Wonder Wrap video we have on our website, if you need visual instruction on how to make these. We also give lots of ideas on what to fill them with.

1. Whisk together all the food ingredients in a bowl. Allow the batter to sit for a few minutes.

2. Heat a stovetop or electric griddle to 275°F (low/medium) and coat lightly with coconut oil spray.

3. Put 2 rounded tablespoons of batter on the heated griddle and immediately spread it as thin as possible, using circular motions with your spoon until it resembles the shape of a wrap or a medium-size tortilla. Cook, turning over after the first side is golden, and continuing to cook the other side until very lightly golden. Continue to make more wraps until the batter is used up.

NOTE: At first, make only one wrap at a time. Once you become a Wonder Wrappin' expert, you can make two at a time to build your stacks of wraps faster.

DF

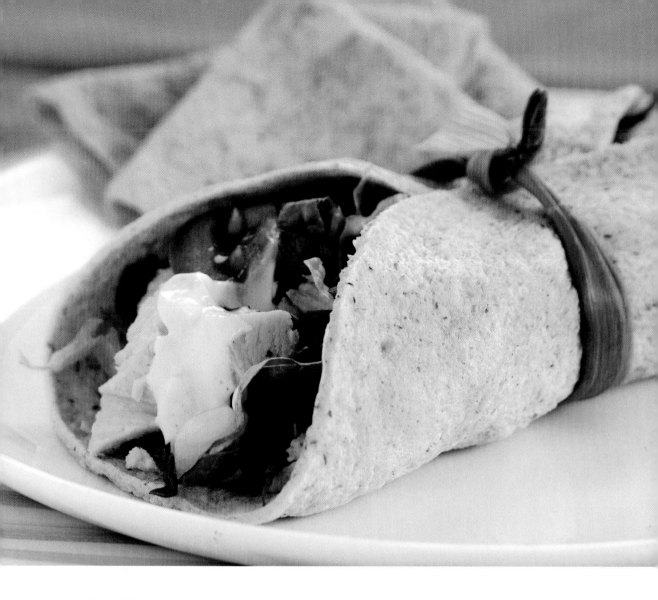

FAMILY SERVE (MAKES 12 TO 18 MEDIUM-SIZE WRAPS)

¼ cup Whole-Husk Psyllium Flakes

2 cups egg whites (carton is easier)

⅛ teaspoon Mineral Salt

⅛ teaspoon each garlic and onion powder

1½ tablespoons nutritional yeast (optional)

Few dashes of hot sauce of choice (optional)

Coconut Oil cooking spray

1. Follow the directions for the single serve, but you may need to refresh the griddle a few more times with coconut oil spray as you make your big batch of wraps.

artisan sourdough bread ⓔ

SERENE CHATS: *If you love an adventure in the kitchen, take a sourdough trip in the time travel machine of your own kitchen. Meander back to early European peasant farms, and smell the fragrant hearth and home of food so honest it was almost poetic, and fed the body, but also the soul. These loaves have a chewy, steamed crust with a moist crumb that carries that characteristic sour tang so beloved by foodies and bread connoisseurs. The long fermentation of true sourdough bread pre-digests much of the starch, lowering the glycemic level drastically and breaking down many of the problems we have today with grains (including significantly lowering the gluten level) for those with sensitive digestive systems.*

I've worked on this recipe for several years now, streamlining the process along the way. I know it looks involved, but it is a whole lot easier to make than it seems on paper. It really is a 1, 2, 3, easy-as-pie recipe that even a Drive Thru Sue would find shockingly simple. You don't need a fancy dough mixer. I do it all by hand (by choice), but if you want to use a mixer that's fine, too. The recipe makes 4 medium loaves. I double the recipe and bake 8 loaves every second day. But if your family is smaller or you are single, you can even halve or quarter the recipe. This bread freezes and thaws beautifully, so don't worry if you need to slice it and store it in the freezer.

First, you catch the wild yeasts in the air to make your starter. Then you make the bread itself. Making the starter takes about a week, but if this first step sounds too involved, just Google "rye starter" and you'll find sources to order it, and you can just jump straight to the bread recipe. But for all my other crazy, adventurous peeps, here's how it works.

7 cups organic rye flour, 1 cup for each day

7 cups room-temperature water (not chlorinated city water), 1 cup for each day

FOR WILD YEAST STARTER

1. Combine 1 cup of rye flour with 1 cup of water in a sterilized nonmetal bowl. To sterilize, pour boiling water over bowl. Cover flour-water mix with a loose mesh material so no bugs can fly in. Put it on a counter where it has room to breathe—don't stuff it in a cupboard.

2. Every day for the next 7 days, add 1 cup water and rye flour to the mix and transfer it to a new sterilized nonmetal bowl. Alternate between two bowls for the seven-day period. Give it a little stir with a nonmetal stirring utensil.

3. If after 7 days your mixture looks a little spongy or bubbly and smells pleasantly sour, then you should congratulate yourself and do a cartwheel, because you are the proud new owner of a Wild Yeast pet! That's it—you did it!

NOTE: If you look after your yeast well, it can live for hundreds of years and you can pass it on to your grandchildren. If it just looks lifeless and half-rotten, then your first yeast attempt may have been unsuccessful. If after a few tries you can't seem to catch any, don't beat yourself up. Many areas are harder to obtain wild yeasts in than others. Order it online and be done with all the fuss. See tips at the end of this recipe for how best to look after your starter pet.

5 cups wild yeast starter

3¼ cups pure water (not chlorinated city water)

3¼ cups organic rye flour

4¾ cups organic spelt flour or kamut flour

1½ tablespoons Mineral Salt

Coconut oil cooking spray

1. Place the 5 cups of starter in a large soup pot (if mixing by hand, like I do) or in your dough mixing machine. If mixing by hand, add the water first, followed by the rye flour and stir everything well. Now add the spelt or kamut and the salt, and stir until well combined. If you have a mixing machine, you can throw all the ingredients in at once. If mixing by hand, get a fat, clean stick (my children found and sanded me one from outside, but you can use whatever kitchen thingy is strong enough to do the job). Plonk the stick in the back section of your pot. Hold it with two hands and lean the pot against your upper body to support it. Move the stick toward you in a forceful motion. Lift it up and place it the back of the pot again, and keep repeating this movement on all quadrants of the pot (like moving through the different numbers on a clock face) for about 10 minutes—makes a nice little workout. Or, be a sane person and turn your machine on the bread kneading cycle for 10 minutes. You may need to add a little more water if the mixture seems too dry. The texture should be smooth and thick, like porridge or oatmeal. It should not be dry like a bread dough that you can knead on a countertop.

2. Lightly coat four bread pans with coconut oil cooking spray. Using a water-moistened small breakfast bowl as a scoop, scoop out the dough from your pot and distribute it evenly among the bread pans.

3. Moisten a knife with water and slash an X on the top of each loaf. Put your bread pans in a place where they can't be disturbed for at least 7 hours, but preferably 12 hours, so the bread can ferment and rise. If it is winter and your home is cold, put them in the warmest spot in the house or in a kitchen cabinet with closed doors and a little pot of steaming water in the cupboard (refill with hot water a few times during the fermentation and rising). On the other hand, if it is summer and your home is excessively warm, this can make your bread rise up and overflow your pans before the full fermentation time has been completed. Try and find a cooler place to let it sit.

4. Preheat the oven to 400°F and place a pan of water on the bottom shelf. Put the loaves in the oven on the middle rack, and bake for 10 minutes, then turn down the temperature to 350°F to complete 2 full hours of baking (another 1 hour and 50 minutes).

5. Remove the loaves from the oven and place a clean dish towel that has been moistened with hot water (and wrung out so it is not dripping) over the top of the loaves still in the pans. After 20 minutes or so (don't time it and get all OCD about it), remove the towel and remove the bread from the pans.

NOTE: Sorry, but this bread will not be ready to cut for a good half-day. It is still firming up inside. The peak of ease for slicing will be in a couple of days, but you can start slicing pieces after a few hours. This bread keeps so well unrefrigerated because it has a lovely protective crust that preserves the moist interior, whose long fermentation time has given it the perfect pH level to resist harmful bacteria. Store the unsliced loaves in an uncovered basket (or with a light mesh over them), and any cut loaves open-side down.

LOOKING AFTER YOUR STARTER PET:

1. Every day feed him 1 cup food (rye flour) and 1 cup of drink (pure water). If you miss a day, then don't think you are a bad pet Mommy, just get back on track. Sourdough pets are easygoing and forgiving, although the more regular you are, the better your bread will rise.

2. Once a month, do basic housecleaning (wash and sterilize the bowl).

3. If you want to go on a "vacay," just give him a meal and put him in the fridge to go to sleep with a loose-fitting lid. You can leave him there like a bear in hibernation for up to a month without another meal. If you want a full-on break from the responsibility of this pet for a longer season, just store him in the freezer indefinitely after a good feed and a kiss goodbye.

4. To wake your sleepy pet, bring him out to room temperature and start to feed him every day until his bubbles and sponginess returns.

5. Don't be alarmed if you see black-purplish water resting on top of your little petty poo. This is called hooch, and it is completely normal after a dormant spell. It just means he is getting hungry. Discard the hooch without being overly perfectionist about it, give him a good stir, and feed him again. Waking a sleepy pet takes a few days to a week of feeding, so be patient with him.

NSI DF

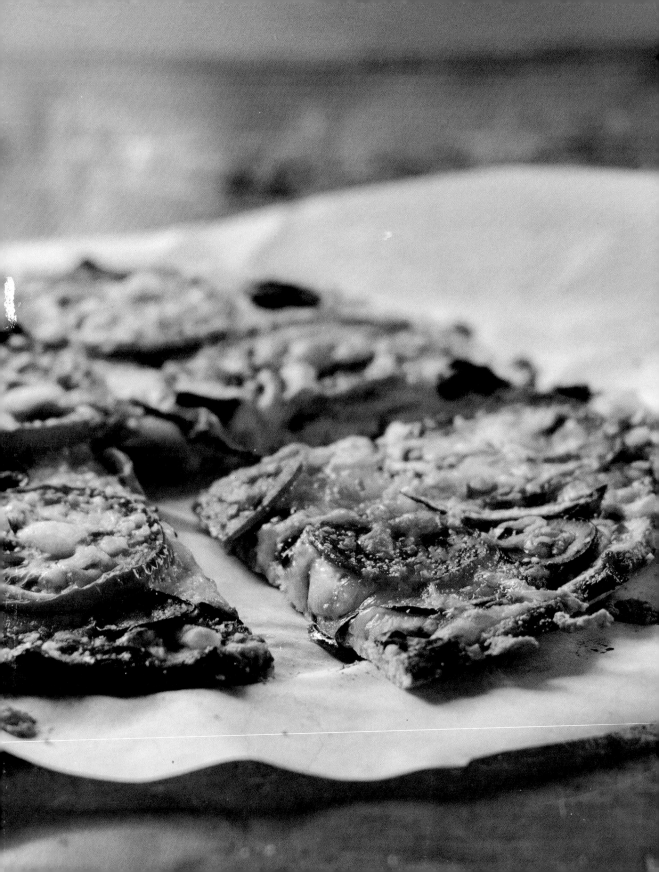

perfect pizza ⓢ

SINGLE SERVE

3 tablespoons Trim Healthy Mama Baking Blend

1 tablespoon finely grated Parmesan cheese (green can kind is fine)

1 stick part-skim mozzarella cheese or slightly less than 1 ounce of part skim cheese (grated)

Pinch of Mineral Salt

Pinch of onion powder

2 large egg whites

¼ teaspoon Italian seasoning mix

FAMILY SERVE VERSION—FEEDS ABOUT 6 HUNGRY PEEPS

1 cup plus 2 tablespoons Trim Healthy Mama Baking Blend

6 tablespoons finely grated Parmesan cheese (green can kind is fine)

5 ounces part-skim mozzarella cheese, grated

¼ teaspoon Mineral Salt

¼ teaspoon onion powder

1½ teaspoons Italian seasoning mix

1¾ cups egg whites (carton or fresh, but carton is quicker here)

PEARL CHATS: I know "perfect" is a boastful title for this pizza crust, but out of all the various plan-friendly crusts I've made, this is my hubby's favorite. He declared it "perfect," so the name stuck. He thinks I'm a genius for coming up with it, and I don't mind basking in the glory! This recipe is made in single and family serve versions. Preparation is basically the same for both.

1. Preheat the oven to 400°F.

2. Put all the ingredients in a bowl and combine well. You should have a very loose, gooey dough. If using carton egg whites in the family-serve version, allow the mix to stand a few minutes so the dough can absorb the whites before it thickens properly.

3. For the single serve, spread the dough out thin on a parchment–lined 9 × 13-inch baking sheet, using the back of a spoon to spread it out as much as possible. You'll find you can keep spreading farther than you thought you could at first; your end result should be about the size of a large dinner plate.

4. For the family serve, divide the dough between 2 parchment–lined 9 × 13-inch baking sheets and use the back of a spoon to spread them both out to the very edges on all sides. (If you're a good spreader you may be able to fill two 11 × 15-inch sheets for even larger, crispier crusts.)

5. Bake the single serve crust for 10 to 12 minutes, and the larger crusts for 13 to 15 minutes (keep an eye on them, as you don't want them too brown).

6. Allow the crusts to cool for a few minutes, then top with sugar-free pizza sauce, then all your favorite toppings. Broil until your toppings are melty and crispy.

rustic pizza

FAMILY SERVE – FEEDS 6 TO 8 (HALVE IF YOUR FAMILY IS SMALLER OR MAKE MORE IF YOU HAVE A VERY LARGE HOUSEHOLD)

¾ cup chia seeds, ground in a blender to make a flour/meal

¾ cup coconut flour

3 tablespoons nutritional yeast

1 tablespoon finely grated Parmesan cheese

1 scant teaspoon Mineral Salt

2 teaspoons onion powder

1 teaspoon smoked paprika or regular

1 teaspoon Liquid Smoke

1 tablespoon cumin seeds (optional)

Handful of pumpkin seeds (optional)

2 tablespoons MCT oil or coconut oil

2 teaspoons aluminum-free baking powder

1¼ cups egg whites (carton or fresh)

¼ cup water

SERENE CHATS: *I "spose" my rustic taste buds were passed down to my children. This is my family's favorite pizza crust. We love to have "Rustic Pizza Night." We fill the table with bowls of toppings, including tomato paste, seasonings, diced chicken sausage, grated Hello Cheese (page 487; that's for me), grated mozzarella (for everyone else), red onions, sliced tomato rings, green and black olives, olive oil, fresh herbs, and so on. I bake the crusts, then each person (who's old enough) rips a piece of crust to suit their appetite, loads it with toppings of their choice, and places it under the broiler for just a few minutes to melt the goodies. Those who want to drizzle olive oil and spices on their slab when it comes out of the broiler do so. Beyond words of yummyness! You can also spread my Cheesy Kale Dip (page 467) on this pizza in place of the tomato paste. We love it!*

Filling wise, eating a piece of this loaded pizza is vastly different from the white crust pizza you might be used to. This is extremely filling, so while the recipe makes just one extra-large crust (or two 9 × 13-inch crusts if you roll it out thin enough), it shouldn't leave anyone hungry. If you do have really big eaters in your home, increase the recipe by half again. I double it, or sometimes even triple it, but I have nine children in the home who are huge eaters—and usually a few hungry nephews and nieces hanging around all too ready to wolf down pieces of this.

Coconut flour and chia seeds are readily found at many grocery stores these days (check Walmart, too), so woot!

1. Preheat the oven to 350°F.

2. Mix all the ingredients well to form a dough ball. Put the dough on one 11 × 15-inch parchment-lined baking sheet or directly on a big pizza stone (or use 2 smaller parchment-lined sheets).

3. Moisten your hands and spread out the dough, or use a moistened rolling pin to get it to reach the edges. This pizza crust is meant to look rustic—don't make it too uniform. The general shape is up to you; how thin or thick you like it is up to you, too. If you want to keep it thin, you'll have a bigger crust for topping. Make sure to push thinner edges in a bit to thicken them so they don't burn.

4. Bake thicker crusts for 35 minutes; if you've made a real thin crust, bake for only 20 minutes, then turn off the oven and leave the crust in for another 15 minutes.

5. Allow the crust to cool for a few minutes, then add your favorite seasonings and toppings. Run the pizza under the broiler for a minute or two, until the toppings are melty and crisp.

NOTE: This basic crust recipe makes fabulous rustic crackers as well. Simply roll it out until very thin onto parchment-lined baking sheets. Bake overnight (right before you hit the sack) at your oven's lowest temperature. The next morning, break it apart into rustic cracker pieces.

NSI (IF OMITTING NUTRITIONAL YEAST) DF

fooled ya pizza

S

2 (16-ounce) bags frozen cauliflower
florets

1½ cups egg whites (carton or fresh)

⅓ teaspoon Mineral Salt

1 teaspoon Italian seasoning mix

⅓ teaspoon garlic powder

4 cups grated part-skim mozzarella
cheese

This pizza crust has been a big hit ever since we shared it in our first book. The "fooled ya" part comes from the fact that most people won't believe there is cauliflower in the crust! We've tweaked the recipe quite a bit, but the original idea comes from Jamie VanEaten, who has a great (funny) blog with lots of yummy S-friendly recipes, at www.yourlight erside.com. This is a family serve recipe. We suggest you make a half-serving the first time so the process feels less overwhelming. A half-serving makes one very large crust that goes completely to the edges of a 9 × 13-inch or even a 10 × 14-inch baking sheet if you spread it thin enough.

1. Preheat the oven to 450°F.

2. Lightly steam the frozen cauliflower. Put it into a colander and press out as much water as you can (important if you want to avoid a soggy crust!). You can also use your hands to squeeze out excess water.

3. Put the pressed cauliflower into a food processor and pulse a few times—not too much. You want to end up with rice-size pieces. Add the egg whites and seasonings and pulse again a few times.

4. Pour the mixture into a large bowl and add the grated cheese, then combine well.

5. Line 2 or 3 cookie sheets (depending on size) with parchment paper. Parchment is very important, as the crusts will stick if you do not use it (do not use wax paper). Divide the dough between the cookie sheets, plopping them into the middle of the sheets and spreading out as thin as possible to the edges, using your hands. Try not to have a thicker middle than sides. And don't let the edges become wispy or they will get too dark when they cook.

6. Bake for 20 minutes. Allow the crusts to cool for a few minutes, then top with your favorites. Broil until the toppings are melty and crispy.

NSI

joseph's pizza crust

WITH **S** OPTION

SINGLE SERVE

½ Joseph's lavash, or 1 large pita cut
   into 2 thin rounds

PEARL CHATS: Sometimes I just can't be bothered making a crust from scratch, and this is when I rely on my "personal choice" items that Serene calls "Frankenfoods." Joseph's low-carb lavash bread works great here, but you can use a Joseph's pita and divide it into two very thin pizza bases by cutting around the circumference, then dividing in two. Low-carb tortillas can also work as thin crusts for pizza. It's important to pre-bake these crusts to make them sturdy enough to hold the toppings, but that only takes a few minutes. We Drive Thru Sue types are best not overdoing these "personal choice" items, though. I stick to half a lavash or one full pita, and have a side salad to help fill me up, but that is not enough for my husband, so I make him a full lavash.

1. Preheat the oven to 400°F.
2. Put the lavash or pita in the oven and pre-bake the crusts for a few minutes, just until they get a little golden brown (watch carefully so they don't burn—you just want them to sturdy up). Or crisp them in the microwave for a minute. Allow to cool for a minute or two.

SERVING IDEAS: If you want to stick to **FP**, spread a thin layer of tomato paste, sprinkle with Italian seasoning, Mineral Salt, and pepper, then top with a small amount of grated part-skim-milk mozzarella (stay within that 5 grams of fat range). Add a little 1% cottage cheese, and spread over, followed by slices of turkey pepperoni and any nonstarchy veggies you desire. For **S** toppings, just top with your usual **S**-friendly favorites, then broil.

NSI

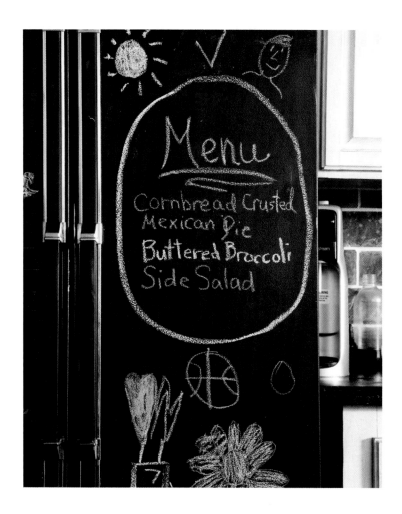

sweet potato fries

FAMILY SERVE – USE A MEDIUM SWEET POTATO MADE INTO FRIES FOR EACH MEMBER OF THE FAMILY BIG ENOUGH TO EAT THAT MUCH

6 medium sweet potatoes, cut into thin julienne strips

1½ tablespoons extra-virgin coconut oil or cooking coconut oil

1 to 1½ teaspoons Mineral Salt

1 teaspoon onion powder

1½ teaspoons paprika (smoked or regular)

Sprinkle of black or cayenne pepper

Such a fun and tasty way to get your E fuel! Enjoy these as a side to a main meal of grilled chicken breast or fish and add a small salad with lean dressing. Or have them as a snack or quick lunch with a Collagen Tea (page 436) or a Trimmy (pages 427–433) for extra protein. As a change of pace, sometimes use 1 tablespoon Trim Bouillon Mix (page 491) in place of the seasonings listed here.

1. Preheat the oven to 375°F.

2. Place the potatoes on one or more large baking sheets. Drizzle on the coconut oil and seasonings, and mix with your hands, making sure all the potatoes are glazed with oil and sprinkled with seasonings.

3. Bake for 30 to 35 minutes, turning once or twice during cooking; broil at the end for a few minutes for a little extra crunch, but be sure to watch they don't burn.

NSI DF

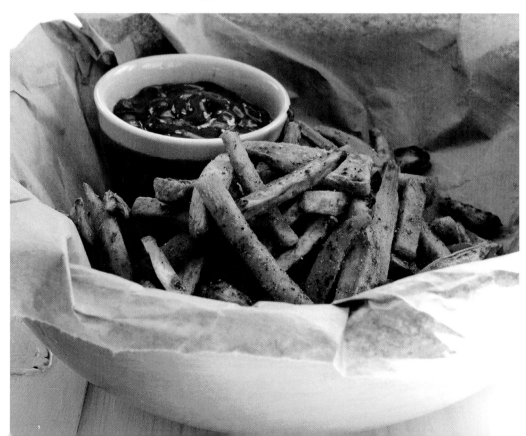

green fries

FAMILY SERVE

2 (16-ounce) bags frozen extra fine
green beans
3 to 4 tablespoons butter (melted) or
coconut oil
Mineral Salt and black pepper to taste
Cayenne pepper to taste (optional)
2 tablespoons nutritional yeast
2 to 3 tablespoons finely grated
Parmesan cheese (optional)

We love these ugly-looking things. The uglier they get, meaning all brown and shriveled, the yummier they taste. They're a great side for all sorts of main meals, but especially burgers. Children don't seem to mind what they look like; ours scarf them up as soon as we take them out of the oven. But if you're unsure of your family's reaction, make a single bag the first time around, instead of a double.

1. Preheat the oven to 375°F.

2. Empty the bags of beans onto two 9 × 13-inch baking sheets. Divide the butter and seasonings between the two trays. Toss the beans with your hands so each green bean gets glazed with oil and coated with seasonings.

3. Bake for 25 to 35 minutes, turning the beans once or twice during cooking, until they are tender and slightly shriveled. They'll be ready when they look crispy in places and have lost their "purtiness"! You can broil at the end for a couple of minutes for an extra crisp result if desired, but keep a watch that they don't burn.

NSI (IF NOT USING NUTRITIONAL YEAST) DF (IF USING COCONUT OIL INSTEAD OF BUTTER AND OMITTING THE CHEESE)

rad hash

SINGLE SERVE

2 teaspoons butter
1 (4-ounce) mini bag matchstick
radishes
2 to 4 tablespoons finely diced onion
1 to 1½ inches smoked sausage,
finely diced

This really is a "rad" side to have at breakfast with fried or scrambled eggs. The matchstick radishes cook up in a jiffy and make you feel as if you are eating savory hash browns. You can find little 4-ounce packets of matchstick radishes at most grocery stores, including Walmart. The thinness of the radishes allows them to cook quickly and the browning lends them more of that hash brown vibe. If you can't find the matchstick variety, finely dice the radishes so they are hash-like.

1. Melt the butter in a medium skillet and add the radishes, onion, and sausage. Cook over medium-high heat, tossing frequently, until the hash is browned and tender. (You can cook the hash in the same pan as you are frying eggs for yourself.)

NSI DF

mashed fotatoes

3 (16-ounce) bags frozen cauliflower florets, or 6 to 8 cups fresh cauliflower florets

3 tablespoons butter

3 tablespoons finely grated Parmesan cheese (optional)

3 tablespoons heavy cream

¾ teaspoon Mineral Salt

¼ teaspoon black pepper

½ to ¾ teaspoon garlic powder (optional)

Turkey or pork bacon bits (optional)

Diced green onions (optional; white and green parts)

This side goes well with just about any S dinner where you would normally use mashed potatoes.

1. Place the cauliflower in a large pot with a little water and steam until tender. Transfer the cauliflower to a colander and push out excess water.

2. Place the cauliflower in a food processor and add the butter, cheese (if using), cream, salt, pepper, and garlic powder (if using). Process to a smooth puree. (You may need to stop the processor to scrape down the sides every now and then.)

3. Scoop out and serve topped with the bacon bits and green onions, if desired.

NSI

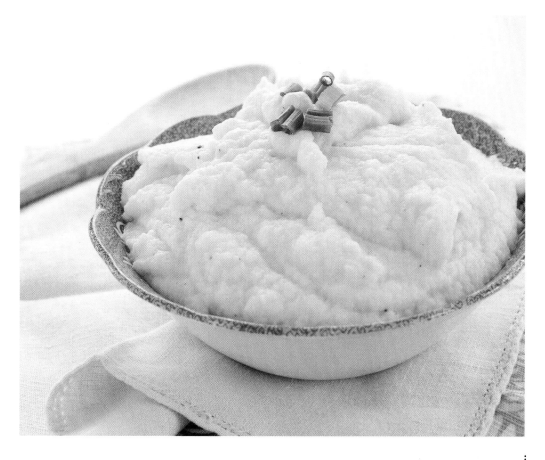

3 pounds pink radishes

1 tablespoon butter, ghee (clarified butter), or coconut oil

1½ teaspoons Mineral Salt

Black pepper to taste

Garlic and onion powder to taste (optional)

Sprinkle of finely grated Parmesan cheese

1 tablespoon nutritional yeast (optional)

¾ to 1 teaspoon Gluccie

¼ to ½ cup Greek yogurt (or sour cream or heavy cream for **S**)

SERENE CHATS: *My five-year-old daughter Breeze named this recipe (and the Princess Icing, page 312). My little girls think they have been to heaven and back when I serve them these mashed taters. You couldn't find a prettier pink, even on the front cover of a Barbie box. But real men will eat them, too, especially when they taste every bit as good as cowboy spuds. Of course, you don't have to call them Princess Taters in front of your man or any male progeny; perhaps if you have boys in your house you could call 'em "piglet taters," as they are the color of a little piggie just born on the farm. Stick some turkey or real bacon bits on top, and the princesses and Barbie dolls will never enter their heads. This recipe makes the standard 6 to 8 very large servings, but you can reduce the ingredient amounts by thirds if you only want a couple of servings. Or, you can make the full batch and freeze leftovers in baggies for your individual sides; they can be quickly heated up.*

1. Place the whole radishes in a medium saucepan with water to cover. Bring to a boil, cover, and reduce the heat to simmer until they are tender.

2. Drain and place the radishes in a blender (not a food processor). Add the butter, seasonings, Parmesan, nutritional yeast (if using), ¾ teaspoon Gluccie, and yogurt or sour cream. Process until smooth. (You may need to do this in two or three batches, but you can put the seasonings in only one batch; sprinkle a little Gluccie into each batch to more evenly distribute it.)

3. Return the puree to the saucepan and stir well to blend the seasonings while you reheat the mixture. You may even need to sprinkle in another ¼ teaspoon Gluccie to thicken the mixture, depending on how much yogurt you had added. Taste and adjust the flavors to "own it."

collagen creamed spinach

MAKES 2 SIDES OR 1 MAIN WITH ADDED CHICKEN BREAST

1 (10-ounce) package frozen chopped spinach

6 tablespoons water

2 teaspoons MCT oil (see Note)

1 tablespoon grated pecorino romano or Parmesan cheese (green can kind is fine; for dairy-free, use Hello Cheese, page 487)

¼ teaspoon Mineral Salt, or to taste

⅛ teaspoon black pepper, or to taste

½ teaspoon onion powder

⅛ teaspoon garlic powder

Cayenne pepper to taste (optional)

½ tablespoon nutritional yeast

1 scoop Integral Collagen

⅛ teaspoon Sunflower Lecithin (optional)

½ cup frozen diced okra, or ⅛ teaspoon Gluccie or just slightly more

SERENE CHATS: *This has to be my all-time favorite veggie side dish. I love it so much that I can eat the entire serving, which here is for two (spinach-loving weirdo that I am). I don't make this side for my children, as they don't appreciate spinach nearly as much, but my husband is crazy about it, too. We happily let our children have bread and a glass of raw milk as their sides while we blissfully eat this, glad they are not interested in stealing our good stuff! You can also have this as a personal side and freeze or refrigerate the leftovers for another time.*

1. Place the spinach in a medium saucepan with the water and bring to a boil over high heat. Cover, turn the heat to low, and simmer until cooked, about 5 minutes. Pour the excess water from the saucepan into a blender, leaving the spinach in the saucepan.

2. Place the oil, cheese, seasonings, nutritional yeast, collagen, lecithin (if using), and okra in the blender and puree until perfectly smooth. (If using Gluccie instead of okra, sprinkle in the Gluccie instead of adding all at once.)

3. Pour the puree into the saucepan with the spinach and, over medium heat, reheat the mixture. Stir, taste, and adjust the seasonings to "own it."

NOTE: You can **S** it up with more MCT oil or a tad of butter or ghee. Actually, a little swirl of raw, pastured, or regular cream added just before serving is a decadent **S** addition. You can add enough diced cooked chicken breast or your favorite lean protein for a main course. The addition of that little extra protein makes this a perfect **FP** main meal.

DF (IF USING HELLO CHEESE, PAGE 487)

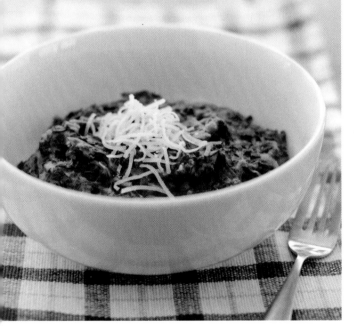

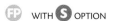
1 medium zucchini (made into noodles using the Troodle or other noodle-maker gadget)

Butter, for serving

Mineral Salt and black pepper, for sprinkling

Coconut oil cooking spray or water (or butter), for cooking

Trim Noodles equals Troodles. Forgive us—or don't, because we are unlikely to stop this ridiculousness of putting two words together to make new names. These zucchini noodles are a fantastic healthy and slimming noodle replacement for the starchy, white fattening kind. Once you start "troodling," you'll easily be able to drop those health-destroying starchy ones from your life. You can use the Troodle maker available on our website or find your own favorite spiral cutter for making these. If you use 4 to 6 zucchini instead of the specified 1, you'll have a Family Serve.

FOR BOILING THE TROODLES

1. Bring a medium saucepan of water to a boil over high heat. Add the Troodles and then allow the water to come back to a boil. Reduce the heat slightly and boil for just a couple of minutes, or until the zucchini noodles release some of their green color into the water. Drain in a colander and press out excess water.

2. Toss the Troodles with a little butter (less than a teaspoon for FP) and salt and pepper, if desired.

FOR SAUTÉING THE TROODLES

1. Spray a medium skillet with coconut oil spray or smear it with a small amount of coconut oil or butter. Add the zucchini noodles and sauté over medium-high heat for just a couple of minutes, or until the Troodles start releasing some of their liquid.

2. Use a slotted spoon to scoop out the Troodles so you don't transfer that excess water onto your plate. Season with a little salt and pepper, if desired.

NSI DF

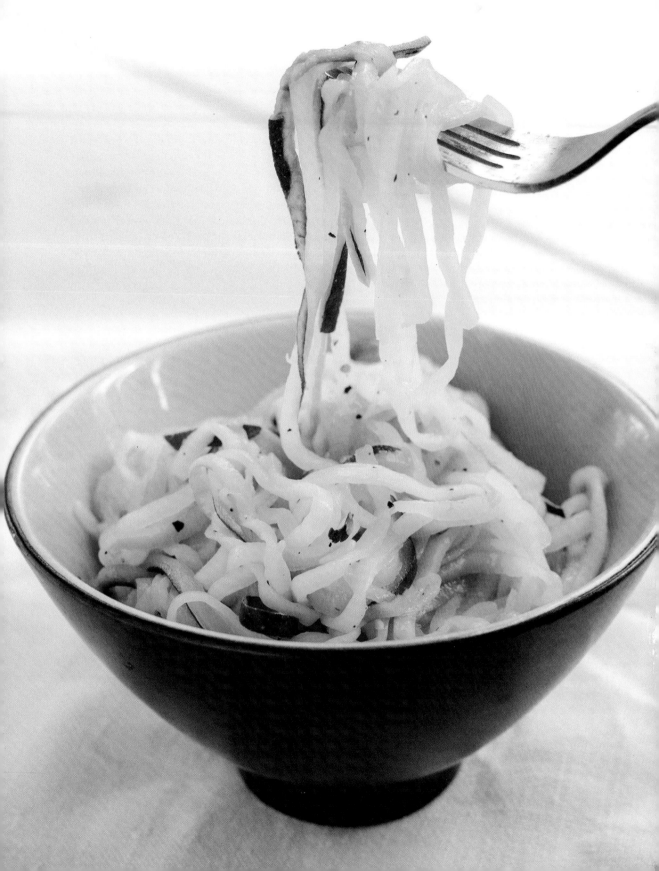

1 large spaghetti squash
1 cup water, if using pressure cooker
 or crockpot
Coconut oil cooking spray, if using
 oven

God's vegetable creations continue to amaze us. Spaghetti squash is such a wonder! Noodles inside a veggie? Incredibly . . . yes! This is another fabulous and healthy replacement for starchy noodles that when cooked you can simply toss with butter and salt and pepper as a simple side or use under any sauce or in many dish creations, such as our Loaded Spaghetti Squash Casserole (page 138). You can choose from three ways to prepare. The pressure cooker gets it done in less than 5 minutes! The crockpot method takes longer but there's less fuss because you don't have to cut the squash in half first.

FOR THE PRESSURE COOKER
This is how you get 'er done in less than five minutes! Cut the squash in half crosswise, pierce the shell in several places, and scoop out the seeds. Lay one half face down and put the other on top, face up. Add the water. Set the timer for 4 to 5 minutes. (Some older spaghetti squash can be tough to cut in half. You could also place the whole pierced squash in the cooker and cook for 10 minutes still a pretty quick option.) Scrape out the spaghetti from each half into a bowl using a fork to "rake it."

FOR THE CROCKPOT
Put the water in the bottom of the crockpot. Pierce the squash in several places, then place in the crockpot and cook on high for 4 to 5 hours or on low for 6 to 8 hours. Cut the cooked squash in half crosswise and remove the seeds. Scrape out the spaghetti into a bowl, using a fork.

FOR THE OVEN
Preheat the oven to 375°F. Cut the squash in half crosswise. Scoop out the seeds and pierce the shell in several places. Place the halves face down in a baking pan that has been lightly coated with coconut oil spray. Bake for 45 minutes or until you can easily pierce the shell with a fork. (Alternatively, you can bake the squash pierced but left whole for 1¼ to 1½ hours.) Scrape out the spaghetti into a bowl, using a fork.

NOTE: If cooking the squash whole, be careful when cutting it in half after cooking; let cool slightly so that you don't burn yourself.

NSI DF

cauli rice

FAMILY SERVE

1 large head cauliflower, trimmed,
  cored, and cut into florets; or
  2 (16-ounce) bags frozen cauliflower
  florets or 2 (16-ounce) bags fresh
  cauliflower crumbles
Coconut oil or butter (for **S**) or chicken
  broth (for **FP**)
Mineral Salt and black pepper to taste

Whenever you would serve rice with a main dish, you can serve this instead. It's perfect with so many main courses, especially those creamy or spicy chicken dishes made in the crockpot. You can keep the rice FP by using just a spritz of coconut oil or sauté it in a more generous amount of coconut oil or butter for S. This recipe makes about 6 servings, but if you are the only one eating it, make the full batch and freeze other portions in baggies.

1. If using fresh cauliflower florets, pulse them in a food processor until they are rice-size pieces. If using frozen cauliflower, lightly steam the veggie and then pulse in a food processor until you have rice-size pieces. The crumbles are already in rice-size pieces.

2. In a large skillet, using a little coconut oil or broth, sauté the riced cauliflower for a few minutes with a sprinkling of salt and pepper.

NSI DF

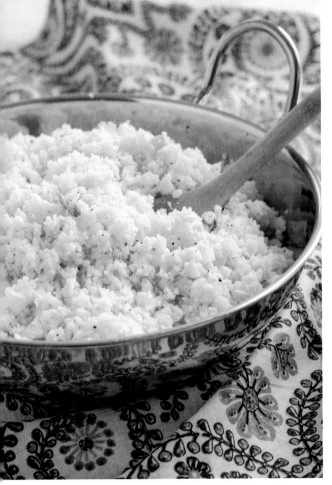

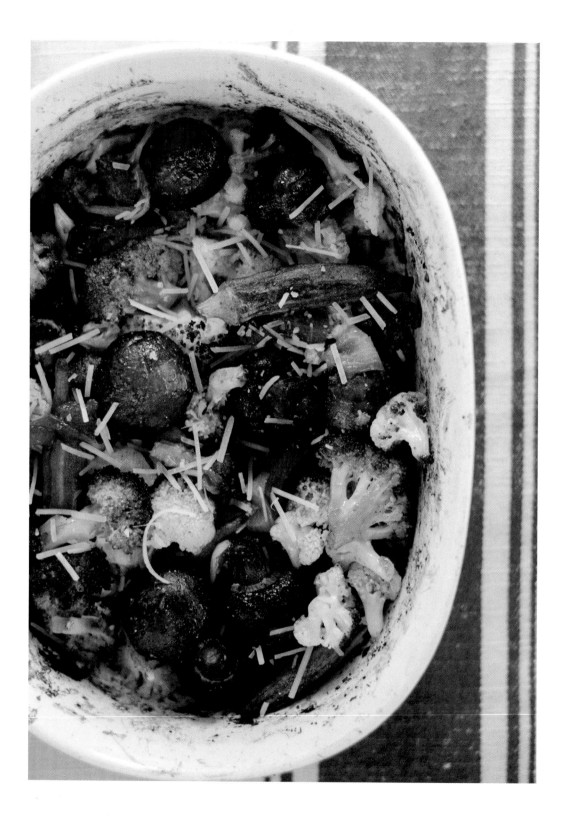

roasted nonstarchies

 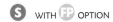

SINGLE SERVE OR FAMILY SERVE

Nonstarchy veggies of choice

Butter or coconut oil, for coating

FOR FLAVORING (OPTIONAL)

Mineral Salt

Black pepper

Nutritional yeast

Paprika

Garlic or onion powder

Ground cumin

Creole seasoning mix

Bragg or Coconut liquid aminos

Finely grated Parmesan cheese

Any nonstarchy veggie you can dream up is wonderful roasted in the oven with healthy fats and seasonings. Roast just one of your favorites or pile in several together in the same roasting tray. The amount of fat you use determines whether you keep your veggies in FP mode or slide into S territory. We like to use ample fat and seasonings on our roasted veggies for family dinners to make sure the whole family enjoys them and so that our children develop a taste for health-promoting vegetables. But sometimes we do keep it light and simply spray the veggies with coconut oil for FP, or just use a teaspoon of fat per serving to stay in FP. The method here works for so many veggies, but just to name a few, here are some tips for roasting them.

- Asparagus, broccoli, Brussels sprouts, zucchini and yellow summer squash, eggplant, fresh mushrooms, and cauliflower can simply be sliced and roasted.

- Cabbage can be cored and cut into thick wedges for "cabbage steaks."

- Radishes can be roasted whole when small; cut the bigger ones in half.

- Onions are better used in small amounts to enhance the flavor of other veggies, rather than roasting a whole onion.

- Turnips should be cut small; unlike radishes that lose their bite when cooked, turnips keep a peppery taste that some people love and others don't.

1. Preheat the oven to 375°F.
2. Place the veggies on a large baking sheet (or sheets), add the butter or coconut oil and seasonings of choice. Mix well with your hands or with a spoon so all the veggies are well seasoned. Bake for 20 to 40 minutes, depending on how small your veggies are cut. You can broil at the end for a few minutes for extra crispiness, but be careful not to burn the tops of the veggies.

NSI DF (IF USING COCONUT OIL INSTEAD OF BUTTER)

deviled eggs

S

FAMILY SERVE

6 to 12 large eggs

3 to 6 tablespoons mayonnaise

Creole seasoning, for sprinkling

Cayenne pepper or paprika, for
  sprinkling

PEARL CHATS: My boys are crazy about these eggs. We enjoy them as a side to Cabb and Saus Skillet (page 58). They also make great snacks or popular potluck contributions. The 6 eggs should be enough for 6 people to each have 2 deviled egg halves as a side item, but my boys eat way more than that so I use 12 eggs or more.

1. Half-fill a medium to large saucepan with water and bring to a boil over high heat. Put the eggs in the boiling water and boil for 10 minutes. Run under cool water to cool the eggs, then peel them when cool enough to handle.

2. Cut each egg down the center lengthwise and scoop the yolks into a bowl. Place the whites on a large plate.

3. Mix the mayo (3 tablespoons for 6 eggs and 6 tablespoons for 12 eggs) with the yolks, then sprinkle ever so lightly with the Creole seasoning (don't use too much or the eggs will taste too salty). Fill the cavities of the whites with the yolk mixture. Sprinkle lightly with cayenne pepper and/or paprika.

NSI DF

not naughty mac 'n cheese

S

FAMILY SERVE

1 family-size package Not Naughty
  Noodles, rinsed, drained, and
  snipped smaller

4 tablespoons (½ stick) butter

4 ounces cream cheese (⅓ less fat
  works well)

1 cup grated cheddar cheese, or more
  to taste

2 to 3 cups diced cooked chicken
  breast (optional; if making this a main
  dish)

Small sprinkle of Mineral Salt and
  black pepper to taste

You can either throw this together in a saucepan or combine ingredients, place in a baking dish, and bake.

1. If preparing on the stovetop, combine all the ingredients in a large skillet, stir well, and heat over medium-high heat until warmed through. If preparing in the oven, preheat the oven to 375°F. Combine all the ingredients in an 8-inch or 7 × 9-inch baking dish. Bake for 15 to 20 minutes, or until heated through.

NSI (IF USING STORE-BOUGHT KONJAC NOODLES)

let 'er rip side salad

SINGLE SERVE

1 to 2 handfuls ripped romaine lettuce leaves
Dressing of choice (see Note)

PEARL CHATS: Forgive the name, but I need to grab your attention for this one. So many of us Drive Thru Sue's don't eat enough salad because making a side salad seems like too much fuss and bother. It doesn't have to be. This is how I keep a lot of salad in my life, even though I have close to a 65 percent Drive Thru Sue nature. The most important thing about salads is the leafy greens. If you're having meat, you need the vitamin C from the greens to make your meal complete. Also, salads fill your plate, so you are not eating an entire plate full of dense, heavy foods—they are the balance to help you find and keep your trim.

So what do you do? You simply rip your lettuce, drop it onto your plate, add your dressing, and you are done, baby! Don't think that is an inadequate salad. You can have some of our fancier salads for full meals, but this is a fantastic way to get more leafy greens into your general life. Don't even want to bother with the step of ripping? Buy prewashed leafy greens, throw some on your plate, add your dressing, and pat yourself on the back. Of course, you can also use this concept for a family serve. Rip enough lettuce so everyone can have some on his or her plate.

1. No additional prep. Simply pile the ripped lettuce on your plate, add the dressing, and enjoy. The end.

NOTE: Don't always douse your salad with store-bought ranch or blue cheese. There is a place for those, but we want you also to enjoy the pure oils and vinegars for your health's sake. Keep that bottle of extra-virgin olive oil handy.

NSI DF

sweet creamy coleslaw

S

FAMILY SERVE – FEEDS BETWEEN 6 AND 8 PEOPLE

4 to 5 cups shredded cabbage (see Note)

2 medium carrots, chopped or grated (see Note)

¼ cup apple cider vinegar

2 teaspoons Super Sweet Blend

Generous ¼ teaspoon Mineral Salt

¼ teaspoon black pepper

1 teaspoon onion powder

¼ to ½ cup mayonnaise

1. Mix the cabbage with the carrots, vinegar, Super Sweet Blend, and seasonings. Stir in the mayonnaise and taste.

NOTE: The cabbage is easily shredded in a food processor. Also, as an alternative to the cabbage and carrot shredding, you can use 1 to 2 (16-ounce) bags of coleslaw mix.

NSI (IF YOU USE YOUR FAVORITE ON-PLAN SWEETENER INSTEAD) DF

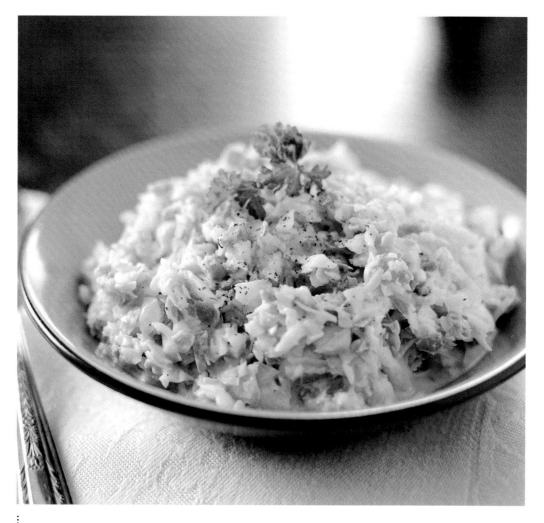

light and lovely coleslaw

4 to 5 cups shredded cabbage

2 medium carrots, chopped or grated

4 tablespoons white wine vinegar

1 tablespoon extra-virgin olive oil

1 teaspoon Super Sweet Blend

1½ teaspoons Dijon mustard

3 pinches Mineral Salt

The Trim Healthy Mama way is to juggle your fuels and calories so your body never stops guessing. For instance, don't always put mayonnaise in your coleslaw; have this lovely light coleslaw sometimes instead. The bright, clean flavors here go so well with so many dishes, from BBQ to burgers.

1. Combine all the ingredients in a medium bowl.

NSI (WITH YOUR FAVORITE ON-PLAN SWEETENER INSTEAD) DF

cauli "potato" salad

2 (16-ounce) bags frozen cauliflower florets, or 1 large head fresh cauliflower, cored, trimmed, and cut into florets

5 hard-boiled large eggs, peeled and chopped

½ medium onion, finely diced

2 celery stalks, thinly sliced

½ cup mayonnaise, or ¼ cup mayonnaise and ¼ cup Greek yogurt

Diced dill pickle (optional)

Creole seasoning to taste (optional)

Handful of turkey or real bacon bits (optional)

Don't be put off by the "cauli" here. This really is fantastic.

1. Lightly steam the cauliflower florets, or roast in the oven with salt and pepper for an even yummier version. Allow the cauliflower to cool, then chop any large florets a bit smaller. Combine with all the other ingredients in a large bowl, then chill.

NSI DF

quinoa salad

FAMILY SERVE – FEEDS BETWEEN 6 AND 8 PEOPLE

3 cups cooked quinoa, cooled
2 ripe tomatoes, diced small
1 medium cucumber, diced
⅓ cup chopped fresh parsley
2 garlic cloves, minced
Juice of 1 large lemon, or more to taste
1 tablespoon extra-virgin olive oil
¾ teaspoon Mineral Salt, or to taste
Sprinkle of black pepper

This salad is fantastic as an E side to grilled chicken or fish. To make this a full meal, all you need do is add diced chicken breast or salmon from a foil pouch. It's also perfect to take on picnics and to parties. You'll have an option to stay on plan, but everyone else will love it, too. The quinoa cooks up quickly—12 to 15 minutes—and 1 cup uncooked yields about 3 cups cooked. To cook quinoa, combine 1 cup dry grain with 2 cups water or broth, bring to a boil, then turn the heat to low, cover tightly, and simmer for 12 to 15 minutes. Fluff with a fork. It's a good idea to make up large batches of quinoa; whatever you don't use for a meal can be stored in the freezer in zippies, in ¾ cup servings for meeting E needs.

1. Mix all the ingredients in a large bowl and chill for 1 hour so that flavors meld.

NOTE: Fresh herbs taste fantastic in this salad. If you have some growing in your garden, try adding some rosemary, basil, oregano—really, whatever you like is going to be delicious and fresh tasting in this salad.

NSI DF

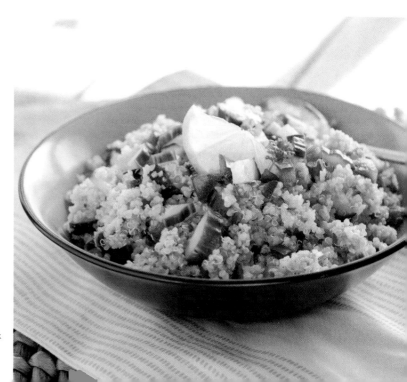

magenta salad

SINGLE SERVES 1 TO 2

(we want you to try this out first but then feel free to quadruple for a side to feed the whole family or to take to luncheons)

1 small to medium beet, peeled
  and grated
⅛ to ¼ cup chopped walnuts
1 teaspoon MCT oil
1 teaspoon tahini (sesame paste)
3 teaspoons rice vinegar, or
  2 teaspoons apple cider vinegar
⅛ teaspoon garlic powder
¼ teaspoon onion powder
⅛ teaspoon Mineral Salt
1 teaspoon dried parsley (optional)

We grew up with this salad. Both our nana and mom loved grated beet salads, and served them often. This bright pink tasty side dish always seemed like a special treat. It was just so pretty that even as children we couldn't resist second helpings.

Those of you familiar with the "Foxy Mama" chapter in the original, self-published *Trim Healthy Mama* book might want to get excited about beets. This veggie is rich in boron, which is super important in the production of sex hormones. High in B vitamins and iron, beets are a wonder food for expecting mamas as they support new cell growth during pregnancy and help replenish iron stores. Beets are also beneficial for those without a bun in the oven, being a powerful liver tonic, a blood purifier, a cancer preventive, and a natural diuretic—they even aid in lowering blood pressure. Beets are a happy veggie, known as a natural relief for depression because they are abundant in betaine. They also contain tryptophan, which is a mood enhancer.

1. Place the grated beet in a medium bowl and add all the other ingredients except the parsley. Toss well, making sure the tahini is blended with the other ingredients. Garnish with the parsley (if using), and dig in.

NSI DF

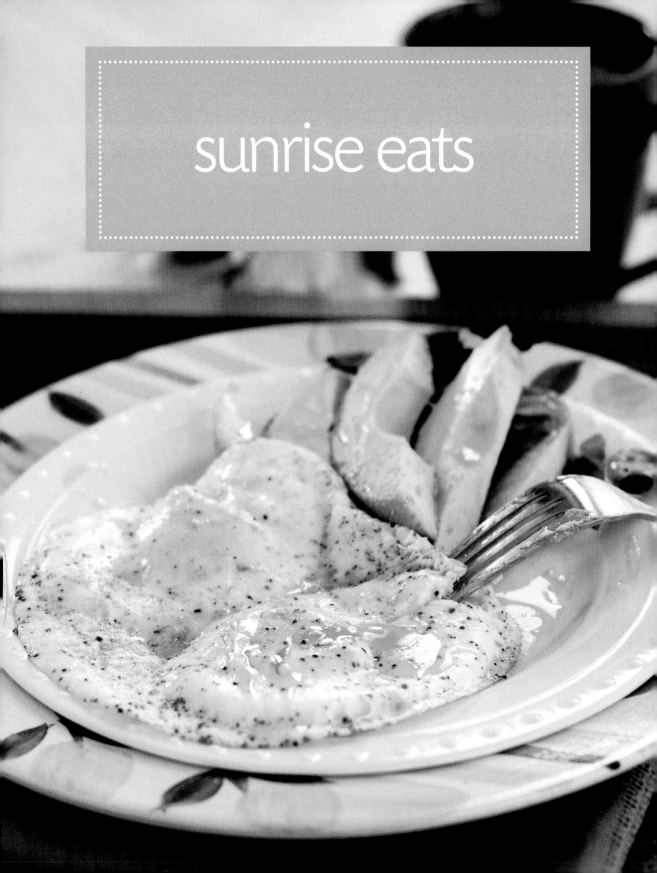

sunrise eats

● = S ● = E ● = FP MORE THAN ONE DOT INDICATES OPTIONS

GOOD MORNING EGGS

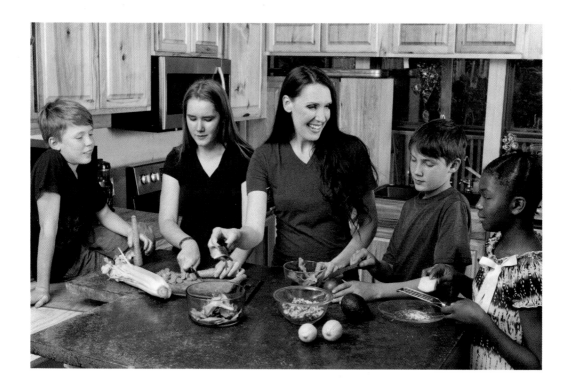

mufflets

FAMILY SERVE (MAKES 16 MUFFLETS)

8 large eggs

1 cup egg whites (from carton or fresh)

¾ cup Seasoning Blend (frozen diced onion, celery, and pepper; see Note)

⅓ cup chopped green onions (white and green parts)

1½ cups grated cheddar cheese

6 to 8 ounces sliced deli turkey meat or ham (such as Hormel Natural)

Generous ¼ teaspoon Mineral Salt

Generous ⅛ teaspoon black pepper

Coconut oil cooking spray

PEARL CHATS: These have all the goodness of an omelet baked in a muffin tin! If you're like me and don't see the point in fussing with extra steps—well, goodie, because there is very little chopping or fussy prep involved here. You can make these ahead of time and freeze in individual portions. Pull a couple out for breakfast (or perhaps three for your husband or you, if you like to eat a larger breakfast), warm them in the microwave for a few seconds (don't look, Serene), and you've got a fast, tasty, protein-rich **S** breakfast. Mufflets are also a great way to feed the whole family for breakfast. Prepare the mix on a Saturday night and put it in the fridge. Sunday morning before church, bake these and you'll have a far less chaotic time getting everybody fed and out the door.

1. Preheat the oven to 350°F.

2. Whisk the whole eggs and egg whites together in a mixing bowl. Add all the other food ingredients and combine well.

3. Coat a 16-cup muffin tin with the coconut oil spray. Use a ¼ cup measuring cup to put ¼ cup of batter into each hole. Bake for 25 to 30 minutes.

NOTE: If you prefer to not use Seasoning Blend, substitute ½ cup chopped green or red pepper and ¼ cup finely diced onion.

NSI

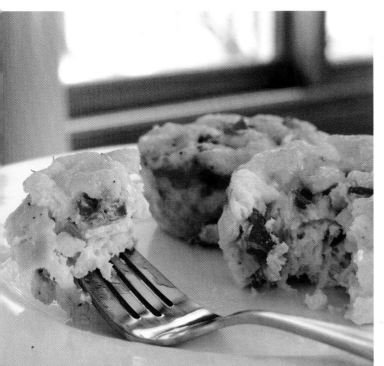

breakfast casserole

FAMILY SERVE – FEEDS 6 TO 8 PEOPLE

1 (8-ounce) package cooked turkey or other breakfast sausage links, chopped

4 slices turkey or other bacon, cooked until crisp and crumbled

8 large eggs, whisked

1 bell pepper, cored, seeded, and diced

2 cups grated Monterey Jack cheese (or other cheese)

2 tablespoons butter

¼ cup finely diced onion

½ cup chicken broth

½ teaspoon Gluccie

¼ cup heavy cream

¼ cup water

Mineral Salt and black pepper to taste

Coconut oil cooking spray

This is a very creamy, know you're eating a doozy of an S type of breakfast. Thanks go to our friend Jennifer Morris for sharing this with us.

1. Preheat the oven to 350°F.
2. Combine the sausage, bacon, eggs, pepper, and 1 cup of the cheese in a large bowl.
3. Melt the butter in a small saucepan. Add the onion, cook until soft, about 2 minutes, then add the broth. Slowly whisk in the Gluccie, stirring until thickened. Add the cream and water, and keep whisking. Add salt and pepper to taste.
4. Stir the sauce into the egg mixture. Lightly coat a 9 × 13-inch baking pan with coconut oil spray and pour the egg mixture into the pan. Top with the remaining cheese. Bake for 35 minutes, or until golden brown on top.

NOTE: The creamy sauce here can be used in any recipe that calls for a "cream of" soup—awesome, huh?

NSI (IF USING XANTHAN TO THICKEN INSTEAD OF GLUCCIE)

nana's fluffy omelet

SINGLE SERVE

2 or 3 large eggs

1½ tablespoons water

1½ tablespoons heavy cream

Mineral Salt and black pepper to taste

Sprinkle of cayenne pepper (optional)

2 to 3 teaspoons butter, coconut oil, or red palm oil (Nana uses red palm oil, which makes her omelets a beautiful golden color)

1 tablespoon finely diced green onion (white and green parts) (optional)

Fillings of choice (such as cheese, veggies, or bacon pieces)

This is our Mother's specialty breakfast. She goes by the name of Nana far more often than Mom these days, as she now has 38 grandchildren. We are all neighbors out here in the Tennessee woods, and we love to walk over to her house on a Saturday morning, knowing this is what she'll be serving. If we turn up in time, we're in for this treat. This omelet is so lovely and fluffy it doesn't need a filling, but you are welcome to put in some cheese or anything else you would like—perhaps spinach or mushrooms.

1. In a medium bowl, whisk the eggs with the water and cream and add the seasonings. Whisk well, until the eggs are light and frothy.

2. Heat the butter or oil with the green onion in a medium skillet over medium heat for 30 seconds or so, until the fat is glistening. Pour in the beaten eggs and add any fillings to the top of the omelet as it forms. When the eggs begin to set, slide your spatula underneath and fold the omelet in half, then cook a bit longer, about 2 minutes. The eggs will firm up in the center but still retain their moisture.

NSI DF (WITHOUT THE CHEESE AND USING ALL WATER IN PLACE OF THE CREAM)

fields of green omcake

S

2 large eggs

⅓ cup egg whites (from carton or fresh)

1 generous teaspoon dried parsley, or ¼ cup chopped fresh parsley

Mineral Salt, black pepper, and cayenne pepper to taste

1 cup finely chopped fresh spinach

1 teaspoon butter or coconut oil spray

1 tablespoon extra-virgin coconut oil or red palm oil

1 to 2 teaspoons nutritional yeast

In the "Higher Learning" chapter of *Trim Healthy Mama Plan,* you can learn about the ultra-slimming benefits of Deep S meals. These satisfying meals use only the purest S fats, like oils and those naturally occurring in meats and eggs, rather than those in dairy or nut fats. Deep S meals also include lots of greens. This Omcake (a cross between an omelet and a pancake) is a beautiful Deep S breakfast full of the detoxifying powers of greens. You won't come away hungry, and it can help your body release stubborn pounds or push you through annoying weight-loss stalls.

1. Whisk the eggs, egg whites, parsley, and seasonings in a medium bowl. Add the spinach and combine well.

2. Set a large skillet over medium heat and lightly coat with coconut oil spray or smear with the butter or oil. Pour the egg mixture into the skillet and cook until the bottom is firm and slightly golden, about 3 minutes. Flip the omcake over and brown on the other side until done, about another 2 minutes.

3. Slide the omcake onto a large dinner plate, then drizzle with the coconut oil or red palm oil and sprinkle on the nutritional yeast.

NSI (WITHOUT THE NUTRITIONAL YEAST) DF (IF NOT USING THE BUTTER)

waffleized breakky sandwich

SINGLE SERVE

1 large egg

1 teaspoon butter

Mineral Salt and black pepper to taste

1 slice cheese of any kind (cheddar works well)

Butter for smearing on waffles (optional)

2 slices turkey or other bacon, or 1 breakfast sausage patty

2 Welcome Back Waffles (page 263), made with egg whites and no sweetener

Down Under (where we grew up), breakfast is shortened to "breakky." So listen up, hearty breakky eaters, this one's for you! Do you like to feel full after eating in the mornings? This breakfast can help you get there, in a big way. Men enjoy this sandwich, too, so try it out on your guy if he's a THM skeptic.

1. Fry the egg in the butter in a large skillet over medium-high heat; season with the salt and pepper. Drop the cheese slice onto the egg and let it melt. Add the bacon or sausage and cook until crisp in the same skillet.

2. Smear the waffles with some butter if desired, then layer them with the cheese-fried egg, and top with the breakfast meat.

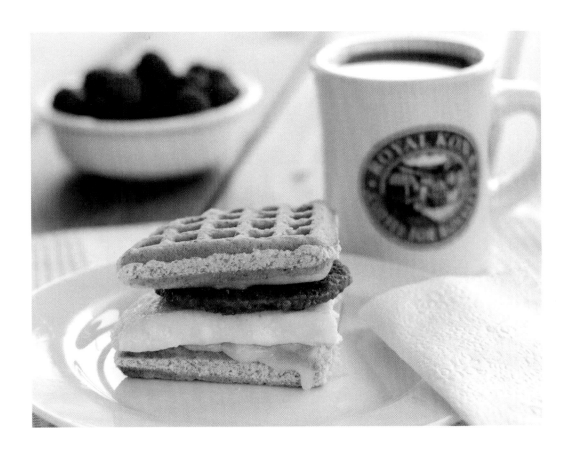

succulent egg sammie

SINGLE SERVE

½ cup egg whites (carton or fresh)

1 tablespoon nutritional yeast

1 tablespoon finely grated Parmesan
cheese (green can kind is fine)

2 teaspoons hot sauce of choice

Mineral Salt and black pepper to taste

Coconut oil cooking spray

2 slices sprouted or traditional
sourdough toast, or 1 split sprouted
muffin (for **E** version); or single
serving of Swiss Bread (page 196)
made into square bread shape (for
FP version)

1 (.75-ounce) light Laughing Cow
cheese wedge, or 1 tablespoon
Laughin' Mama Cheese (page 484)

1 ripe tomato, sliced

Keep changing up your fuels, Mamas! Are you in an S mode
rut? Snap out of it! You will barely believe this is an E or a
FP sandwich, 'cause the moist tomato and the crisp protein
source make this a hearty morning meal.

1. In a small bowl, whisk the egg whites with the nutritional
   yeast, cheese, hot sauce, and seasonings.

2. Lightly coat a medium skillet with coconut oil spray and set
   it over medium-high heat. Pour the eggs into the skillet and
   cook until the underside is golden brown, about 3 minutes.
   Flip, then cook until perfectly firm and slightly crisp.

3. Smear the bread or muffin with the cheese, then make layers
   with the tomato slices and fried egg whites.

NSI (IF LEAVING OUT NUTRITIONAL YEAST) DF (IF USING HELLO
CHEESE, PAGE 484)

eggatable scramble

ⒻⓅ

SINGLE SERVE

½ cup egg whites (carton or fresh)

1 tablespoon finely grated Parmesan
cheese (green can kind is fine)

Mineral Salt and black pepper to taste

¼ to ½ teaspoon onion powder

2 teaspoons nutritional yeast

Coconut oil cooking spray

½ large tomato, diced

½ green, yellow, or red bell pepper,
cored, seeded, and diced

½ cup sliced button mushrooms

We know we have gone beyond what is funny about putting
two words together to make a recipe title, nevertheless it
still pleases us. Eggatable Scramble is so much more fun to
say than simply "Vegetable and Egg Scramble." Since this is
not a boring recipe, it should not have a boring name.

1. Whisk the egg whites with the Parmesan, salt and pepper,
   onion powder, and nutritional yeast in a small bowl until
   light and fluffy.

2. Coat a small skillet with coconut oil cooking spray and set it
   over medium-high heat. Put the tomato, pepper, and mushrooms in the skillet and toss for a couple of minutes. Add the
   egg mixture and toss together with the vegetables until the
   whites firm up, 3 to 5 minutes.

NSI (IF LEAVING OUT NUTRITIONAL YEAST)

big fried-egg trick

SINGLE SERVE

2 teaspoons coconut oil, butter, or red palm oil

2 large eggs

½ cup egg whites (carton or fresh)

Italian seasoning and onion powder to taste

Sprinkle of nutritional yeast or a pinch of Mineral Salt

Hot sauce of choice

Grated Parmesan cheese to taste

Here's how to get full on a fried-egg breakfast without needing any sides. It's true that you can sometimes have three full eggs for breakfast if you want (we've even been known to eat four on occasion), but once you've got two eggs on your plate, you've got all the nutrition from the yolks that you need. This is a way to celebrate the slimming and succulent simplicity of eggs without overdoing a good thing and heading into calorie abuse.

1. Melt the coconut oil in a small skillet over medium-high heat. Crack the whole eggs into the hot skillet and pour the egg whites around the eggs. Sprinkle on the seasonings, hot sauce, and cheese. Cook until the whites have set and the underside is crispy. Flip to seal in a soft yolk or cook all the way through, if you prefer solid yolks.

2. Slide the eggs out onto a large dinner plate. (If you're not successful at getting it all out without breaking, know that it still tastes the same—no worries.)

NSI (IF LEAVING OUT NUTRITIONAL YEAST) DF (IF LEAVING OUT PARMESAN)

breaggy fry up

SINGLE SERVE

1 tablespoon butter or coconut oil

2 or 3 large eggs, or 2 eggs and
  1 cooked sausage link, sliced

Single-serve batch Swiss Bread
  (page 196), cubed or crumbled (you'll
  probably only need to use one of the
  Swiss Bread rolls and save one for a
  later snack)

Sprinkle of nutritional yeast

Grated Parmesan cheese (optional;
  green can kind is fine)

Hot sauce of choice

Mineral Salt and black pepper to taste

Nothin' better than crispy bread morsels, eggs, and buttah— all fried up together in one big group hug. We personally think Breaggy Fry Up is an absolutely stellar name for this recipe, but we're not sure we would think the same if we had begun the book with this chapter. Perhaps upon perusing the recipe names in this particular chapter, it's possible to detect a hint of insanity from the authors. We're not pleading inno- cent. We saved the writing of the "Good Morning Eggs" sec- tion for last because we thought it would be the easiest. The writing process took months and months for us (in fact, at this point, during our last week of writing, Serene has only five weeks to go before she has her baby!). We have been in uncontrollable fits of laughter, imagining possible reviews of this book, such as: "The recipe titles look like they have been written by kindergarteners high on Kool-Aid." Or, "Sadly, the entirety of the book is based around collagen—a product they sell! Shameless." Or more likely this one, "Every recipe uses okra!"

Our imagined response is that okra is "stellar," too, and so is this recipe—so enough of our nonsense . . . go make it!

1. Heat the butter in a small skillet over medium-high heat, add eggs, and scatter the bread cubes and sausage (if using) around and on the eggs. Sprinkle with the nutritional yeast, Parmesan (if using), hot sauce, and seasonings. Cook until set and crispy on the underside, 3 to 4 minutes. Flip in one piece (hopefully) and cook for 1 to 2 minutes to seal in the soft yolks or cook them until they are firm, if preferred, an additional couple of minutes.

2. Slide the eggs onto a plate in one large group hug (but if that does not work, imagine these directions as telling you that a broken Breaggie Fry Up is preferable). You're good to go.

NOTE: In place of Swiss Bread you can use 1 piece sprouted or sourdough bread for an **S** Helper or 2 pieces for a Crossover—yum!

DF (IF USING COCONUT OIL INSTEAD OF BUTTER AND OMITTING THE CHEESE)

eggs and avs

SINGLE SERVE

Coconut oil cooking spray

2 or 3 large eggs

Mineral Salt and black pepper to taste

½ avocado, cut into chunks

1 tablespoon extra-virgin olive oil

Grated light cheese, like pecorino romano or Parmesan (avoid a heavy cheese like cheddar)

2 teaspoons nutritional yeast

Boost your health with the raw fats of avocado and extra-virgin olive oil in this breakfast. It's a fantastic start to a pregnant or nursing woman's day (or anyone's day, for that matter), crowned with Chocolate Beauty Milk (page 440) on the side. Since this is a pure S meal, preggies and nursers might want a Crossover later in the day.

1. Lightly coat a small skillet with coconut oil cooking spray. Place the skillet over medium-high heat and crack the eggs into the skillet. Sprinkle the eggs with the salt and pepper and cook to your preference.

2. Put the avocado chunks on one side of a dinner plate and your cooked eggs alongside them. Drizzle both the avocado and eggs with the olive oil and then sprinkle with the cheese and nutrional yeast. Enjoy all the drippy goodness!

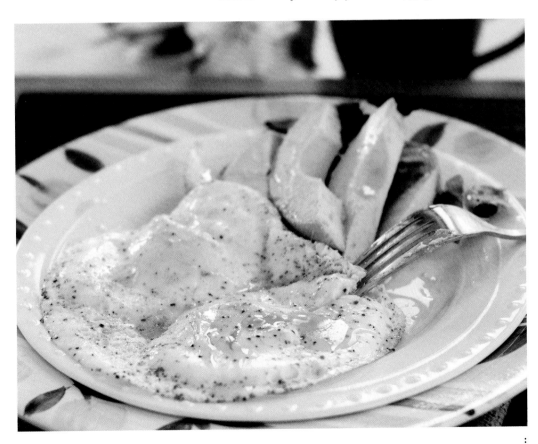

GOOD MORNING GRAINS

Get your healthy, energizing grains in! Breakfast is an ideal time to do that. We enjoy just a teaspoon or so of Super Sweet Blend or a doonk or two of stevia in our bowl of morning grains (like oatmeal), as we prefer them only mildly sweet. This is our own budget-friendly approach; you might prefer to use Gentle Sweet if you like a more sugary taste in your breakfast grain dishes. If so, simply use Gentle Sweet in double the amounts called for, then add more if needed.

sweet dreams oatmeal bowls

The following oatmeal recipes take the madness out of your morning by allowing you to do the prep the night before. Simply heat up your delicious bowl of goodness the next morning, and then on with your day you go!

SWEET DREAMS PEACHY CREAM OATMEAL

SINGLE SERVE – MAKES 1 BOWLFUL

½ cup old-fashioned rolled oats
½ cup unsweetened almond or
   cashew milk
½ cup water
½ cup diced fresh or frozen peaches
1 to 1½ teaspoons Super Sweet Blend
Pinch of Mineral Salt
½ scoop Pristine Whey Protein, or
   1 scoop Integral Collagen
A dollop of 1% cottage cheese or
   0% plain Greek yogurt (optional)

Mix all the ingredients (except for the cottage cheese or Greek yogurt) in a small saucepan or a microwave-safe bowl. Store overnight in the fridge. In the morning, simmer on low heat for 3 to 4 minutes, until creamy, or heat in a microwave, then add optional cottage cheese or Greek yogurt.

NSI (IF YOU HAVE YOUR FAVORITE ON-PLAN SWEETENER, OMIT THE WHEY PROTEIN AND PAIR WITH 1% COTTAGE CHEESE OR 0% GREEK YOGURT FOR PROTEIN) DF (IF USING COLLAGEN INSTEAD OF WHEY PROTEIN)

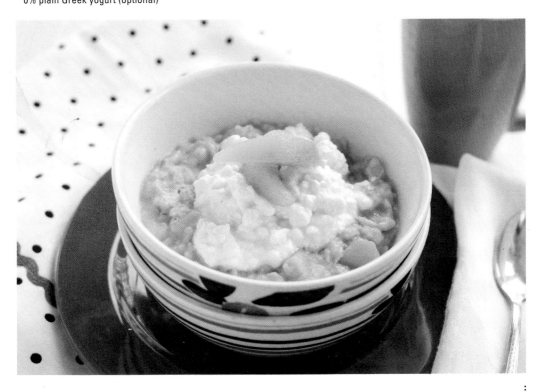

SWEET DREAMS APPLE CINNAMON OATMEAL

SINGLE SERVE – MAKES 1 BOWLFUL

Use the same ingredients as in the master recipe, except substitute ½ cup diced or grated apple for the peaches, and include ½ teaspoon ground cinnamon.

SWEET DREAMS PB AND J OATMEAL

SINGLE SERVE – MAKES 1 BOWLFUL

Use all the same ingredients as in the master recipe, except leave out the fruit, add 2 tablespoons Pressed Peanut Flour or 1 teaspoon natural-style peanut butter, and 1 tablespoon all-fruit jelly. Also, add 2 extra pinches of salt.

very good !

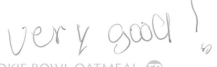

SWEET DREAMS COOKIE BOWL OATMEAL FP
....

SINGLE SERVE – MAKES 1 BIG BOWLFUL

¼ cup old-fashioned rolled oats

¾ cup water

2 generous pinches Mineral Salt

¼ cup unsweetened almond or
cashew milk

½ teaspoon Gluccie, or 2 teaspoons
Just Gelatin

1 heaping tablespoon unsweetened
cocoa powder

4 to 5 teaspoons Gentle Sweet

1 tablespoon Pressed Peanut Flour, or
1 teaspoon natural-style, sugar-free
peanut butter

½ tablespoon chia seeds

PEARL CHATS: My husband is not an oatmeal fan, but he is a No-Bake Cookies (page 316) lover. I figured if I could imitate the flavors of that cookie in a bowl of oatmeal, I could get him to eat some. It worked! He actually smiles when I serve this to him. He much prefers Gentle Sweet in this breakfast. You have the choice to either use Gluccie or gelatin here as a thickener.

1. Put the oats, ½ cup of the water, and the salt in a small saucepan and bring to a swift boil over medium-high heat. Reduce the heat, cover, and simmer for about 2 minutes.

2. While the oats are simmering, combine the almond milk, Gluccie, cocoa, Gentle Sweet, remaining ¼ cup water, and the peanut flour in a blender and blend well for at least 1 minute. (If using the gelatin instead, just combine in a bowl and whisk well.)

3. Stir the puree into the oats off the heat and mix well.

4. Pour into a large cereal bowl or a 2-pint jar. Add the chia seeds and stir well. Cover and store overnight in the fridge.

5. The next morning, stir well, then eat the oatmeal cold (it's actually better that way) or warm up for a minute or two in the microwave or a saucepan.

DF

E

8 cups grain of choice (steel-cut oats, old-fashioned rolled oats, hulled barley, brown rice, or farro)

½ cup rye sourdough starter (see page 207), or ½ cup whole rye flour

1 tablespoon Mineral Salt

SERENE CHATS: *I love to soak my grains for the extra creamy texture it brings, the characteristic tang, the release of extra nutrition, and because it makes them easier to digest this way. With nine children still living at home and one more on the way, I soak bulk amounts over the weekend so that I can cook them all up on Monday morning and have a giant pot of deliciously fermented, chewy grains to serve for breakfast the whole week. We go into fine detail on whether or not soaking is a must for grains in* Trim Healthy Mama Plan. *Our official stance is—drum roll—you sure don't have to do it, but you might just wanna!*

I store the leftover cooked grains after Monday morning's breakfast in gallon-size zippies in the fridge, and then each morning (bar weekends, when my children fry up eggs on toast), the one child assigned as my breakfast helper puts enough soaked grains for all the children in a pot, pours boiling water over, and reheats them in a snap. Into their own bowls of oatmeal my children stir in butter, pour in some raw milk, and add a little honey and a doonk of stevia, cinnamon, and vanilla, then they chow down. If my husband and I are choosing to eat grain that morning, I take our portion and make one of the creamy grains with it (see pages 252–253).

*Fermented or soured foods are naturally preserved by the flourishing of good bacteria and the killing off of bad microbes. These soaked grains are always just as fresh a full week later as when I first prepared them. I think if there were any left over, they would last another week, but I haven't been able to test this, with all the hungry mouths in my home. This recipe has been halved from what I make, but it still yields a lot. At the end of the week, if you still have leftovers you can freeze them in little single-serve portions to quickly thaw for creamy grains later on. Feel free to halve this recipe if you have a smaller household or are living alone, but I still recommend making enough so that you have this yummy **E** option available all week and also have plenty to freeze.*

1. Place the grain, starter (or rye flour), and enough warm water to cover in a large pot. Cover with a loose-fitting lid or tea towel, and place in a warm environment. (Don't stress about this. I usually just place it on the warming center on my stove for a few hours and then remove it to sit on my counter next to my stove, where it will collect some warmth from the cooking environment at meal times.)

2. After 24 hours, drain the grain through a colander and add fresh warm water and fresh starter or flour. Cover loosely and leave for an additional 24 hours (see Note), then drain again.

3. Put the soaked grain and the salt in a large pot and add enough water to cover to the first knuckle of your middle finger, when your finger touches the top of the grains. Bring to a boil over high heat. As soon as it boils, cover with a fitted lid. Turn the heat all the way down to low, and simmer, stirring occasionally, until the grain is deliciously tender and chewy (approximately 30 minutes, depending on type of grain used).

NOTE: It is not absolutely necessary to soak all grains for 48 hours. It does make them more tangy and digestible, but 24 hours is sufficient for many grains. Steel-cut oats need the full time for healthy culturing. Rolled oats will not stand up to 48 hours of soaking; their outer shells are no longer intact, so a 24-hour soak is sufficient.

NSI DF

creamy grains

BERRY CREAMY GRAINS

SINGLE SERVE

¾ cup any cooked plan-friendly grain (brown rice, quinoa, whole barley, farro, or old-fashioned or steel-cut oats), or purist soaked and cooked versions of any plan-approved grain (see page 250)

½ scoop Pristine Whey Protein (optional; see Note)

1 cup hot (not quite boiling) water

1 teaspoon extra-virgin coconut oil, butter, or ghee (clarified butter)

¼ to ½ teaspoon ground cinnamon

3 pinches Mineral Salt

½ teaspoon vanilla extract

1 scoop Integral Collagen

1 teaspoon Just Gelatin

1½ teaspoons Super Sweet Blend, or 2 to 3 doonks Pure Stevia Extract

½ teaspoon Sunflower Lecithin (optional)

¼ to ½ cup frozen or fresh blueberries or a berry mix

1. Place the grain in a small saucepan. Add the whey (if using), but do not turn the heat on yet.

2. Blend the water, coconut oil, cinnamon, salt, vanilla, collagen, gelatin, Super Sweet Blend, and lecithin (if using) until smooth. Pour over the grain and stir well, breaking up any grain clumps and dissolving the whey. Add the berries and turn on the heat to medium-low. Bring to a perfect soothing hotness to eat; don't boil hard and destroy the fragile whey micro-fractions. Pour into a large cereal bowl and enjoy.

NOTE: Adding the half scoop of whey will give roughly 25 grams of protein together with the collagen and gelatin.

DF (IF NOT USING THE WHEY PROTEIN)

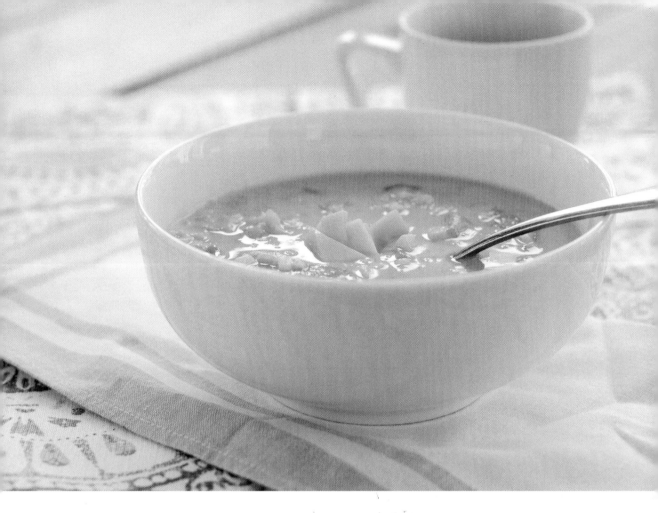

BANANA CREAMY GRAINS Ⓔ

SINGLE SERVE

Use all the same ingredients as in the master recipe except substitute ground cinnamon with a little nutmeg. Stir in ¼ teaspoon pure banana extract and top with ½ a sliced banana. Delish!!

MANGO CREAMY GRAINS Ⓔ

SINGLE SERVE

Use all the same ingredients as in the master recipe, except omit the cinnamon. Add ¼ to ½ cup frozen or fresh mango cubes (can be pulsed in a food processor to thaw more quickly in the hot water).

stovetop crunch granolas

Miss a nice bowl of crunchy cereal with milk? These quickie recipes offer all that satisfaction. Katie is a Trim Healthy Mama who came up with this idea and shared it in the community. We ran with it and created some of our favorite flavors. Once it cools, you pour this into a cereal bowl and douse it with unsweetened almond or cashew milk (or Foundation Milk, page 439), then stir in a couple tablespoons of Pristine Whey Protein or Integral Collagen for extra protein. Or, you can enjoy it with a Trimmy Light (page 430) or a Collagen Tea (page 436) for added protein.

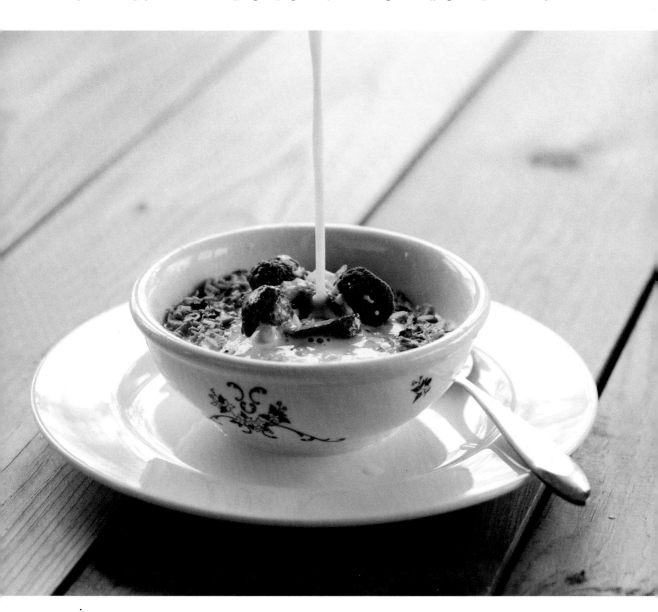

CHOCOLATE NUT CRUNCH GRANOLA

SINGLE SERVE

½ cup old-fashioned rolled oats (plus 1 to 2 tablespoons more, if desired)

1½ teaspoons Super Sweet Blend, or 3 to 4 teaspoons Gentle Sweet

Pinch of Mineral Salt

1 teaspoon unsweetened cocoa powder

1 to 2 teaspoons Pressed Peanut Flour (see Note)

Dash of vanilla extract

Coconut oil cooking spray

Unsweetened almond, cashew, or flax milk for pouring over granola

1. Mix all the food ingredients well in a medium bowl.

2. Coat a medium skillet with coconut oil spray, and place over medium heat. Add the oat mixture and cook until oats are lightly browned, stirring frequently, for 5 to 7 minutes. The cocoa does get a bit black while cooking and looks a little burned, but it still tastes great so just keep stirring and don't worry too much about that.

3. Transfer to a bowl and let cool (the longer it cools the crunchier it gets). Add unsweetened milk with optional protein powder and enjoy.

NOTE: Alternatively, you could increase the cocoa to 1½ teaspoons and omit the peanut flour, and have chocolate granola. The recipe can be doubled or even quadrupled, if desired.

NSI (IF YOU USE YOUR FAVORITE ON-PLAN SWEETENER INSTEAD) DF

PUMPKIN CRUNCH GRANOLA

SINGLE SERVE

Use all the same ingredients as in the master recipe, but omit the cocoa and peanut flour, and add ¾ teaspoon pumpkin pie seasoning.

APPLE PIE CRUNCH GRANOLA

SINGLE SERVE

Use all the same ingredients as in the master recipe, but omit the cocoa and peanut flour, and add ¾ teaspoon apple pie seasoning. Add half a peeled, diced fresh apple, if desired.

crockpot oatmeals

Wake up to a hearty hot breakfast all ready and waiting. Feed the whole family or just yourself, and refrigerate or freeze any leftovers. Sometimes people shy away from cooking oatmeal in their crockpot because it can get either too mushy or too dried out. This is especially true when cooking old-fashioned rolled oats. There is a remedy for this, however. Put your oats and other ingredients in a heat-safe ceramic or glass bowl in the crockpot and surround it with water. This water bath allows the oats to cook more slowly.

Steel-cut oats hold up much better in the crockpot and are the usual favorite for cooking this way. It requires using almost double the liquid than what old-fashioned oats need, so less grain is required. It is less important to use a water bath when cooking steel-cut oats, but you can still do it and see if you like the results better. Don't rule old-fashioned oats out—they can turn out super yummy, too; it's all about your personal preference. The following recipes include some unsweetened almond or cashew milk, but if your budget is tight, using all water to cook the oats won't be a problem at all.

APPLE CINNAMON CROCKPOT OATMEAL

FAMILY SERVE – SERVES 6 (HALVE INGREDIENTS IF YOUR FAMILY IS SMALLER)

3 cups old-fashioned rolled oats, or 1½ cups steel-cut oats

3½ cups water

3 cups unsweetened almond or cashew milk

3 large apples, peeled, cored, and diced

2½ tablespoons Super Sweet Blend

1½ teaspoons vanilla extract

2 teaspoons ground cinnamon

1 teaspoon grated nutmeg (optional)

⅓ teaspoon Mineral Salt

3 scoops Pristine Whey Protein (optional)

1. Put all the ingredients in a heat-safe bowl that can fit into your crockpot. Stir well and place the bowl in the cooker. Add enough water to come halfway up around the bowl.

2. Turn on to low heat right before hitting the sack. Cook all night. In the morning, stir well before serving.

NSI (IF YOU SUBSTITUTE YOUR FAVORITE ON-PLAN SWEETENER AND LEAVE OUT THE WHEY PROTEIN) DF (IF YOU LEAVE OUT THE WHEY PROTEIN)

CHOCY NUT CROCKPOT OATMEAL

FAMILY SERVE – SERVES 6 (HALVE INGREDIENTS IF YOUR FAMILY IS SMALLER)

Use the same ingredients as in the master recipe, except omit the apples and cinnamon, increase the Super Sweet Blend to ¼ cup (however, you may prefer the taste of Gentle Sweet in double amounts in this version), and add ⅓ cup Pressed Peanut Flour and ⅓ cup unsweetened cocoa. Use ½ teaspoon salt.

BANANA BREAD CROCKPOT OATMEAL

FAMILY SERVE – SERVES 6 (HALVE INGREDIENTS IF YOUR FAMILY IS SMALLER)

Use the same ingredients as in the master recipe, but omit the apple and cinnamon and include 2 to 3 large sliced bananas. Include 1½ teaspoons pure banana extract and 1½ teaspoons grated nutmeg.

CHERRY ALMOND CROCKPOT OATMEAL

FAMILY SERVE – SERVES 6 (HALVE INGREDIENTS IF YOUR FAMILY IS SMALLER)

Use the same ingredients as in the master recipe, but omit the apples and cinnamon and add 2 to 3 cups frozen cherries and 2 teaspoons almond extract.

PANCAKES, WAFFLES, CREPES, AND DONUTS

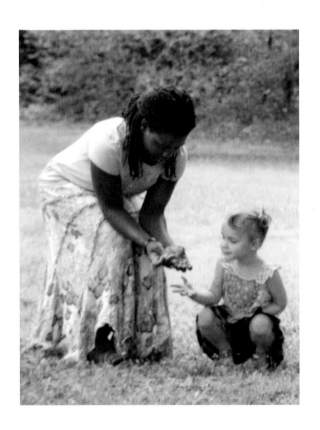

trim healthy pancakes or waffles

SINGLE SERVE — MAKES 3 PANCAKES

double

⅓ cup old-fashioned rolled oats

⅓ cup low-fat cottage cheese

⅓ cup egg whites (carton or fresh)

1 teaspoon Super Sweet Blend

⅓ teaspoon vanilla extract

Generous ½ teaspoon aluminum-free
baking powder

Coconut oil cooking spray

**FAMILY SERVE— MAKES 18
PANCAKES (SEE NOTE)**

2 cups old-fashioned rolled oats

2 cups low-fat cottage cheese

2 cups egg whites (carton is easier,
but can use fresh)

6 teaspoons Super Sweet Blend

2 teaspoons vanilla extract

4 teaspoons aluminum-free baking
powder

Coconut oil cooking spray

These make for a great energizing breakfast topped with your choice of berries, fruit, all-fruit jelly, Greek yogurt, or Slim Belly Jelly (page 478) or Pancake Syrup (page 480). Trim Healthy Pancakes use everyday, inexpensive ingredients, so it's easy to make up a quick batch for yourself or feed the whole family. Our children are big fans of these pancakes. But even if it is only you eating them, it's a good idea to try your hand at making a family batch, especially if you work outside the home. You can put some of the pancakes in the fridge for a quick grab-and-go breakfast and freeze the rest (using coffee filters or wax paper to separate the pancakes). The best success in making these pancakes is achieved using a nonstick griddle and a light spray of coconut oil. The preparation is the same for both single- and family-serve quantities. As waffles, they can be made in an electric waffle maker; follow the manufacturer's instructions.

1. Put the oats in a blender and blend until they turn into a powder. Turn off the blender and add the cottage cheese, egg whites, Super Sweet Blend, vanilla, and baking powder. Blend well, then allow the mixture to sit for a few minutes to let it thicken up.

2. Lightly coat a nonstick griddle or nonstick fry pan with coconut oil spray and heat over low/medium heat. Ladle desired-pancakes-size amounts onto the griddle and cook until golden brown, about 3 minutes. Flip and brown the other side, an additional minute or two. When making the family-serve version, keep the pancakes warm in a 200°F oven as you make additional ones.

NOTE: When making the family batch, enjoy 3 pancakes for your serving.

NSI (IF USING YOUR FAVORITE HANDY ON-PLAN SWEETENER)

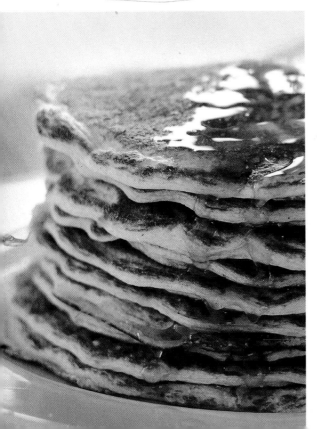

These taste every bit as good if not better than the master recipe of Trim Healthy Pancakes, but it is especially important to use coconut oil cooking spray and a nonstick griddle or they will stick. These pancakes are thinner than the others, but their wonderful taste makes up for their lack of fluff. Use the same ingredients as for the master single-serve version, but omit the cottage cheese and replace with ⅓ cup unsweetened almond or cashew milk, 1 teaspoon apple cider vinegar, 2 teaspoons Integral Collagen, and 2 teaspoons Just Gelatin. Prepare as follows.

1. Blend the oats as instructed, then add all the other ingredients. Allow the mixture to thicken in the fridge for 15 minutes before using, or make up the batter the night before.

2. Coat an electric nonstick griddle with coconut oil spray and heat to 250°F. These must start off at a low temperature to cook all the way through. Pour the pancake batter onto the griddle and cook for 3 minutes, then turn the temperature up to 275°F. Cook the pancakes until golden brown on the first side, another 2 to 3 minutes. Flip and brown on the other side, another couple of minutes, but don't take the pancakes off the heat too early—these pancakes take a total of 9 to 10 minutes to cook. It may take a little practice to get these right, but they are worth it.

D F

giant blueberry baked pancake

FAMILY SERVE – MAKES 6 VERY GENEROUS SERVINGS

2 cups old-fashioned rolled oats

2 cups low-fat cottage cheese

2 cups egg whites (carton is easier, but can use fresh)

6 teaspoons Super Sweet Blend

2 teaspoons vanilla extract

4 teaspoons aluminum-free baking powder

2 cups frozen or fresh blueberries (see Note)

Coconut oil cooking spray

Don't have time to fuss with pancakes in the morning? Enjoy all the goodness without the work. This idea can save many a frazzled Mama on a busy morning. Bake it once a week and you'll have multiple breakfasts sitting in the fridge waiting for you. Top with more blueberries or your favorite E-friendly pancake toppings. This is simply the Trim Healthy Mama pancake recipe with added blueberries, but by baking it you attain a completely different result, more cake than pancake.

1. Preheat the oven to 350°F.

2. Put the oats in a blender and blend until they turn to a powder. Turn off the blender and add the cottage cheese, egg whites, Super Sweet Blend, vanilla, and baking powder. Blend well. Add the blueberries to the blender jar, but do not blend; just stir them into the batter.

3. Lightly coat a 9 × 13-inch baking dish with coconut oil spray. Pour the batter into the pan and bake for 35 minutes, or until golden brown on top .

NOTE: Since we're already in **E** mode here, you can also use other frozen fruits, like cherries, peaches, or even pineapple or mango in place of the blueberries.

NSI (IF YOU USE YOUR FAVORITE ON-PLAN SWEETENER) DF

bring on da buttah pancakes

S

⅓ cup Trim Healthy Mama Baking
Blend

1 large egg

¼ cup unsweetened almond or
cashew milk

1 teaspoon Super Sweet Blend

Generous ½ teaspoon aluminum-free
baking powder

Dash of vanilla extract

Butter or coconut oil cooking spray

**FAMILY SERVE — MAKES
18 SMALL PANCAKES**

2 cups Trim Healthy Mama Baking
Blend

6 large eggs

1½ cups unsweetened almond or
cashew milk

2 tablespoons Super Sweet Blend

4 teaspoons aluminum-free baking
powder

2 teaspoons vanilla extract

Butter or coconut oil cooking spray

Want some melted butter on your pancakes and a side of bacon? Okay, here you go. The preparation is the same for both single-serve and family-serve quantities.

1. Mix all the ingredients except the butter in a bowl, stirring with a whisk or a fork.

2. Grease a griddle or large skillet with butter. Ladle in some of the batter and cook the pancake on one side, about 3 minutes, and then flip and continue to brown on the other side, an additional couple of minutes.

DF

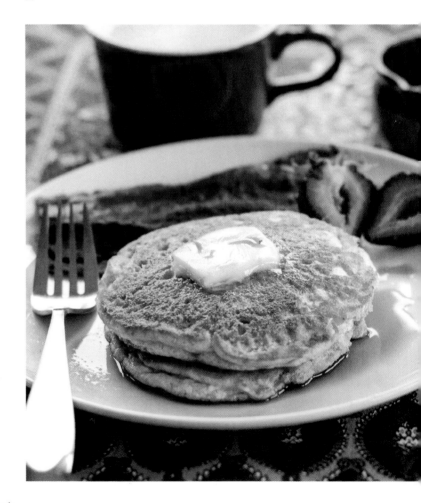

welcome back waffles

⅓ cup Trim Healthy Mama Baking
  Blend
1 large egg
3 tablespoons unsweetened almond or
  cashew milk
1 teaspoon melted butter or coconut oil
1 teaspoon Super Sweet Blend
Generous ½ teaspoon aluminum-free
  baking powder
Dash of vanilla extract
Coconut oil cooking spray or butter

The Trim Healthy Mama lifestyle is all about treating yourself to goal weight with healthy versions of those foods that once robbed your vigor and expanded your waistline. No need to miss out on waffles! Welcome them back into your life with a smile. This is a similar recipe to the pancake recipe (opposite), but the batter is a little thicker and sturdier and we added a tad more fat so the waffles have a slight crispness.

1. Mix all the ingredients except the cooking spray in a bowl, using a whisk or a fork. Using a spatula, scrape the batter into a coconut-oil-sprayed waffle iron (see manufacturer's instructions) and spread out carefully to fill the waffle form.

2. Cook until golden brown and cooked through, according to manufacturer's instructions.

NOTE: If you want to make a breakfast sandwich with 2 waffles (as in the Waffleized Breakky Sandwich, page 241), omit the egg, vanilla, and sweetener. Use ¼ cup egg whites in place of the egg, since you'll be using a whole egg in your sandwich. You can also add any savory flavorings of your choice, like grated Parmesan cheese, onion or garlic powder, or crumbled dried rosemary.

DF (IF USING COCONUT OIL INSTEAD OF BUTTER)

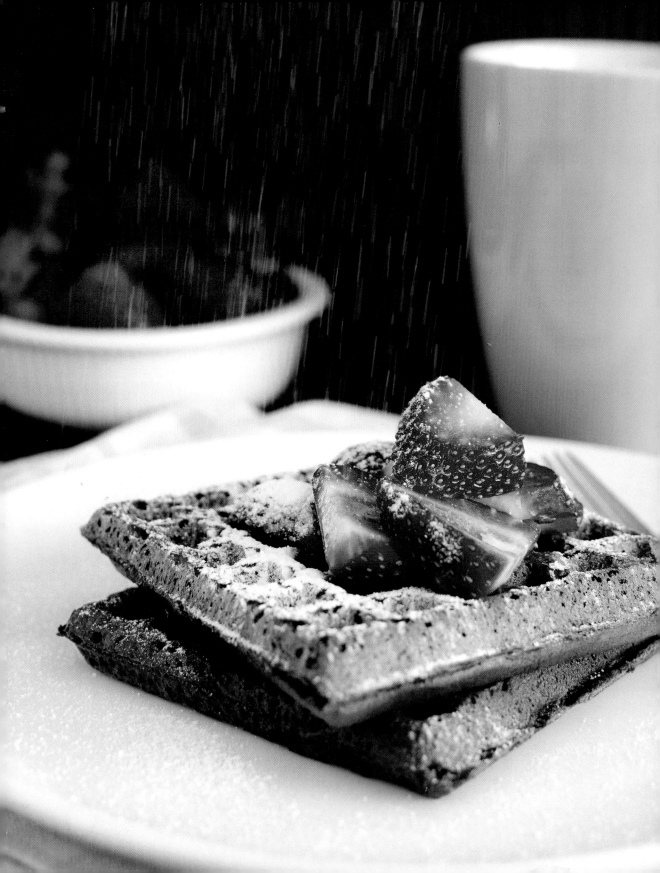

chocolate waffles with strawberries

good – thin batter

⅓ cup old-fashioned rolled oats, ground into flour

1 generous tablespoon unsweetened cocoa powder

2 large egg whites

¼ cup unsweetened almond or cashew milk

5 teaspoons Gentle Sweet

Pinch of Mineral Salt

Dash of vanilla extract

½ teaspoon aluminum-free baking powder

Cocnut oil cooking spray

FAMILY SERVE — MAKES 12 LARGE WAFFLES

2 cups old-fashioned rolled oats, ground into flour

6 generous tablespoons unsweetened cocoa powder

1¾ cups egg whites (from carton is easier, but can use fresh)

1½ cups unsweetened almond or cashew milk

½ cup Gentle Sweet

2 to 3 doonks Pure Stevia Extract

6 pinches Mineral Salt

1½ teaspoons vanilla extract

4 teaspoons aluminum-free baking powder

Coconut oil cooking spray

It's perfectly fine to eat a sweet chocolaty breakfast. These guiltless E waffles are packed with nutrition, and the nice slow-burning carbs give you energy for your morning. If you have a child or teenager with weight problems who is addicted to sugar-laden breakfasts, serve these waffles. Watch your child's health and weight start to turn around. The preparation is the same for the single-serve and family-serve portions.

1. Place the ground oats in a bowl and add the cocoa, egg whites, almond milk, Gentle Sweet, salt, vanilla, and baking powder. Blend well.

2. Prepare your waffle iron according to the manufacturer's instructions. Pour the batter onto the hot coconut-oil-sprayed waffle iron and cook according to manufacturer's instructions.

SERVING IDEA: Top the waffles with Handy Chocolate Syrup (page 479), 0% Greek yogurt, and sliced strawberries, or simply sprinkle with Gentle Sweet and sliced strawberries.

NSI (IF YOU USE YOUR FAVORITE ON-PLAN SWEETENER) DF

french toast in a bowl

SINGLE SERVE

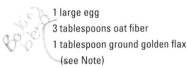

1 large egg

3 tablespoons oat fiber

1 tablespoon ground golden flax (see Note)

½ teaspoon aluminum-free baking powder

¼ cup water

1 tablespoon softened butter

¾ teaspoon Super Sweet Blend

Unsweetened almond or cashew milk

2 teaspoons natural-style peanut butter

Pancake Syrup (page 480) or sugar-free syrup

This recipe comes from one of Trim Healthy Mama's most popular bloggers. She is an extremely talented young woman of 19. At 18, Briana began churning out amazing THM recipes that had the community begging her for more. This simple breakfast or snack recipe has been one of her biggest hits, and no wonder—because who doesn't love French toast? Now, those of us with a Drive Thru Sue mindset can have it in a couple minutes. You can top this with Pancake Syrup (page 480), but if you're a Drive Thru Sue and are all about ease, buying a sugar-free pancake syrup won't hurt your progress too much.

Briana is also known for her on-plan ice cream recipes. You can find many more of Briana's Trim Healthy Mama recipes at her blog www.brianathomasblogspot.com.

1. Combine the egg, oat fiber, flax, baking powder, water, butter, and Super Sweet Blend in a ceramic bowl and microwave for 90 seconds or until almost cooked through.

2. Douse the "toast" with the almond milk to moisten (like what happens when you dip bread slices in an egg-and-milk mixture to fry, only the steps are turned around here). Smear with the peanut butter and drizzle with the syrup.

NOTE: The flax and oat fiber may be substituted with 4 tablespoons Trim Healthy Mama Baking Blend.

chocolate monkey crepes

3 tablespoons Trim Healthy Mama
   Baking Blend

⅓ cup egg whites (carton or fresh)

¼ cup unsweetened almond or
   cashew milk

Pinch of Mineral Salt

¾ teaspoon Super Sweet Blend

½ teaspoon pure banana extract

Coconut oil cooking spray

½ large banana (or 1 small banana),
   sliced

⅓ to ½ cup 0% Greek yogurt

Handy Chocolate Syrup (page 479)

Fruit for topping, such as strawberries
   (optional)

Fat-free Reddi-wip (optional)

Here's a delish way to eat bananas in a safe, protein-rich breakfast.

1. Place the Baking Blend, egg whites, almond milk, salt, Super Sweet Blend, and extract in a small bowl and mix with a whisk. Allow the batter to sit for 3 to 5 minutes.

2. Lightly coat an electric griddle with coconut oil spray and set to 275°F. When the griddle is hot, pour one third of the batter onto the griddle. Spread out thinly with a spatula and cook until browned on bottom, 2 to 3 minutes. Flip and brown on the other side, about 2 more minutes.

3. Repeat until all 3 crepes are made.

4. Lay each crepe flat on a dish, fill each with some of the banana slices, yogurt, and a swirl of chocolate syrup. Roll up the crepes and top with the remaining banana slices, added optional fruit, a drizzle more of the chocolate syrup, and if you're not a staunch purist, an optional squirt of the Reddi-wip.

DF

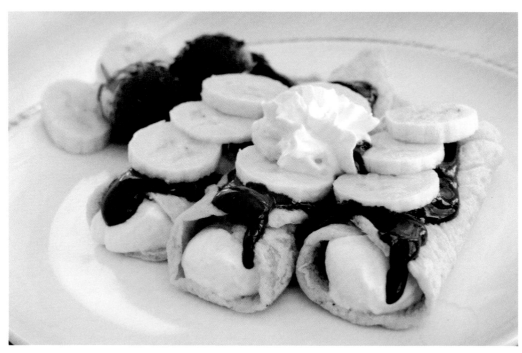

donuts

These are not your cut-out type of donuts; the recipe makes a loose batter that you pour into a donut form and bake in the oven or use an electric donut maker. They cook up quickly and are delicious with the suggested toppings. Here is the basic recipe and three ways to move them to a new level.

BASIC DONUTS

FAMILY SERVE

Coconut oil cooking spray (optional)

3 large eggs

⅓ cup sour cream (for dairy-free, use canned full-fat coconut milk)

2 teaspoons vanilla extract

¼ cup water or unsweetened almond or cashew milk

6 to 7 tablespoons melted butter or coconut oil

1 cup Trim Healthy Mama Baking Blend

1 teaspoon aluminum-free baking powder

⅛ teaspoon Mineral Salt

½ cup Gentle Sweet, or ¼ cup Super Sweet Blend

1. Preheat the oven to 350°F if you are baking the donuts. Lightly coat a donut form with coconut oil cooking spray. If using an electric donut maker, consult the manufacturer's instructions for preheating and grease well.

2. In a large bowl, whisk together the eggs, sour cream, vanilla, water, and ¼ cup melted butter. Add the Baking Blend, baking powder, salt, and Gentle Sweet and stir to combine.

3. Pour the batter into the prepared donut form and bake for 15 to 20 minutes, until golden on top. Or, follow the manufacturer's instructions for cooking the donuts in an electric donut maker; usually the donuts cook for 5 to 7 minutes, until brown.

4. Remove the donuts from the form or maker, and brush with the remaining 2 to 3 tablespoons melted butter.

DF (IF USING FULL-FAT COCONUT MILK INSTEAD OF SOUR CREAM AND GHEE INSTEAD OF BUTTER)

POWDERED CINNAMON SUGAR DONUTS

FAMILY SERVE

Prepare the master recipe. Mix ¾ teaspoon ground cinnamon with 3 tablespoons Gentle Sweet. Roll the butter-brushed donuts in the mixture.

CHOCOLATE DRIZZLED DONUTS

FAMILY SERVE

Prepare the master recipe. Drizzle the butter-brushed donuts with Handy Chocolate Syrup (page 479).

JELLY DONUTS

FAMILY SERVE

Prepare the master recipe. Top the butter-brushed donuts with Slim Belly Jelly (page 478). Or, serve with up to 1 teaspoon store-bought all-fruit jelly for each donut.

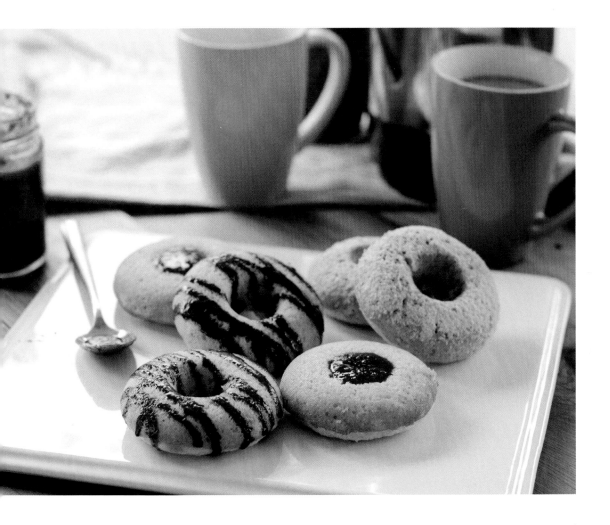

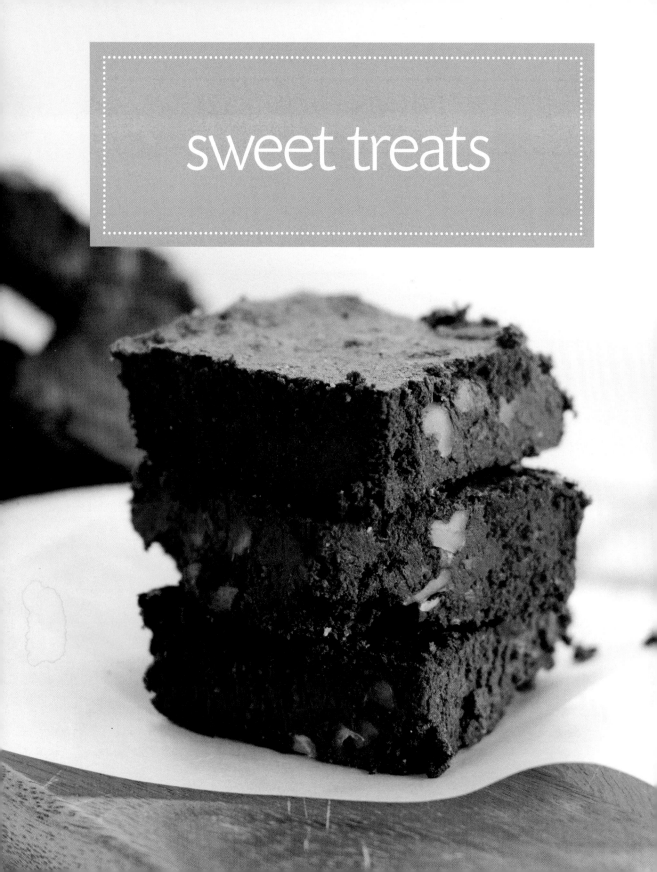

sweet treats

● = S   ● = E   ○ = FP   MORE THAN ONE DOT INDICATES OPTIONS

● = S   ● = E   ● = FP   MORE THAN ONE DOT INDICATES OPTIONS

QUICK SINGLE MUFFINS

PEARL CHATS: Just so you know how different we are, Serene has never made a single-serve muffin or cake in her entire journey as a Trim Healthy Mama. She sticks to the family-serve cakes and muffin recipes because she doesn't use a microwave and can't be bothered baking in the oven for just one serving. I, on the other hand, am a single-serve muffin and cake freak! I love the ease, the sheer lack of fuss and time it takes to create these incredible indulgences. I make them for my breakfast or for a yummy afternoon snack.

Much to Serene's chagrin, I still often use my microwave for these treats, but I do sometimes bake a single-serve muffin or two in the oven or I put the batter in a waffle maker. Enjoy your unique THM journey, and don't let your sister beat up on ya! (Oh, man, she saw this. I'm in trouble . . . here she comes, all pregnant, too; she's feisty when she's pregnant. . . .)

volcano mud slide muffin

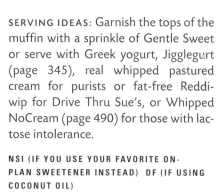

1 large egg

1 tablespoon extra-virgin coconut oil
or butter

Dash of vanilla extract

2 tablespoons unsweetened cocoa
powder

1 heaping tablespoon golden flax meal

4½ to 5 teaspoons Gentle Sweet

Pinch of Mineral Salt (omit if using
butter)

Generous ½ teaspoon aluminum-free
baking powder

2 tablespoons water

My, oh my, what a dark, deeply mysterious, fantastically oozy and chocolaty muffin this is. Since we're dealing with a chocolate baked good here, Gentle Sweet gives the best result. The trick is not to overnuke or overbake. Keep things a little molten for the win!

1. Preheat the oven to 350°F if baking the muffin.

2. Put all the ingredients in a large coffee mug or into a well-greased ramekin and mix well. Microwave the coffee mug for 40 to 50 seconds or bake the ramekin for 8 to 10 minutes, until the muffin is mostly cooked through but still slightly gooey at the middle of the top. You can eat this straight out of the mug or ramekin. No need to remove.

SERVING IDEAS: Garnish the tops of the muffin with a sprinkle of Gentle Sweet or serve with Greek yogurt, Jigglegurt (page 345), real whipped pastured cream for purists or fat-free Reddi-wip for Drive Thru Sue's, or Whipped NoCream (page 490) for those with lactose intolerance.

NSI (IF YOU USE YOUR FAVORITE ON-PLAN SWEETENER INSTEAD) DF (IF USING COCONUT OIL)

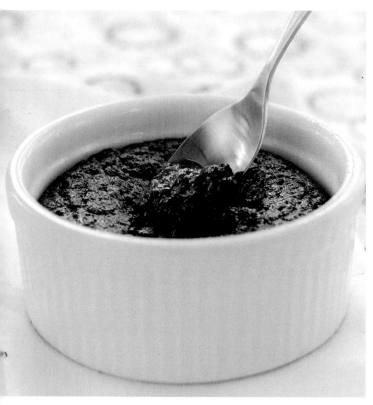

brainy blueberry muffin

S

Coconut oil cooking spray (optional)

1 large egg

2 tablespoons water

1 tablespoon coconut oil or butter

¼ cup Trim Healthy Mama Baking Blend

2 teaspoons Super Sweet Blend

1 small pinch Mineral Salt (omit if using butter)

Generous ½ teaspoon aluminum-free baking powder

2 tablespoons fresh or frozen blueberries

It's a fact that blueberries have many health benefits, including protecting your brain and, yes, even making you smarter! Eating blueberries in a muffin has to be one of the most delicious ways to become a brainiac, but the problem is that most blueberry muffins are loaded with sugar and empty carbs. Blood sugar spikes then kill off the brain cells—where's the smarts in that? Here's the clever way to eat a blueberry muffin and keep that blood sugar stable!

1. Preheat the oven to 350°F if baking the muffins. Lightly coat an 8-cup muffin tin with coconut oil spray.

2. Whisk the egg in a small bowl or, if microwaving, in a large coffee mug. Add the remaining ingredients and mix well. If baking, divide the batter between 2 muffin holes and fill the remaining holes with water (gives a nice steaming effect); bake for 15 to 17 minutes. Or, microwave in the mug for 1 minute 20 seconds.

SERVING IDEA: Top with a pat of buttah!

DF (IF USING COCONUT OIL INSTEAD OF BUTTER)

frosted cinnamon muffin

SINGLE SERVE – MAKES 1 LARGE MUFFIN IN A MUG OR RAMEKIN IN THE OVEN

FOR THE MUFFIN

1 large egg

1 tablespoon water

1 tablespoon extra-virgin coconut oil
or butter

Dash of vanilla extract (optional)

3 tablespoons golden flax meal

1½ teaspoons ground cinnamon

2 teaspoons Super Sweet Blend, or
4 teaspoons Gentle Sweet

Pinch of Mineral Salt (omit if using
butter)

Generous ½ teaspoon aluminum-free
baking powder

FOR THE FROSTING

1 tablespoon ⅓ less fat cream cheese

1 heaping tablespoon plain Greek
yogurt

¼ teaspoon vanilla extract, or a squirt
of lemon juice

2 teaspoons Gentle Sweet, or ½ to
¾ teaspoon Super Sweet Blend,
ground in a coffee grinder

If you're new to the plan and do not have any Trim Healthy Mama Baking Blend, don't worry. You can still eat these muffins. You'll be able to find ground golden flax at your local grocery store and then you can make this cinnamon goodness that is not stingy with the frosting!

1. Preheat the oven to 350°F if baking.

2. Make the muffin. Put all the ingredients in a large coffee mug for the microwave or ramekin for the oven and stir well. Microwave for 1 minute or bake in the ramekin for 15 minutes, or until no longer gooey on top.

3. Make the frosting. Mix the ingredients with a fork and spread on top of the muffin or get fancy and pipe it on.

NSI (IF YOU USE YOUR FAVORITE ON-PLAN SWEETENER) DF (IF USING COCONUT OIL INSTEAD OF BUTTER)

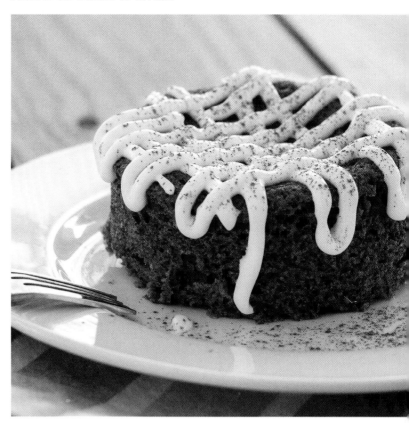

banana nut muffin

SINGLE SERVE – MAKES 1 LARGE MUFFIN IN A MUG OR 2 SMALLER MUFFINS IN THE OVEN

Coconut oil cooking spray (optional)

1 large egg

2 tablespoons plus 1 teaspoon water

½ teaspoon pure banana extract

¼ cup Trim Healthy Mama Baking Blend

4 teaspoons Gentle Sweet, or
  1½ teaspoons Super Sweet Blend (this has the best taste with Gentle Sweet)

1 rounded tablespoon crunchy natural-style peanut butter (sugar-free)

½ teaspoon aluminum-free baking powder

PEARL CHATS: This is one of my husband's favorite breakfasts!

1. Preheat the oven to 350°F if baking the muffins. Lightly coat an 8-cup muffin tin with coconut oil spray.

2. If baking, whisk the egg in a small bowl; if microwaving, whisk it in a large coffee mug. Add all the other ingredients and mix well. If baking, divide the batter between 2 holes of the muffin tin and fill the other holes with water (for a nice steaming effect); bake for 15 minutes, or until no longer gooey on top. Or microwave for 1 minute in the mug.

SERVING IDEA: Top the muffins with a pat of buttah!

DF (WITHOUT THE BUTTER TOPPING)

lemon poppy seed muffin   Ⓢ

Coconut oil cooking spray (optional)

1 large egg

2 tablespoons golden flax meal

1 tablespoon coconut flour

2 tablespoons lemon juice

1 tablespoon butter or coconut oil

½ teaspoon poppy seeds

Pinch of Mineral Salt

2 teaspoons Super Sweet Blend,
   or 3 to 4 teaspoons Gentle Sweet
   (see Note)

½ teaspoon aluminum-free baking
   powder

2 to 3 drops essential lemon oil
   (optional but really makes this
   muffin sing!)

Here's another great recipe from Gwen Brown, who has an awesome blog full of delicious THM recipes (www.gwens-nest.com). Enjoying this muffin for breakfast is one of Gwen's favorite ways to start her day and part of the reason she lost 45 pounds to get to goal weight. She pairs it with stevia-sweetened Greek yogurt mixed with fresh lemon juice and the berry syrup on her blog, which is similar to our Slim Belly Jelly (page 478), but made with the minimum amount of Gluccie. Both coconut flour and golden flax meal are easily found, rather inexpensively, at most grocery stores these days, so go ahead and give this a try.

1. Preheat the oven to 350°F if baking the muffins. Lightly spray an 8-cup muffin tin with coconut oil cooking spray.

2. Combine all the ingredients in a coffee mug if microwaving or in a small bowl if baking. Stir with a fork. Mix really well to make sure that the ingredients are evenly incorporated. Cook in the microwave for 50 seconds or so (this muffin is much yummier a little underdone versus overdone). Or spoon the batter into 3 of the muffin holes and fill remaining cups with water (for nice steaming effect) and bake for 12 to 14 minutes, until muffins are almost done but still slightly gooey on top.

NOTE: Feel free to quadruple the recipe to make a dozen breakfast muffins in the oven. Ultra-frugal Mamas can get away with using just 2 or 3 doonks Pure Stevia Extract instead of the sweeteners listed for the single serve.

NSI (IF YOU USE YOUR FAVORITE ON-PLAN SWEETENER) DF (IF USING COCONUT OIL INSTEAD OF BUTTER)

Coconut oil cooking spray (optional)

1 large egg

2 tablespoon plus 1 teaspoon water

1 tablespoon coconut oil or butter

¼ cup Trim Healthy Mama Baking Blend

4 teaspoons Gentle Sweet

Pinch of Mineral Salt

1½ tablespoons stevia-sweetened chocolate chips or chopped 85% dark chocolate

1. Preheat the oven to 350°F if baking the muffins. Lightly coat an 8-cup muffin tin with coconut oil spray.

2. Mix all the ingredients in a large coffee mug for microwaving or in a small bowl if using the oven. Microwave for 1 minute 15 seconds. Or divide the batter and place in 2 muffin holes, then fill the remaining holes with water (for a nice steaming effect) and bake for 15 to 17 minutes, or until just done on top.

3. Top the muffin with a pat of buttah!

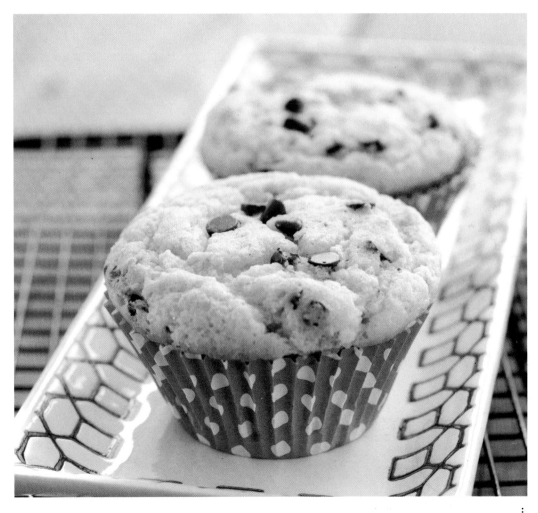

apple cinnamon swirl muffin

SINGLE SERVE – MAKES 1 LARGE MUFFIN IN A MUG OR 2 SMALLER MUFFINS IN THE OVEN

Coconut oil cooking spray (optional)

3 tablespoons Trim Healthy Mama Baking Blend

2 tablespoons old-fashioned rolled oats

¼ cup egg whites (from carton or fresh)

1 generous tablespoon unsweetened applesauce

4 teaspoons Gentle Sweet

Generous ½ teaspoon aluminum-free baking powder

½ apple, peeled, cored, and diced (other half retained)

¾ teaspoon ground cinnamon or apple pie spice

This muffin makes the perfect filling and energizing breakfast (if you eat the other half of your apple), and it's friendly to those with dairy allergies. Enjoy with a Healing Trimmy (see pages 430–433) or Collagen Tea (page 436), both of which contain some extra protein, and you are good to go. Or, if your body loves dairy, include some Greek yogurt or Jigglegurt (page 345) on the side or on top of your muffin. Drive Thru Sue's may want to include a squirt or two of fat-free Reddi-wip to top the muffin. Please don't forget to eat the other half of your apple while your muffin is cooking—you need all those good carbs for an energizing breakfast.

1. Preheat the oven to 350°F if baking the muffins. Lightly coat an 8-cup muffin tin with coconut oil spray.

2. Mix all the ingredients except the apple and cinnamon in a large coffee mug for microwaving or a small bowl if baking the muffins. Fold in the diced apple. Sprinkle the cinnamon on top of the batter, and then carefully fold the batter over the top and around it just a few times (it should not be fully mixed in).

3. Microwave for 1 minute, 20 seconds in the mug, or divide the batter into 2 muffin holes of the muffin tin and fill the other holes with water (for a nice steaming effect). Bake for 15 minutes or until just cooked through. You can also use a large ramekin for the oven, but bake a few minutes longer.

DF

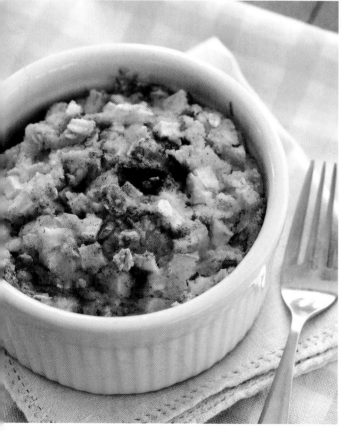

strawberry muffin

Coconut oil cooking spray (optional)

2 large frozen or fresh strawberries, or 3 smaller ones

3 tablespoons Trim Healthy Mama Baking Blend

1½ teaspoons Super Sweet Blend

¼ cup egg whites (from carton or 2 large eggs)

½ teaspoon strawberry extract (optional)

1 rounded tablespoon low-fat cottage cheese or plain 0% Greek yogurt

½ teaspoon aluminum-free baking powder

Keep juggling those THM fuels, never forgetting about your Fuel Pulls. This is a nice way to get an FP snack or dessert into your snack or dessert rotation. The strawberry pieces keep this muffin moist even though it is FP. Top it with a little 0% Greek yogurt or fat-free Reddi-wip if you are a Drive Thru Sue.

1. Preheat the oven to 350°F if baking the muffins. Lightly coat an 8-cup muffin tin with coconut oil spray.

2. If using frozen strawberries, take them out of the freezer to thaw slightly while you mix your other ingredients.

3. Combine the Baking Blend, Super Sweet Blend, egg whites, extract (if using), cottage cheese, and baking powder in a large coffee mug for microwaving or in a small bowl if baking. Cut the strawberries into small pieces with a sharp knife. Add to the batter. Microwave for 1 minute 40 seconds, or divide the batter into 2 of the muffin holes and fill the other holes with water (for a nice steaming effect). Bake for 15 to 17 minutes, or until just cooked through.

NOTE: Enjoy this recipe as a dessert, a snack, or breakfast.

NSI (IF YOU USE YOUR FAVORITE ON-PLAN SWEETENER)

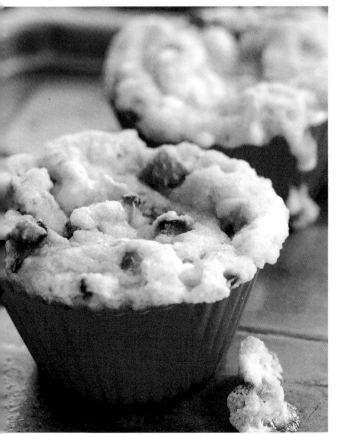

FAMILY MUFFINS

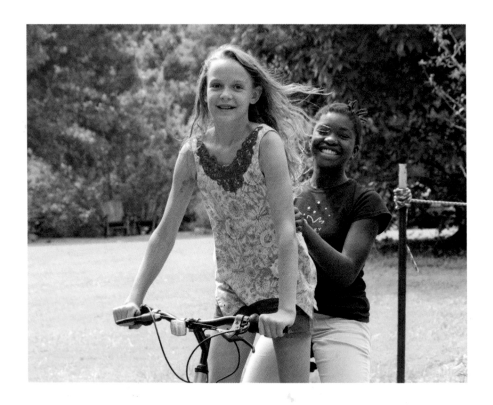

chocolate banana muffins

Coconut oil cooking spray

2 cups old-fashioned rolled oats, ground into flour in a blender

½ cup unsweetened cocoa powder (equal mix of extra-dark and regular is the bombiest)

¾ cup Gentle Sweet

⅓ teaspoon Mineral Salt

1½ teaspoons aluminum-free baking powder

½ teaspoon baking soda

3 large egg whites, lightly beaten (fresh is best)

1 cup plain 0% Greek yogurt (for dairy-free, use unsweetened applesauce)

½ cup water

1½ teaspoons vanilla extract

1 large banana or 2 small bananas, cut into small pieces about the size of your pinky nail

Ultra-moist and chocolaty with a hint of banana, these muffins are amazing!!! Have two for your breakfast, keeping to less than 1 teaspoon of butter spread on top or squirt on a little fat-free Reddi-wip if you are not a purist.

1. Preheat the oven to 350°F. Lightly coat a 12-cup muffin tin with coconut oil spray.

2. Combine all the ingredients except the banana in a large bowl. Fold in the banana pieces gently. Spoon the batter into the muffin holes, making sure to get some banana pieces in each muffin. Bake for 16 to 18 minutes .

NSI (IF YOU USE YOUR FAVORITE ON-PLAN SWEETENER INSTEAD)
DF (IF YOU USE UNSWEETENED APPLESAUCE INSTEAD OF YOGURT)

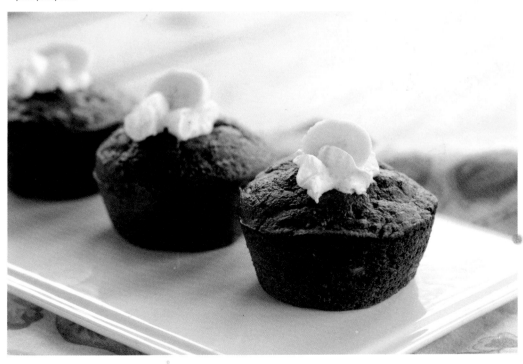

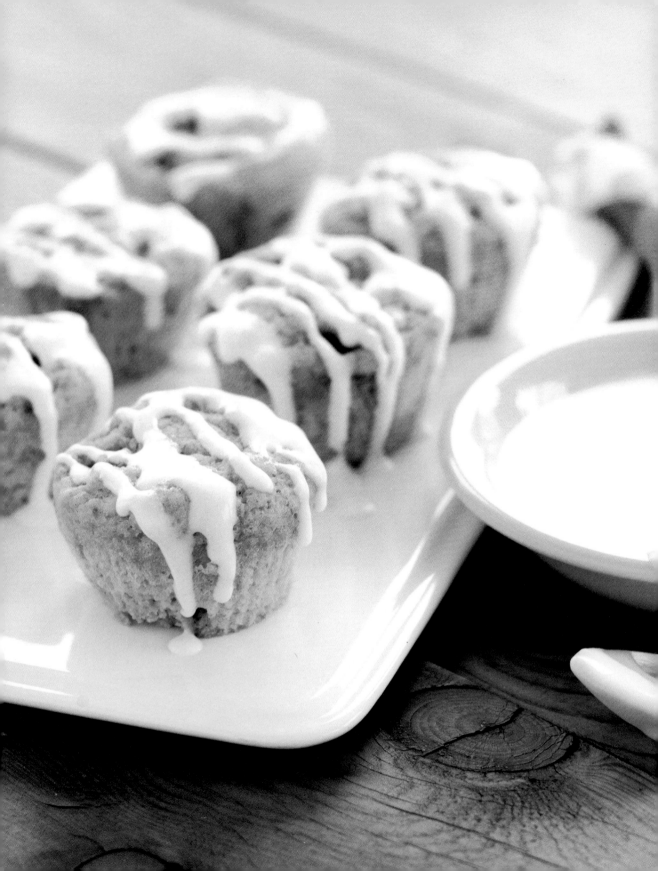

glosted raspberry muffins

S

FOR THE MUFFINS

12 paper muffin cup liners or coconut oil cooking spray

3 large eggs plus ½ cup egg whites (carton or fresh)

½ cup plus 2 tablespoons unsweetened almond or cashew milk

4 tablespoons melted coconut oil or butter

2 teaspoons raspberry or vanilla extract

1½ cups Trim Healthy Mama Baking Blend

3 tablespoons Super Sweet Blend, or ½ cup Gentle Sweet

1½ teaspoons aluminum-free baking powder

½ teaspoon baking soda

1¾ cups fresh or frozen raspberries, cut in halves

FOR THE GLOSTING (CROSS BETWEEN A GLAZE AND A FROSTING)

2 tablespoons butter

3 tablespoons cream cheese (⅓ less fat works well)

2 tablespoons unsweetened almond or cashew milk

¾ teaspoon raspberry or vanilla extract

2 to 2½ tablespoons Gentle Sweet

A "glosting" is a delicious, drippy, messy, lick-your-fingers cross between a glaze and a frosting. If there is no name for things, one must make up fitting names, we think. Our Luscious Lemon Cake (page 289) also has a glosting that's to die for—or we should say, to live for! We enjoy glosting on so many THM treats.

1. Preheat the oven to 375°F. Insert paper liners into the cups of a 12-cup muffin tin or lightly coat with coconut oil spray. (The liners make removing the muffins, which are very moist from the raspberries, an easier task.)

2. Make the muffins. In a large bowl, whisk together the eggs and egg whites, almond milk, coconut oil, and extract, then incorporate the Baking Blend, Super Sweet, and baking powder and soda. Whisk until you have a smooth batter. Allow the batter to sit and thicken a little, 2 to 3 minutes, then fold in the raspberries and combine gently.

3. Fill the muffin cups with batter and bake for 20 to 25 minutes, or until the tops are just done. If you've used frozen berries, the baking may take a bit longer.

4. While the muffins are cooling, make the glosting. Combine the butter and cream cheese in a small bowl. Whisk until smooth, then add 1 tablespoon of the almond milk and the extract. Whisk until completely smooth, then add the rest of the milk followed by the Gentle Sweet. Keep whisking until combined properly.

5. Drizzle the glosting all over the tops of the muffins, allowing some to drop down the sides to make muffins a drippy, delicious mess.

just peachy muffins

Coconut oil cooking spray

1 cup old-fashioned rolled oats
(left whole)

1½ cups old-fashioned rolled oats,
ground into flour

¼ teaspoon Mineral Salt

2 teaspoons aluminum-free baking
powder

1 teaspoon baking soda

¾ cup Gentle Sweet

1 cup plain Greek yogurt (or
unsweetened apple sauce for
dairy-free)

1 cup egg whites (carton or fresh)

2 teaspoons vanilla extract

2 cups diced fresh or frozen peaches

1. Preheat the oven to 350°F. Lightly coat a 12-cup muffin tin or two 8-cup muffin tins with the coconut oil spray.

2. Pour all the ingredients into a large bowl and blend with a fork—you don't even need an appliance for this! Spoon the batter into the muffin holes and bake for 20 to 25 minutes, or until a knife inserted in the center comes out clean.

NSI (IF YOU USE YOUR FAVORITE ON-PLAN SWEETENER) DF (IF YOU SUBSTITUTE UNSWEETENED APPLESAUCE FOR THE YOGURT)

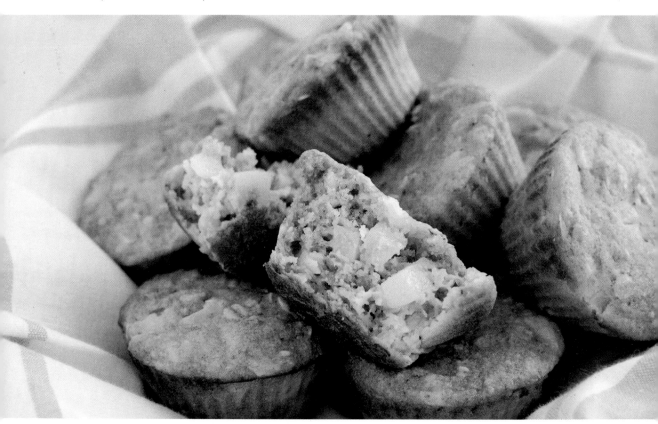

chocolate chai-glazed cinnamon muffins

FOR THE MUFFINS
Coconut oil cooking spray
3 large eggs and 3 egg whites
¾ cup plus 1 tablespoon water
1 teaspoon vanilla extract
2 cups golden flax meal
1 teaspoon aluminum-free baking
   powder
1 teaspoon baking soda
4 tablespoons ground cinnamon
4 to 5 tablespoons Super Sweet Blend
   or double amounts of Gentle Sweet

FOR THE CHAI CHOCOLATE GLAZE
1 batch liquid Skinny Chocolate (page
   377), melted
1 teaspoon ground cinnamon, or
   3 to 4 drops of a chai blend of pure
   essential oils

Golden flax meal can be found at almost any grocery store, so this recipe is dedicated to our Mamas determined not to use special ingredients. You will need your favorite on-plan sweetener, but many grocery stores also have something there that can work, too. Be sure to drink plenty of water when you eat these muffins, owing to the high fiber of the flax flour. The muffins plus good water intake equal great bowel function.

1. Preheat the oven to 350°F. Lightly coat a 12-cup muffin tin with coconut oil spray.

2. Make the muffins. In a large bowl, whisk together the eggs and egg whites, water, and vanilla. Gradually add the flax meal, baking powder, baking soda, cinnamon, and Super Sweet Blend. Continue to whisk until the mixture is smooth.

3. Spoon the mixture into the muffin holes and bake for 20 to 25 minutes, or until tops are just done.

4. As the muffins are cooling, make the glaze. Combine the melted Skinny Chocolate and cinnamon or chai essential oils. Spoon the glaze over the muffin tops, then put them in the fridge so the glaze hardens.

NSI (IF YOU USE YOUR FAVORITE ON-PLAN SWEETENER INSTEAD) DF

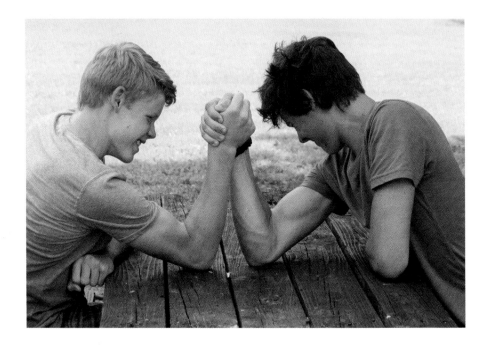

luscious lemon cake

S

SINGLE SERVE

FOR THE CAKE

1 large egg

2 tablespoons lemon juice

1 teaspoon butter or coconut oil

3 tablespoons Trim Healthy Mama
Baking Blend

3 teaspoons Super Sweet Blend

½ teaspoon aluminum-free baking
powder

FOR THE GLOSTING (CROSS BETWEEN
A GLAZE AND A FROSTING)

1 teaspoon softened butter

2 teaspoons cream cheese

1 to 1½ teaspoons Gentle Sweet, or
½ to ¾ teaspoon Super Sweet Blend,
ground in a coffee grinder

1 to 2 teaspoons lemon juice (or more
if you are a lemon freak)

PEARL CHATS: Of all our single-serve cakes, this might have to take first place as my favorite. It is so fluffy and buttery (even though it does not have a lot of butter), and the crumb resembles that of a boxed cake. It has that perfect balance of sweet and tangy. Super Sweet Blend works well in this particular cake as it offsets the tartness of the lemon, so that is great if you are on a tight budget. But if you are a loyal Gentle Sweet user, just double up on the amount called for. To Serene's dismay, I actually prefer the microwave version.

1. Preheat the oven to 375°F if using it to bake the cake.

2. Make the cake. In a small greased microwave-safe/oven-safe glass dish, beat the egg well with a fork, then add the remaining ingredients and stir well. Microwave for 1 minute 20 seconds or bake for 15 minutes, or until top is just done.

3. Make the glosting. Mix the butter and cream cheese with a fork in a small bowl until smooth, then add the sweetener and lemon juice.

4. Pour the glosting onto the top of the still warm cake and get your fork ready to enjoy!

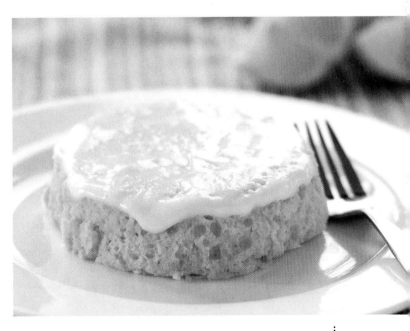

pineapple upside down cake

Coconut oil cooking spray

½ (8-ounce) can crushed pineapple or pineapple tidbits

⅓ cup old-fashioned rolled oats, ground into flour in a blender

2 teaspoons Super Sweet Blend

1 teaspoon Just Gelatin

2 teaspoons Integral Collagen

Generous ½ teaspoon aluminum-free baking powder

¼ cup egg whites (from carton or 2 large eggs)

1 tablespoon unsweetened almond milk

1 teaspoon apple cider vinegar

A delicious and fast way to get more E's into a Drive Thru Sue's life! This cute mini-cake makes a quick, breakfast or a nice afternoon snack with a Trimmy Light (page 430). Purists can use the oven baking option instead of the microwave. The cake comes close to your full 45 grams of carbs for an E meal, so it's best not eaten as a dessert after an E meal. Drive Thru Sue's can use a *little* bit of fat-free Reddi-wip on top of this cake, but it is so moist and full of flavor that it doesn't really need it.

This cake is great for our allergen-free Mamas, as it is both gluten- and dairy-free. If you're budget conscious and prefer to not use any special ingredients, try the NSI option following; however, heads up, allergen-free Mamas: that version does include some dairy.

1. Preheat the oven to 350°F if using it to bake the cake. Lightly coat a large coffee mug, oven-safe ramekin, or small baking dish with coconut oil spray.

2. Drain the excess juice from the pineapple and put in the bottom of the coffee mug or ramekin (doesn't matter if a little juice remains). Mix the remaining ingredients in a small bowl until smooth and pour over the pineapple.

3. Microwave the mug for 2 minutes 15 seconds, or bake the ramekin or small dish in the oven for 15 to 20 minutes, or until top is just done.

4. Place a small plate over the top of the mug/ramekin/baking dish, and flip upside down. The cake should plop out nicely with the pineapple on top.

NSI (FOR A BUDGET-FRIENDLY OPTION, OMIT THE GELATIN, COLLAGEN, ALMOND MILK, AND VINEGAR, AND REPLACE WITH 1 HEAPING TABLESPOON LOW-FAT COTTAGE CHEESE OR PLAIN GREEK YOGURT) DF

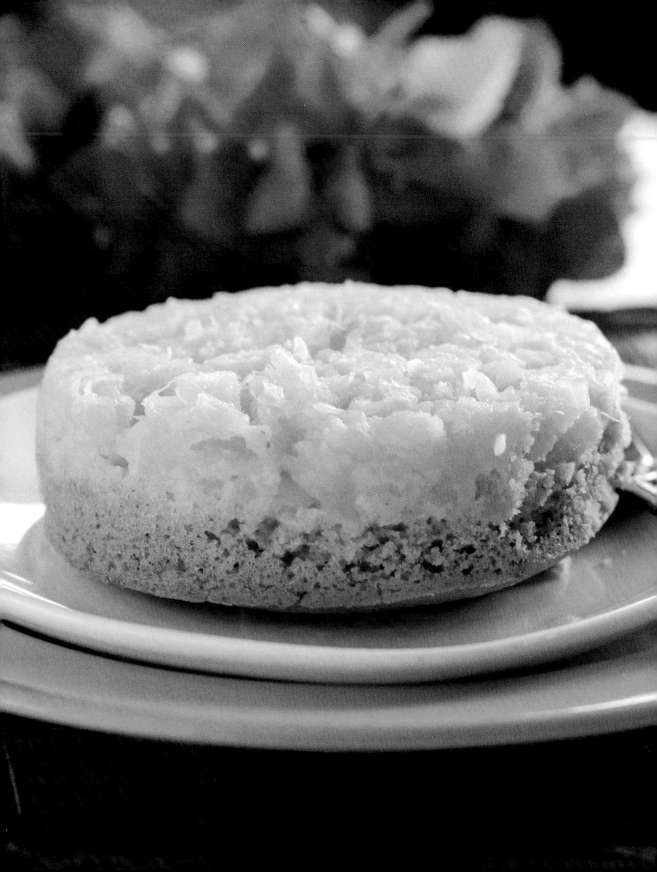

peanut puff cake

(S)

FOR THE CAKE

Coconut oil cooking spray (optional)

2 tablespoons Pressed Peanut Flour

1 tablespoon Trim Healthy Mama
Baking Blend (see Note)

3½ teaspoons Gentle Sweet

¼ cup egg whites (from carton or
fresh)

2 tablespoons plain 0% Greek yogurt

2 tablespoons unsweetened almond or
cashew milk

2 pinches Mineral Salt

½ teaspoon aluminum-free baking
powder

FOR THE FROSTING

2 teaspoons natural-style sugar-free
peanut butter

1 teaspoon Pressed Peanut Flour

1 heaping tablespoon plain 0% Greek
yogurt

Pinch of Mineral Salt

1 teaspoon water

1½ teaspoons Gentle Sweet

Scratch that itch for peanutty flavor with this yummy little cake that is not stingy on the frosting!

1. Preheat the oven to 375°F if using it to bake the cake. Lightly coat a small oven-safe glass dish with coconut oil spray.

2. Make the cake. Mix the cake ingredients in a small bowl until smooth. Transfer to a wide-bottom coffee mug if microwaving or the greased dish if using the oven. Microwave the mug for 1 minute 30 seconds, or bake the dish in the oven for 15 to 17 minutes, or until top is just done.

3. Make the frosting. Combine the ingredients in a small bowl and use to frost the cake.

NOTE: You can substitute a mix of coconut, almond, or flax flour for the Baking Blend.

glazed chocolate coconut cake

S

SINGLE SERVE

FOR THE CAKE

Coconut oil cooking spray (optional)

1 large egg

1 heaping tablespoon unsweetened dark cocoa powder

2 tablespoons plain Greek yogurt

1 tablespoon unsweetened shredded coconut

4 teaspoons Gentle Sweet

½ teaspoon aluminum-free baking powder

Dash of coconut or vanilla extract

Pinch of Mineral Salt

1 to 2 tablespoons water

FOR THE COCONUT GLAZE

¾ teaspoon unsweetened almond or cashew milk

1½ teaspoons Gentle Sweet

1 rounded teaspoon finely shredded unsweetened coconut (see Note)

¼ teaspoon coconut or vanilla extract

Dawn is a Trim Healthy Mama having great success on the plan. She tweaked the original Chocolate Cake in a Mug recipe from our first book by adding unsweetened shredded coconut and Greek yogurt (for added moisture), and that version was a huge hit in the community. We decided to top Dawn's version with a yumsers coconut glaze, and the delish factor just shot through the roof. You can read about Dawn's THM progress and see more of her recipes at www.ohsweetmercy.com. No special ingredients are needed here if you have your favorite on-plan sweetener handy.

1. Preheat the oven to 350°F if using it to bake the cake. Lightly coat a small baking dish with coconut oil spray.

2. Make the cake. Whisk the egg in a mug or small bowl. Add the remaining ingredients and mix well. Microwave the mug for 60 to 90 seconds, or transfer to the greased dish and bake for 15 to 20 minutes in the oven, or until top is just done.

3. Make the glaze. Mix the ingredients until smooth, then pour over the top of the cake.

NOTE: If the coconut is not fine enough for the glaze, you can grind it briefly in a coffee grinder.

NSI (IF YOU USE YOUR FAVORITE ON-PLAN SWEETENER INSTEAD)

mini white cake with butter cream frosting

FOR THE CAKE

Coconut oil cooking spray (optional)

1 large egg

2 tablespoons unsweetened almond or
cashew milk, or water

1 teaspoon butter or coconut oil

3 tablespoons Trim Healthy Mama
Baking Blend

2½ teaspoons Super Sweet Blend,
or 5 teaspoons Gentle Sweet

½ teaspoon vanilla extract

½ teaspoon aluminum-free baking
powder

FOR THE BUTTERCREAM FROSTING

2 teaspoons softened butter

2 teaspoons ⅓ less fat cream cheese

2 teaspoons Gentle Sweet, or
¾ teaspoon Super Sweet Blend,
ground in a coffee grinder

¼ teaspoon vanilla extract

Life is not all about chocolate, after all. (We thought it was, for a minute.) Sometimes you just want white cake, right? Enjoy this with the simple buttercream frosting or leave that off and use the cake as a shortcake with sliced fresh strawberries and whipped stevia-sweetened cream on top—how fabulous! Or try the Whipped NoCream (page 490) as the topping on your shortcake. You can get adventurous with this basic cake recipe, adding ½ to 1 teaspoon pumpkin pie spice and substituting a heaping tablespoon of pumpkin puree for the water—and you have a pumpkin cake.

1. Preheat the oven to 375°F if using it to bake the cake. Lightly coat a microwave-safe/oven-safe dish with coconut oil spray.

2. Make the cake. In a small bowl, beat the egg well with a fork, then add the remaining ingredients and stir well. Pour into the greased dish. Microwave for 1 minute 20 seconds, or bake in the oven for 15 minutes, or until top is just done.

3. Make the frosting. Whisk together the ingredients in a small bowl until smooth. Frost the cake.

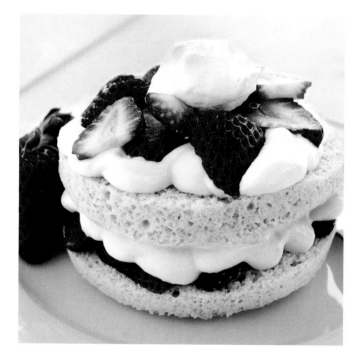

FAMILY CAKES

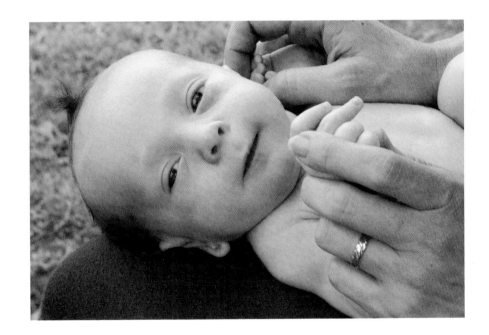

trimtastic chocolate zucchini cake

S

FAMILY SERVE

FOR THE CAKE

Coconut oil cooking spray

1 medium zucchini (about
   1⅓ to 1½ scant cups)

4 large eggs

4 tablespoons (½ stick) butter

¾ cup Trim Healthy Mama Baking
   Blend

¾ cup Gentle Sweet

⅛ teaspoon Pure Stevia Extract,
   or to taste

1½ teaspoons vanilla extract

1 teaspoon aluminum-free baking
   powder

1 teaspoon baking soda

2 pinches Mineral Salt

4 tablespoons unsweetened cocoa
   powder

⅓ cup stevia-sweetened chocolate
   chips or chopped 85% dark
   chocolate

FOR THE CHOCOLATE CREAM FROSTING

½ cup heavy cream

2 tablespoons unsweetened cocoa
   powder

3½ tablespoons Gentle Sweet

Dash of vanilla extract

You're new to plan. You're weaning yourself off sugar. You're craving chocolate, NOW! You feel yourself about to cave to the cupcakes at the bakery down the road. There's no time to mess around with recipe experiments in such dire circumstances. This is an emergency! Make this cake and you'll be comforted with the fact that, yes, you can be a Trim Healthy Mama for the rest of your life. It's so moist, so chocolaty, and since it uses Gentle Sweet, you won't get any weird bitter taste.

So easy—all the ingredients go in your food processor. Zucchini makes baked goods moist and delish, but many recipes get all fussy with it. They make you shred it, then salt it, then squeeze out the water—grrrr. Who has time for all that? Let's make use of the great moisture zucchini brings and just throw it in the food processor. It's the THM way to take the easy road.

1. Preheat the oven to 350°F. Lightly coat an 8-inch square baking pan with coconut oil spray.

2. Make the cake. Trim the zucchini, chop into a few pieces, and process in a food processor so it is not mush but broken down well into very tiny pieces. Add the remaining cake ingredients and process until well combined.

3. Pour the batter into the prepared pan and bake for 35 to 40 minutes, or until golden brown on top.

4. While the cake is cooling inside the tray, make the frosting. Blend all the ingredients in a blender until thickened (or shake in a tightly sealed jar for a minute or two until thickened). Spread onto the cake inside the tray.

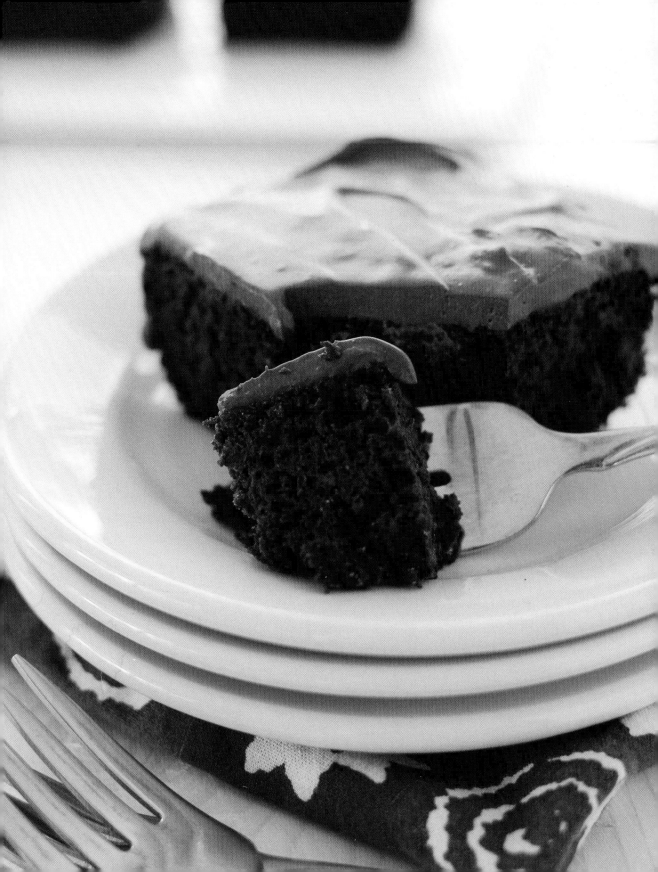

Coconut oil cooking spray

2 large bananas

2 cups old-fashioned rolled oats, ground into flour in a blender

½ cup old-fashioned rolled oats (left whole)

Scant ¼ teaspoon Mineral Salt

2 teaspoons aluminum-free baking powder

1 teaspoon baking soda

½ cup Gentle Sweet

2 to 3 doonks Pure Stevia Extract

1 cup plain Greek yogurt

1 cup egg whites (carton or fresh), lightly beaten

1 teaspoon vanilla extract

1 teaspoon banana extract (optional)

With each bite of this rustic cake you'll help to bury the myth that you can't eat bananas as a Trim Healthy Mama. You sure can, Mate! You just have to do it smartly. Take care of your blood sugar levels and don't go over half a large or one small banana per serving. You're well within that range here, and with the addition of oats, you have a nice rounded E breakfast or snack.

This cake requires no special ingredients (if you have your favorite on-plan sweetener handy)—which is worth several happy dances in itself. Our favorite result comes with Gentle Sweet, but Super Sweet Blend works fine in half this amount or use your own favorite on-plan sweetener. Individual pieces freeze well, so it's perfect for grab-and-go breakfasts. Enjoy this with a dollop of Greek yogurt or Jigglegurt (page 345) or the FP version of NoGurt (page 343). Or Drive Thru Sue's may want a squirt of fat-free Reddi-wip. Our children (and husbands) love this topped with pats of butter for a Crossover, and since we're at goal weight, we gotta admit that we enjoy it that way now and then, too.

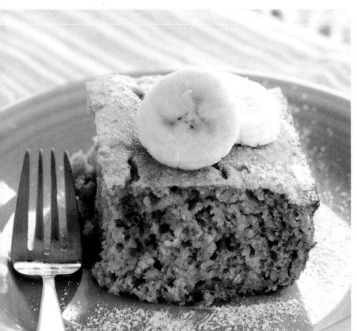

1. Preheat the oven to 350°F. Lightly coat an 8-inch square baking pan or a 9 × 13-inch baking dish with coconut oil spray.

2. Mash the bananas in a large bowl with a fork. Add all the other ingredients and blend well. Pour the batter into the prepared pan and bake for 35 to 40 minutes, or until golden brown on top. Leave the cake in the pan to cool.

NSI (IF YOU USE YOUR FAVORITE ON-PLAN SWEETENER)

lemon curd layer cake   ⓢ

FAMILY SERVE

FOR THE CAKE

Coconut oil cooking spray

1⅓ cups oat fiber (see Note)

⅓ cup Gentle Sweet

2 teaspoons vanilla extract

2 large eggs plus 4 egg whites
   (yolks saved for the curd)

⅔ cup plus 2 tablespoons
   unsweetened almond or cashew milk

2 tablespoons coconut oil or butter

1½ teaspoons aluminum-free baking
   powder

½ teaspoon baking soda

FOR THE LEMON CURD

½ cup (1 stick) butter

⅓ cup fresh lemon juice

4 large egg yolks (from whites above)

5 tablespoons Gentle Sweet

FOR THE FROSTING

½ cup heavy cream

2 tablespoons Gentle Sweet

¼ teaspoon lemon extract

Tangy and creamy, the lemon curd here makes this cake pure bliss for lemon lovers. Oat fiber (not to be confused with oat bran or oat flour) is an inexpensive low-glycemic flour, so it makes this cake budget friendly, too.

1. Preheat the oven to 350°F. Lightly coat an 8-inch square baking pan with coconut oil spray.

2. Make the cake. Put all the cake ingredients in a food processor and process for about 1 minute. Pour into the prepared pan and bake for 20 to 25 minutes, or until lightly golden. Allow the cake to cool.

3. Meanwhile, make the lemon curd. Melt the butter in a small saucepan. Turn the heat to medium-low and add the remaining ingredients. Heat slowly, whisking well, until the mixture begins to thicken. Once the curd reaches a slow simmer, whisk constantly for about 2 minutes as it thickens more. Take it off the heat and place in the refrigerator.

4. Remove the cake from the pan and cut horizontally into 3 layers. Put the bottom layer on a cake stand or large plate and spread half the curd on it. Add the middle cake layer, and spread it with the remaining curd. Add the top layer.

5. Make the frosting. Combine the ingredients in a blender or beat with an electric egg mixer until smooth. Use to frost the top of the cake.

NOTE: You can find oat fiber at www.trimhealthymama.com or at other online health stores.

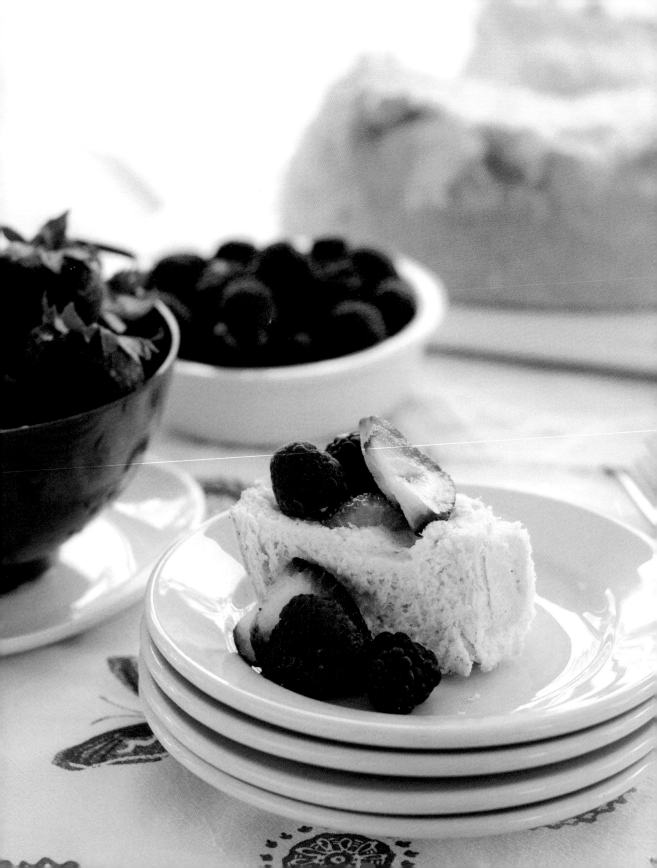

butterfly wings cake

FAMILY SERVE

½ teaspoon aluminum-free baking powder

½ cup Gentle Sweet

½ cup Pristine Whey Protein

2 tablespoons Whole-Husk Psyllium Flakes, ground in a coffee grinder

6 large egg whites

½ teaspoon cream of tartar, or ¼ teaspoon xanthan gum

Spread your wings, Mama, you're transforming! This cake is usually called angel food, but since the butterfly represents your Trim Healthy Mama metamorphosis into a healthier and more vibrant you, this title fits. With each bite of this light and airy, whimsical cake you can think of yourself rising out of the chains of extra weight and above the health problems that once held you down.

This is perfect with a topping of Slim Belly Jelly (page 478), a smear of store-bought all-fruit jelly, or just topped with fresh berries to stay in FP mode. But for an S, oh my, this makes a fantastic strawberry shortcake with real whipped cream and sliced fresh strawberries. Or, try it with the glosting from the Glosted Raspberry Muffins (page 285) or Whipped NoCream (page 490)!

1. Preheat the oven to 325°F. Line the bottom of a 10-inch tube cake pan or springform pan with parchment, cutting out for any spacer in the middle.

2. In a medium bowl, whisk the baking powder, sweetener, protein powder, and ground psyllium until combined. In a separate large bowl, beat the egg whites and cream of tartar or xanthan with an electric egg beater or mixer on high until soft peaks form. Gently stir in the dry mixture one spoonful at a time until well incorporated.

3. Pour the batter into the ungreased cake pan, spreading evenly. Bake for 30 minutes, or until golden brown on top.

4. Allow to cool fully (see Note) before cutting around the sides to release the cake and remove it.

NOTE: This cake will rise well, but it is normal for it to deflate somewhat as it cools. Some people have success turning their angel-type cakes baked in a tube pan upside down to cool before removing from the pan. You can try this if you want.

chocolate truffle cakes

This is a triple-offer recipe. You get three versions with one basic recipe: Mint Chocolate Truffle, Espresso Chocolate Truffle, or Raspberry Chocolate Truffle. Hmmm, what a hard choice. Poor you! All versions of this cake are a treat to your taste buds, and are incredibly healing to your body, so take your pick or try them all.

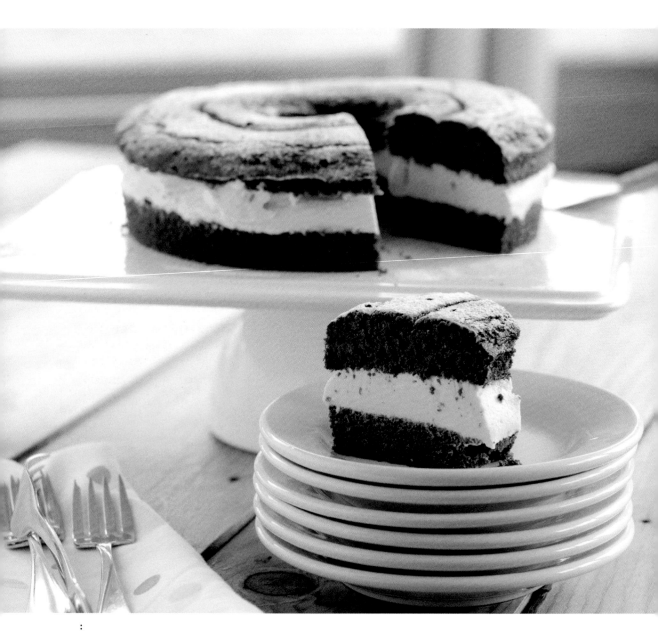

MINT CHOCOLATE TRUFFLE CAKE

FOR THE MINT TRUFFLE LAYER

1 cup hot (not quite boiling) water

1½ tablespoons Just Gelatin

8 fresh spinach leaves (you won't
   taste them)

¾ cup extra-virgin coconut oil

1½ cups frozen diced okra

6 tablespoons Gentle Sweet, plus
   additional for sprinkling

2 to 3 doonks Pure Stevia Extract

1½ to 2 teaspoons mint extract, or
   1 to 2 drops pure essential mint oil
   (to taste)

Pinch of Mineral Salt

2 scoops Integral Collagen

½ scoop Pristine Whey Protein
   (optional)

FOR THE CAKE

Coconut oil cooking spray

1 cup plus 3 tablespoons Trim Healthy
   Mama Baking Blend

½ cup unsweetened cocoa powder, or
   ¼ cup regular cocoa and ¼ cup
   extra-dark

Up to 6 pinches Mineral Salt (only
   2, if using butter)

1½ teaspoons aluminum-free baking
   powder

½ teaspoon baking soda

¾ cup Gentle Sweet, plus more for
   sprinkling on top

⅛ teaspoon Pure Stevia Extract

5 large eggs

¾ cup egg whites (carton or fresh)

½ cup extra-virgin coconut oil or ½ cup
   (1 stick) butter

1 teaspoon vanilla extract

½ cup water

The generous mint truffle layer in this rich chocolate cake is
enough to make any mint lover swoon. But it's not just for
taste. It's a superhero healer in disguise and a good fit if you
have to be dairy-free. It's a tweak on the filling for Secret Silk
Pie (page 330). If you are not a mint lover, try the espresso or
raspberry truffle versions instead.

1. Make the truffle layer. Put the hot water, gelatin, and spinach
   leaves in a blender and puree until smooth and the spinach
   is completely broken down. Add the coconut oil and blend
   again.

2. Add the okra and blend until completely smooth. Add the
   remaining truffle ingredients except the optional whey powder and blend until well combined and perfectly smooth.
   Add the whey and blend for only 10 more seconds. Pour the
   truffle mix into a shallow dish and refrigerate.

3. Preheat the oven to 350°F. Lightly coat a 10-inch Bundt pan
   with coconut oil spray.

4. Make the cake. Combine the Baking Blend, cocoa, salt, baking powder and soda, and sweeteners in a medium bowl.
   Combine the whole eggs and egg whites, coconut oil, vanilla,
   and water in a food processor or blender and process for 20
   seconds. Add the dry mixture and pulse to combine (don't
   overprocess).

5. Pour the batter into the prepared pan and bake for 35 minutes. Put a dish of water in the oven while baking to create
   a steaming effect. Cool the cake, then remove from the pan.

6. Place the cake on a cake stand or large plate and horizontally
   slice it in half, lifting the top half off. Spread a thick layer of
   the mint truffle on the bottom layer, then put the top back
   on. Sprinkle the cake with a light dusting of Gentle Sweet.
   Keep cake refrigerated.

DF (IF LEAVING OUT THE WHEY PROTEIN)

ESPRESSO CHOCOLATE TRUFFLE CAKE

FAMILY SERVE

Everything is the same as in the master recipe, except substitute ½ cup very strongly brewed coffee for the water in the cake ingredients. For the truffle layer, omit the mint extract and the spinach and replace with 1 to 2 teaspoons coffee extract. Add 4 rounded tablespoons of cocoa and 1 cup of strongly brewed coffee in place of the hot water.

RASPBERRY CHOCOLATE TRUFFLE CAKE

FAMILY SERVE

Everything is the same as in the master recipe, except with the option of adding 1 cup frozen or fresh raspberries to the cake batter, and baking it for 5 more minutes. For the truffle layer, make a batch of Raspberry Tart Icing (see page 312) and use that for the middle layer of the cake.

glazed crumb cake

FAMILY SERVE

FOR THE TOPPING

2 tablespoons Trim Healthy Mama
Baking Blend

1 teaspoon ground cinnamon

⅓ cup finely chopped walnuts or
pecans

2 very rounded tablespoons softened
or melted butter (for dairy-free, use
coconut oil)

2 teaspoons Super Sweet Blend, or
¼ cup erythritol

½ teaspoon blackstrap molasses
(optional)

FOR THE CAKE

Coconut oil cooking spray

¼ cup old-fashioned rolled oats,
ground into flour in a blender

1¼ cups Trim Healthy Mama Baking
Blend

½ cup Gentle Sweet

4 doonks Pure Stevia Extract

1½ teaspoons aluminum-free baking
powder

¼ teaspoon baking soda

2 teaspoons ground cinnamon

2 large eggs plus ½ cup egg whites
(carton or fresh)

½ cup plain 0% Greek yogurt

1 teaspoon vanilla extract

½ cup melted butter or coconut oil

⅓ cup water or unsweetened almond
or cashew milk

FOR THE GLAZE

2 tablespoons cream cheese (⅓ less
fat works well)

1 tablespoon room-temperature butter

1 tablespoon plus 1 teaspoon
unsweetened almond or cashew
milk, or water

4 teaspoons Gentle Sweet

½ teaspoon vanilla extract

1. Make the topping. In a small bowl, combine the ingredients for the topping with your hands so you end up with small crumbs or pulse in a food processor. Set aside.

2. Preheat the oven to 350°F. Lightly coat a 7 × 9-inch or 8-inch square baking pan with the coconut oil spray.

3. Make the cake. Place the oat flour in a large mixing bowl and add all the other cake ingredients, whisking well. Pour the batter into the prepared pan, then sprinkle on the topping. Bake for 35 to 40 minutes, or until golden brown on top.

4. Make the glaze. In a small bowl, whisk together the cream cheese, butter, and 1 teaspoon of the milk or water. Whisk until completely smooth, then add the remaining table-spoon of milk or water. Whisk again, then add the sweetener and vanilla. Stir well. Drizzle this glaze over the still-warm cake in its dish in a random fashion.

DF (IF USING COCONUT OIL INSTEAD OF THE BUTTER)

time for lime cake or cupcakes

FOR THE CAKE

Coconut oil cooking spray

2 large eggs plus ⅔ cup egg whites (carton or fresh)

6 to 8 large fresh spinach leaves

1 (15-ounce) can great northern beans, rinsed and drained, or 1½ cups cooked white beans, drained

½ cup Trim Healthy Mama Baking Blend, or 6 tablespoons oat fiber or coconut flour

½ cup Gentle Sweet

2 tablespoons extra-virgin coconut oil

⅓ cup plain Greek yogurt or cottage cheese

¼ cup fresh lime juice

3 to 4 drops essential lime oil (optional)

1½ teaspoons aluminum-free baking powder

½ teaspoon baking soda

FOR THE FROSTING

4 ounces ⅓ less fat cream cheese

3 large fresh spinach leaves

2 tablespoons fresh lime juice

3 drops essential lime oil

½ cup heavy cream

8 teaspoons Gentle Sweet

Made into cupcakes, this cake is a bright, fun treat for parties. But don't wait for a party. This moist, sweet, and citrusy cake with its creamy lime frosting makes a great afternoon snack, or even a breakfast with a Healing Trimmy (see pages 430–433). A few spinach leaves give it a lovely light green hue, but there is no spinach taste—we promise! And you don't have to use any special flours to make this cake; an 80-cent can of beans will do. And you can find coconut flour at most grocery stores these days.

The optional lime oil really, really makes it! Thankfully, pure essential lime oil is one of the least expensive oils. If you don't have an oil dealer as a friend (and who doesn't know an essential oil dealer these days?), you can buy it for about $7 at health food stores. We also suggest it in the Creamy Key Lime Shake (page 408) and for the Key Lime Pie (page 326), so it won't sit on your shelf forever.

1. Preheat the oven to 350°F. Lightly coat an 8-inch square baking pan with the coconut oil spray if making the cake, or line the holes of a 12-cup muffin tin with paper liners.

2. Make the cake. Put the whole eggs, egg whites, and spinach in a blender and blend on high until the spinach is completely broken down; you don't want any little bits of leaf or stalk. Add all the other cake ingredients, then blend well for 30 seconds or so.

3. Pour the batter into the prepared baking pan and bake for 30 to 35 minutes, or for 25 minutes in the muffin tin for the cupcakes.

4. While the cake or cupcakes cool, make the frosting. Put the cream cheese, spinach, lime juice, and lime oil in a blender and process until pureed and smooth. Add the cream and sweetener, and blend another minute or so.

5. Once cool, frost the cake in the pan or remove the cupcakes from the muffin tin and frost cupcakes in the liners. Place the cake or cupcakes in the refrigerator overnight or for a few hours before eating (this takes away any beaniness).

NSI (IF USING COCONUT FLOUR IN PLACE OF BAKING BLEND AND YOUR FAVORITE HANDY ON-PLAN SWEETENER)

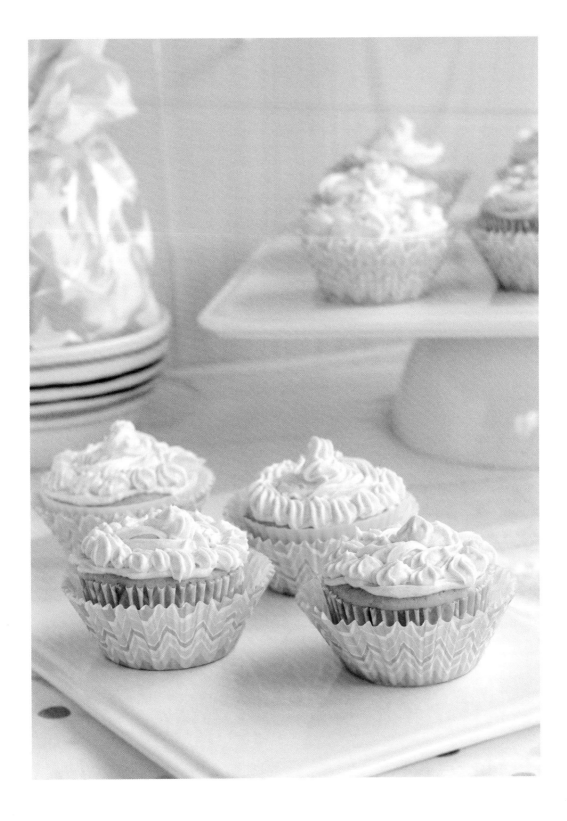

raspberry frosted special agent cake

FAMILY SERVE

S

FOR THE CAKE

Coconut oil cooking spray

1 (15-ounce) can black beans, rinsed and drained, or 1½ cups cooked beans, drained

2 large eggs plus ⅔ cup egg whites (carton or fresh)

4 tablespoons cocoa powder

1½ teaspoons aluminum-free baking powder

½ teaspoon baking soda

2 tablespoons coconut oil or butter

2 teaspoons vanilla extract

⅓ cup plain 0% Greek yogurt or cottage cheese or ricotta

5 tablespoons Super Sweet Blend

2 to 3 doonks Pure Stevia Extract (if more sweetness is desired)

FOR THE FROSTING

8 ounces cream cheese (⅓ less fat works well)

¼ cup (½ stick) butter

3 to 4 teaspoons Super Sweet Blend, or 2 to 2½ tablespoons Gentle Sweet

⅓ cup pureed fresh or frozen raspberries

The special agent in this recipe is once again beans! Don't worry, the amount used here (and in the Time for Lime Cake or Cupcakes, page 306) still leaves you in S territory (fewer than 6 carbs or ¼ cup beans for a generous serving). You'll want to bake, frost, then refrigerate this cake for several hours before eating; that's the trick for no hint of beaniness. You'll have a moist, luscious cake that is so perfect and pretty with the raspberry topping.

1. Preheat the oven to 350°F. Lightly coat an 8-inch square baking pan or a 9-inch round cake pan with coconut oil spray.

2. Make the cake. Put all the cake ingredients in a food processor and process until completely smooth, a couple of minutes. Pour the batter into the prepared pan and bake for 30 to 35 minutes. Allow the cake to cool in the pan.

3. Make the frosting. Put all the frosting ingredients into a blender and process until completely smooth and until the raspberries are fully pureed and incorporated. Frost the cake in the pan or remove and frost—your choice—then place in the refrigerator overnight, or at least a few hours before eating.

NSI (IF YOU USE YOUR FAVORITE ON-PLAN SWEETENER)

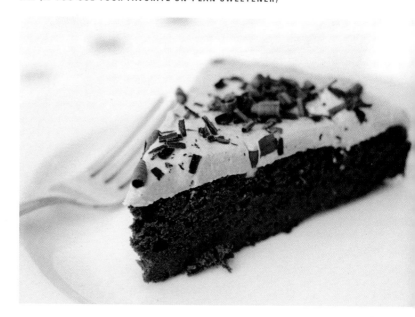

FOR THE ICING

1 (15-ounce) can full-fat coconut milk

2 large omega-3 eggs

1 tablespoon vanilla extract

½ cup unsweetened cocoa powder

4 teaspoons Super Sweet Blend, or
8 teaspoons Gentle Sweet, or to
taste

¾ cup extra-virgin coconut oil

FOR THE CAKE

Coconut oil cooking spray

1 cup coconut flour

½ cup golden flax meal

½ cup unsweetened cocoa powder

⅓ cup Super Sweet Blend or double
amounts Gentle Sweet

2 teaspoons aluminum-free baking
powder

2 teaspoons baking soda

10 large eggs

½ cup extra-virgin coconut oil

1½ (15-ounce) cans full-fat coconut
milk or light coconut milk

1 teaspoon vanilla extract

This makes a very large, moist layer cake that works well for birthdays or other festive occasions. You can find coconut flour, golden flax meal, and canned coconut milk at most grocery stores these days (even Walmart and Target), so that means no special ingredients are needed and it is also dairy-free! That means you can make this cake sooner rather than later. This cake is loaded with the best fats the earth has to offer.

1. Make the icing. Pour the coconut milk into a blender. Add all the remaining ingredients and blend well. Transfer the icing to the refrigerator, where it will thicken and set as hard as butter (might take a few hours).

2. Preheat the oven to 350°F. Lightly coat two 8-inch square baking pans with coconut oil spray.

3. Make the cake. Put the flour, flax meal, cocoa, Super Sweet Blend, and baking powder and soda in a large mixing bowl and whisk together. Blend the eggs, coconut oil, coconut milk, and vanilla in a blender, then add to the mixing bowl. Combine all the ingredients well, then let the batter sit for 5 minutes.

4. Divide the batter between the prepared pans and bake for 30 to 35 minutes. Let the cake layers cool, then remove them from the pans and place one cake on a stand or large plate.

5. Allow the icing to soften a little at room temperature so it becomes spreadable. Spread a thick layer on one of the cakes, then top with the other cake. If there's enough icing left, you can put a thin layer on the sides and top of the cake, if desired.

NSI (IF YOU USE YOUR FAVORITE ON-PLAN SWEETENER)   DF

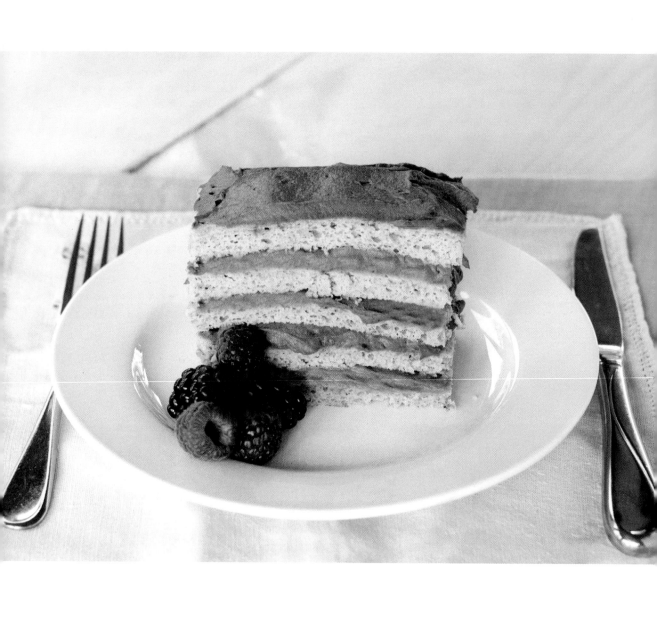

Coconut oil cooking spray

¾ cup Trim Healthy Mama Baking Blend

1½ tablespoons Whole-Husk Psyllium Flakes

2½ tablespoons Gentle Sweet

2 doonks Pure Stevia Extract

1½ teaspoons aluminum-free baking powder

8 ounces radishes, diced but not peeled

½ teaspoon Gluccie

2 tablespoons coconut oil

3 large eggs plus 6 egg whites

2 teaspoons vanilla extract

¼ teaspoon Sunflower Lecithin (optional)

Princess Icing (recipe follows) or Raspberry Tart Icing (recipe follows)

Imagine a world where someone who needs to lose weight or find renewed health is told to eat a large slab of cake for dinner. That world is not just in fairy tales—it's your world now. One where cake whittles the waistline and floods the body with vitality and vigor.

This cake has all the healthy components of a well-rounded S meal. It contains veggies (although you'd never know it), a balanced amino-acid protein profile, prebiotic cleansing fiber, and superfoods, including thermogenic fat of the healthiest kind. Go ahead—don't just have a little piece for dessert; eat a big ol' one for dinner! Pair it with some Tummy Tucking Ice Cream (page 363) and you'll feel full and satisfied. You haven't spoiled your dinner, you've perfected it. Live a little and don't stick cake on the dessert menu only (although we guess you are allowed to eat this as a dessert, too).

The cake is pleasantly sweet but not so sickly sweet that you couldn't eat your fill of it. Depending on which of the two icings you choose, you get either a double dose of carefully chosen, nutrient-dense, and weight-reducing veggies or a serving of high-antioxidant red raspberries. The Princess Icing is soft and sweet, the Raspberry Tart Icing is bursting with tangy berry flavor. And Mamas with food sensitivities, take notice! This cake is completely gluten- and dairy-free!

1. Preheat the oven to 350°F. Lightly coat a large baking sheet or 2 smaller ones with the coconut oil spray.

2. Place the Baking Blend, psyllium flakes, Gentle Sweet, stevia extract, and baking powder in a large bowl. Put the radishes, Gluccie, coconut oil, eggs and egg whites, vanilla, and lecithin (if using) in a blender and process to a smooth puree. Add the puree to the dry ingredients in the bowl and mix well, until smooth.

3. Spread the batter on the baking sheets until ⅓ to ½ inch thick, as if you were making focaccia. Bake for 30 minutes. When cooled, slice into 2 by 4-inch rectangles that can be stacked one on top of the other.

4. Spread whichever icing you choose on each layer, then top with the remaining layers. Ultimately, the number of tiers you end up with will depend on how many layers you use to form a cake.

PRINCESS ICING

1 cup diced radishes

1 small egg-size chunk of raw beet

½ cup water

2¼ teaspoons Just Gelatin

½ cup extra-virgin coconut oil

¼ teaspoon Gluccie

⅛ teaspoon Sunflower Lecithin (optional)

3 teaspoons vanilla extract

1 scoop Integral Collagen

3 teaspoons Super Sweet Blend

3 pinches Mineral Salt

So-named so by Breeze, Serene's five-year-old daughter, because this is a lovely pink color. She managed to get two Princess titles in this book (Princess Taters, page 220).

1. Place the radishes, beet, and water in a small saucepan set over high heat and bring to a boil. Cover, lower the heat, and simmer until the veggies are soft.

2. Drain off the cooking water into a ½ cup measure and top it off with hot water (some of the original water may have evaporated during cooking time). Place in a blender, add the gelatin and coconut oil, and blend well. Add the radishes and beet, as well as the Gluccie, lecithin (if using), vanilla, collagen, Super Sweet Blend, and salt. Blend until smooth. Pour the puree into a shallow pan and place in the freezer for just a few minutes, then move to the refrigerator to set.

NOTE: We usually double this icing recipe, as it freezes and thaws well for future use. This way we always have a quick icing on hand and it makes Cake for Dinner an easy meal to prepare.

RASPBERRY TART ICING

½ cup hot (not quite boiling) water

2¼ teaspoons Just Gelatin

½ cup extra-virgin coconut oil

1 cup frozen raspberries

3 to 4 teaspoons Super Sweet Blend, or to taste

2 pinches Mineral Salt

2 teaspoons lemon juice

2 drops essential lemon oil (optional)

¼ teaspoon Sunflower Lecithin (optional)

¼ teaspoon Gluccie

1 scoop Integral Collagen

½ teaspoon vanilla extract

1. Place the hot water, gelatin, and coconut oil in a blender and blend until smooth. Add all the other ingredients and blend until smooth. Taste to adjust sweetness.

2. Pour the icing into a shallow container and place in the freezer to chill for just a few minutes, then move to the refrigerator to set.

NOTE: We usually double this recipe, as it can be kept in the freezer for future use and thawed when needed.

DF

BROWNIES AND COOKIES

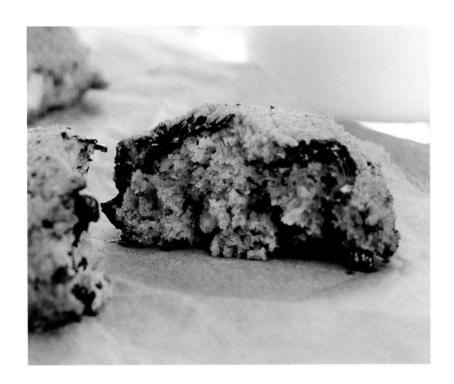

cry-no-more brownies ⓢ

Coconut oil cooking spray

4 ounces unsweetened chocolate

¾ cup (1½ sticks) butter

¾ cup Gentle Sweet

3 to 4 doonks Pure Stevia Extract

1 teaspoon vanilla extract

2 pinches Mineral Salt

½ cup Trim Healthy Mama Baking Blend

½ to ¾ cup coarsely chopped walnuts or pecans (optional)

¾ cup frozen diced okra (see Note)

3 large eggs

Wipe away your grieving tears over the loss of brownies. We'll admit that healthy versions too often do not taste like the real thing, with their weird, catch-in-your-throat texture and bitterness. It's enough to make you cry. Well, cry no more, Mama, 'cause the brownies you have been pining for . . . are back! Not only will they soothe a real sweet tooth but they will also soothe your stomach lining with their healing ingredients and lower your blood sugar levels. They'll help you keep the weight off, not on. Yeehah!!

1. Preheat the oven to 350°F. Lightly coat an 8-inch square or 7 × 9-inch baking pan with coconut oil spray.

2. Place the chocolate and butter in a small ceramic bowl and set above a saucepan of simmering water to melt.

3. Combine all the remaining ingredients except the okra and eggs in a large mixing bowl. Place the eggs and okra in a blender and process until smooth. (If you're using a full cup of okra, you may need to let the okra thaw a bit first or blend in a couple of batches to get it smooth.)

4. Add the puree to the bowl along with the melted butter and chocolate. Carefully stir to combine ingredients; the secret to moist brownies is not overstirring at this point. Pour the batter into the prepared pan and bake for 30 to 35 minutes.

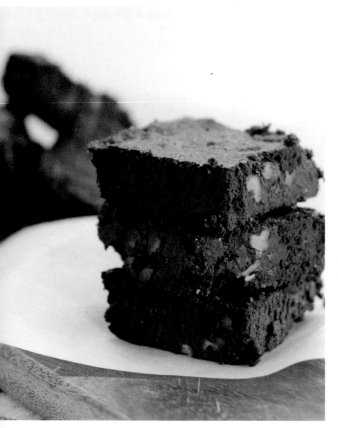

NOTE: Serene uses a full cup of okra, and her most determined okra-hating son asked for these brownies for his birthday after he tried them. That's top secret, so don't tell him. Also, these brownies are perfect left out of the refrigerator and usually get gobbled up before you could think of preserving them, but they get super fudgy when refrigerated so that is another great option.

DF (IF USING COCONUT OIL IN PLACE OF BUTTER)

double peanut fudge swirl brownies

MULTIPLE SERVE

FOR THE BROWNIES

Coconut oil cooking spray

½ cup unsweetened cocoa powder

½ cup Pressed Peanut Flour

1 large egg

¼ cup water

¼ cup melted butter

Pinch of Mineral Salt

⅓ cup Gentle Sweet

2 doonks Pure Stevia Extract

1 teaspoon aluminum-free baking
   powder

½ teaspoon baking soda

FOR THE PEANUT SWIRL

¼ cup natural-style, sugar-free
   peanut butter

¼ cup heavy cream

¼ cup Gentle Sweet

Pinch of Mineral Salt

2 tablespoons water

If you are wild about the flavor of peanut butter and chocolate together, these brownies do not disappoint.

1. Preheat the oven to 350°F. Lightly coat an 8-inch square baking pan with coconut oil spray.

2. Make the brownies. In a large bowl, combine all the brownie
   ingredients and stir until smooth. Pour the batter into the
   prepared pan.

3. Make the swirl. In a small bowl, mix all the ingredients until
   smooth.

4. Spoonful by spoonful, drop the swirl onto the brownie batter. Swirl in carefully, drawing lines through the brownie
   batter. You should be able to see beautiful swirl patterns.

5. Bake the brownies for 20 minutes. Allow to completely cool,
   then refrigerate for best results. These taste the best after a
   whole night in the fridge.

no-bake cookies

MULTIPLE SERVE — MAKES ABOUT 18 COOKIES

½ cup extra-virgin coconut oil (or cooking coconut oil, the tasteless kind, if preferred)

2 cups unsweetened coconut flakes (we prefer big flakes for this)

6 tablespoons Pressed Peanut Flour

¼ cup unsweetened cocoa powder

2 tablespoons natural-style, sugar-free peanut butter

4 to 5 teaspoons Super Sweet Blend, ground in a coffee grinder, or 10 teaspoons Gentle Sweet

4 pinches Mineral Salt

DF

PEARL CHATS: A yummy and simple version of those sweet, peanut buttery, impossibly good cookies your aunt brings to the family reunion. Well, perhaps your aunt doesn't, but my husband's aunt does. And while nothing can compete with those, my daughter Meadow came up with this simple but healthy substitute.

1. Warm the coconut oil to liquid if it is solid, then combine with the remaining ingredients in a large bowl. Scoop out rounded tablespoons and mound them on a parchment-lined baking sheet. Freeze until solid.

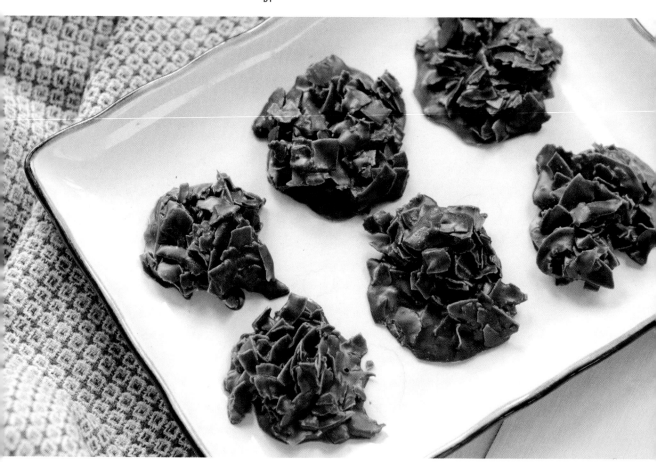

banana meringues

4 large egg whites

¼ teaspoon xanthan gum

2 teaspoons banana or vanilla extract

1½ teaspoons Super Sweet Blend, ground in a coffee grinder

4 teaspoons erythritol

You need an **FP** cookie or two in your life. You don't have to muster up any portion control here and no special ingredients are needed other than your sweetener. These are ultra-**FP** and perfect for when you want to eat something sweet, but you've already had a big, heavy meal. We tried so many versions of these cookies and had to come to the conclusion that Gentle Sweet does not work here; xylitol pulls in too much moisture, so they never crisp up. Super Sweet Blend tastes a little bit strong on its own, so the best bet is to use a combination of Super Sweet Blend and erythritol (or buy a store-bought blend of these). Best to make these cookies in the late evening. If you let them dry overnight in the oven, they will stay crisp for weeks!

1. Preheat the oven to 225°F. Line a couple of baking sheets with parchment.

2. Put the egg whites, xanthan gum, and banana extract in a glass, ceramic, or metal bowl. Start beating the egg whites with an electric mixer until they begin to thicken. Slowly add both the sweeteners a little at a time. Continue beating until the whites are so stiff that you can turn the bowl upside down and the peaks will not fall out, 7 to 10 minutes.

3. Drop spoon-size dollops of batter onto the prepared baking sheets. Or you can get fancy and put the batter in a quart-size zippy bag, cut a hole in the corner, and squeeze out pretty shapes. Bake for 20 to 25 minutes, or until just golden brown. Turn off the oven and let the meringues dry in the oven overnight or for 7 to 8 hours.

NSI (IF YOU USE YOUR FAVORITE ON-PLAN SWEETENER) DF

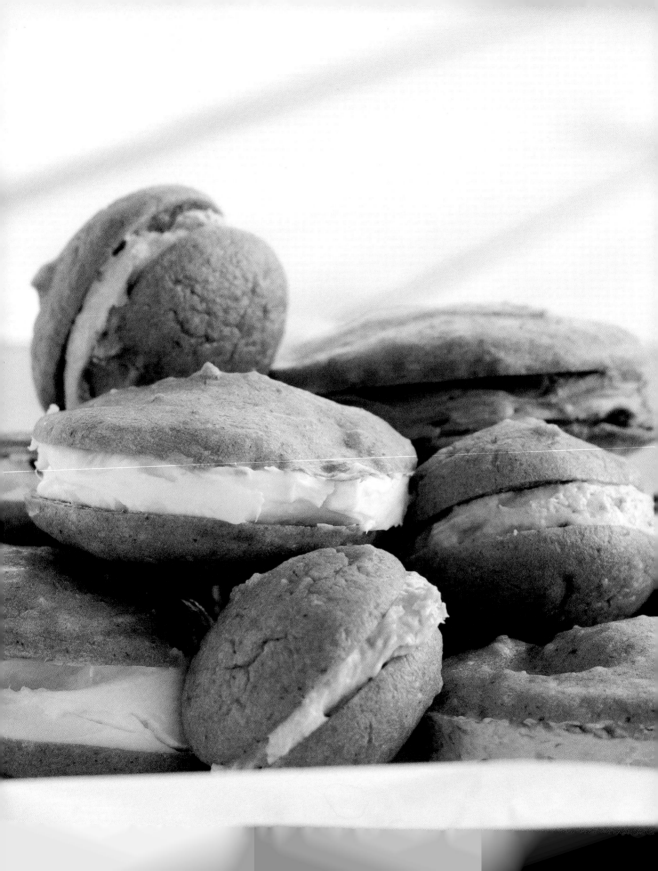

peanut gems

Coconut oil cooking spray

1 cup Pressed Peanut Flour

½ cup egg whites (from carton or fresh), lightly beaten

1½ teaspoons aluminum-free baking powder

6 tablespoons water

1 teaspoon Whole-Husk Psyllium Flakes

4 teaspoons Super Sweet Blend

6 pinches Mineral Salt

1 tablespoon ghee (clarified butter) or melted butter

½ teaspoon butter extract (optional)

Yay for anything peanut! This super-quick, throw 'em together recipe is a winner when eaten warm straight from the oven or used as yummy cookie sandwiches (see below for all our ideas). These "awsies" (short for "awesome") are always gobbled up as quick as we can make them in our homes. You might want to double the batch if you have hungry, eager mouths around you and want any left over.

1. Preheat the oven to 350°F. Lightly coat a couple of baking sheets with coconut oil spray.

2. Combine all the ingredients in a bowl. Drop by rounded teaspoonfuls onto the prepared baking sheets and bake for 15 minutes. Cool on a rack. Stuff the sandwiches (see "Suggested Cookie Sandwich Ideas" below) and chill or freeze.

DF (IF USING GHEE)

SUGGESTED COOKIE SANDWICH IDEAS (THESE ARE S OPTIONS)

- Stuff stiffly whipped heavy cream or Whipped NoCream (page 490) between them and chill (or freeze, then let thaw a few minutes before eating).

- Stuff with extra-thick Slim Belly Jelly (page 478) and whipped cream, then chill (or freeze, then let thaw a few minutes before eating).

- Whip together the following ingredients in a food processor for a decadent creamy filling with just a hint of cinnamon: ½ cup extra-virgin coconut oil, ⅓ cup organic pastured or regular butter, ¼ cup plain 0% Greek yogurt, 2 tablespoons ⅓ less fat cream cheese (or substitute 2 tablespoons additional Greek yogurt plus ⅛ teaspoon Gluccie), 1 teaspoon vanilla extract, 2 pinches Mineral Salt, 1 teaspoon Super Sweet Blend (or 2 teaspoons for "sweeties"), and ½ teaspoon ground cinnamon.

believe it or not chocolate chip cookies

(Makes 24 cookies; nope we're not going to tell you how many to eat; that would be putting you on a diet. You'll learn to tune in to hunger and full signals as time goes on.)

Coconut oil cooking spray

½ cup (1 stick) butter

6 large egg yolks, lightly beaten

1 teaspoon blackstrap molasses (optional)

2 teaspoons vanilla extract

¾ cup Gentle Sweet

1 to 2 doonks Pure Stevia Extract (optional)

1½ cups Trim Healthy Mama Baking Blend

½ teaspoon Mineral Salt

2 teaspoons aluminum-free baking powder

⅓ cup chopped walnuts or pecans

⅓ cup stevia-sweetened chocolate chips or chopped 85% dark chocolate

When people ask you how you're getting so trim, you can just tell them about these decadent cookies and all the other "very undiety stuff" you get to eat. They can believe it or not. (This recipe is another great way to use up those extra egg yolks you don't want to throw away.)

1. Preheat the oven to 350°F. Lightly coat a couple of baking sheets with the coconut oil spray.

2. Mix the butter, egg yolks, molasses (if using), and vanilla in a large bowl until well combined (you can use a stand mixer, a food processor, or mix by hand). Add the Gentle Sweet, stevia (if using), Baking Blend, salt, and baking powder, and blend until smooth, then stir in the nuts and chocolate chips.

3. Drop the dough by small amounts onto the prepared baking sheets and bake for 12 to 15 minutes.

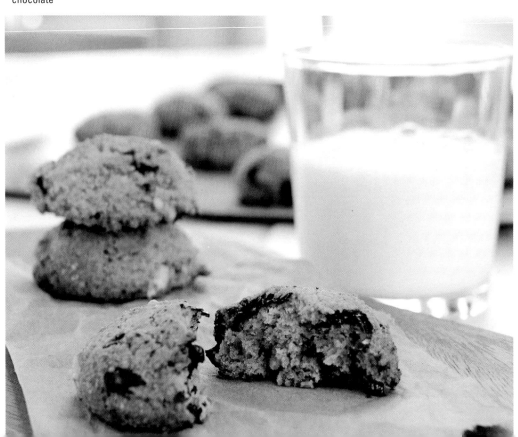

MULTIPLE SERVE — MAKES 20 TO 25 COOKIES

Coconut oil cooking spray

1 cup Trim Healthy Mama Baking Blend

⅔ cup unsweetened cocoa powder

1 teaspoon baking soda

½ teaspoon Mineral Salt

¾ cup Gentle Sweet

4 doonks Pure Stevia Extract

1 cup melted butter, ghee (clarified butter), or coconut oil

2 large eggs, lightly beaten

1 to 1¼ cups frozen diced okra

2 teaspoons vanilla extract

¾ cup chopped walnuts (optional)

⅓ cup chopped stevia-sweetened chocolate or 85% dark chocolate (optional)

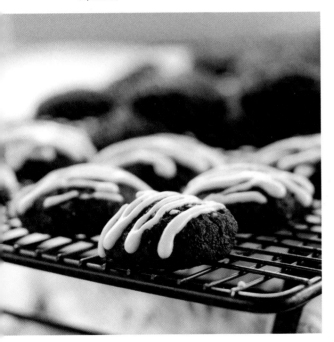

Pure yumserness! Moist morsels of cookie crumb, tantalizing every taste bud while also going to bat for your health, rather than destroying it—now that is what we call a TREAT! After trying these you'll never want one of those sugar-laden junky ones again (well, here's hoping). Oh, and SHHHHHH!!!! These are part of our secret line of foods that is "Mum's the word" when it comes to a revolutionary health ingredient. Oh, by the way, we don't just try and hide this special ingredient in these recipes and hope to get away with it. No, it actually contributes to the moist and pleasant texture. It is a recipe helper, not just a health helper. These are even more amazing with the glosting on top from **Glosted Raspberry Muffins (page 285).**

1. Preheat the oven to 350°F. Lightly coat a couple of baking sheets with the coconut oil spray.

2. Place the Baking Blend, cocoa, baking soda, salt, Gentle Sweet, and stevia in a large mixing bowl and whisk well.

3. Place the melted butter, eggs, okra, and vanilla in a blender and blend on the lowest setting to break up the okra. Switch to the highest setting and blend until everything is completely broken down and creamified. Add the puree to the mixture in the bowl and stir in the nuts (if using) and chocolate (if using).

4. Drop by rounded teaspoons onto the prepared baking sheets and bake for 15 minutes.

5. Cool the cookies on a rack, then place in the refrigerator to let their perfect moisty morsel texture set properly before you experience their ultimate amazingness. If desired, top with Glosting (page 285).

DF (IF USING COCONUT OIL)

PIES, CHEESECAKES, AND COBBLERS

Let's give you some piecrust options first, then we'll bring on the fillings—oh, and cheese-cakes, too! Cheesecakes might have the word "cake" in them, but they're much more like a pie in our minds so they must live here and will have to learn to play well with the others.

simple simon pressed crusts

The following no-bake piecrusts are as easy as Simon says "Pat your head!" If you want a thick crust, use the full recipe as your base. If you want a thinner crust, use only part of the recipe, depending on how big you want to make a crust (often just half is enough for a thin crust in an 8 × 8-inch dish); you make the full amount and then simply roll the leftover into quick treat balls that you can store in your fridge (or freezer) in zippies for snacks. You can always add more sweetener, or even some cocoa, extracts, or flavorings to the Simple Simon treat balls, but you may have to add more coconut oil if you use cocoa powder, as it tends to be drying.

SIMPLE SIMON ALMOND PRESSED CRUST

MULTIPLE SERVE

2 cups almond meal

2 tablespoons extra-virgin coconut oil

5 pinches Mineral Salt

1 to 2 teaspoons Super Sweet Blend, ground in a coffee grinder (see Note), or 2 to 4 teaspoons Gentle Sweet

1. Place all the ingredients in a food processor and process long enough for the almond meal to release some of its oil, then combine with the coconut oil to make moist, pressable dough. Press into the bottom of your dish and chill until firm.

NOTE: These recipes call for ground Super Sweet Blend; we suggest grinding some in a coffee grinder ahead of time and keeping it in a zippered bag for uses like these crusts. But if you don't care about being such a tightwad budgeter (as we are), use Gentle Sweet.

NSI (IF YOU USE YOUR FAVORITE ON-PLAN SWEETENER) DF

SIMPLE SIMON COCONUT PRESSED CRUST

MULTIPLE SERVE

2 cups unsweetened shredded
coconut or larger coconut flakes

2 tablespoons MCT oil (see Note)

3 pinches Mineral Salt

1 to 2 teaspoons Super Sweet Blend,
ground in a coffee grinder

This will be sure to please you if you are a macaroon lover. Coconut calories are also easier for your body to burn than those from almond meal.

1. Grind the coconut flakes in a blender to make a fine meal. Transfer to a food processor and add the remaining ingredients. Process long enough so that the natural oil in the coconut and the MCT oil combine and form a soft dough. Press into the bottom of a Pyrex and chill until firm.

NOTE: The reason we use MCT oil here is that the coconut sets harder than almond meal. If you only have coconut oil, the recipe still works but it sets up more crisp, a little harder to cut through—but hey, that might be what you like, so have at it. Also, this crust is delicious rolled into balls and eaten as a "macaroony" treat.

SIMPLE SIMON PEANUT PRESSED CRUST

MULTIPLE SERVE

1 cup peanut flour

3 tablespoons melted butter, ghee
(clarified butter), or coconut
cooking oil

2 tablespoons water

1 to 2 teaspoons Super Sweet Blend,
ground in a coffee grinder, or 2 to
4 teaspoons Gentle Sweet

5 pinches Mineral Salt

A peanut junky's dream to use with any filling that suits the flavor of peanuts.

1. Place all the ingredients in a food processor and process until you can press the mixture between your fingers and the dough holds its shape. Flatten into the bottom of a Pyrex dish and chill to firm up, then use as a base to the peanut-crusted pie of your dreams.

NOTE: Children and peanut-loving Mamas: You'll love this rolled into balls, and when chilled in the fridge, eaten as little protein bites.

traditional piecrust

MULTIPLE SERVE — MAKES 1 STANDARD 10-INCH CRUST

1 cup Trim Healthy Mama Baking Blend
5 tablespoons cold butter
2 teaspoons Super Sweet Blend
2 large egg yolks
1 tablespoon cold water

This is a prebaked piecrust that is wonderful with sweet treats like the Key Lime Pie (page 326), but also great with savory pies. For the latter, simply omit the sweetener and make a nice crust for your quiche or other savory goodies.

1. Preheat the oven to 350°F.

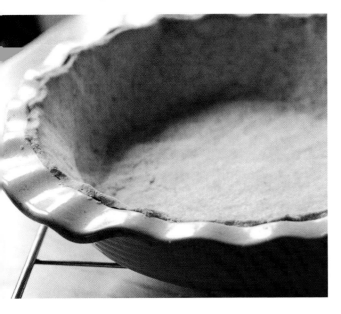

2. Place the Baking Blend, butter, and sweetener in a food processor and process to coarse meal. Add the egg yolks and pulse to mix well. Add the cold water and pulse again. You should be able to press the mixture together and have it stick. If it doesn't, add a little more cold water.

3. Immediately roll out the dough between 2 sheets of wax or parchment paper according to the size of your pie pan. Remove the paper and invert into your pan while slowly peeling off the bottom paper. If part of the crust breaks, that is okay; gently press it back together to fit into your pan.

4. Bake the crust for 10 to 15 minutes, or just until slightly toasted. Let cool before filling.

nut baked crust

MULTIPLE SERVE — MAKES 1 STANDARD 10-INCH CRUST

1 cup almond flour
1 large egg white
1½ teaspoons Super Sweet Blend, ground in a coffee grinder

This is a little simpler than the Traditional Piecrust (above), even though it is also prebaked. This one also can be used for savory recipes if the sweetener is removed.

1. Preheat the oven to 350°F.

2. Combine all the ingredients in a medium bowl, then press into a pie pan.

3. Bake for 10 minutes. Let cool until ready to fill.

NSI (IF YOU USE YOUR FAVORITE ON-PLAN SWEETENER) DF

S

FOR THE FILLING

1 tablespoon Just Gelatin

¼ cup cold water

1 cup low-fat cottage cheese

12 ounces cream cheese (⅓ less fat works well)

2½ tablespoons Super Sweet Blend

2 doonks Pure Stevia Extract (optional)

⅓ cup lime juice (from Key Limes or any old limes)

8 to 10 fresh spinach leaves (optional; see Note)

2 to 3 drops essential lime oil or lime extract (optional)

¼ cup hot (not quite boiling) water

Traditional Piecrust, prebaked (page 325)

FOR THE TOPPING

½ cup heavy cream

2 to 3 teaspoons Super Sweet Blend

There's a lot of joy to be found in a piece of Key lime pie, and that joy only piles higher when you know it is also good for you. You can make this without a crust if you want to get very simple, but we love it with the Traditional Piecrust. Any of the other crusts are suitable options as well. Super Sweet Blend works here for a budget-friendly option, but if you prefer Gentle Sweet, then just double the amount of sweetener. Hey, we know traditional key lime pies are not supposed to be green, but the addition of the few spinach leaves make such a fun limey color we cannot help ourselves. Leave them out if you want.

1. Make the filling. Sprinkle the gelatin onto the cold water and set aside to soften. Place all the remaining filling ingredients except the hot water in a blender and process until completely smooth (you don't want any spinach bits floating around). Add the hot water to the gelatin, stir, and then add to the blender. Process again until smooth. Taste the filling and adjust the sweetness to your liking.

2. Pour the mixture into the cooled piecrust. Chill in the refrigerator for 2 hours or until set.

3. Make the topping. Beat the cream and sweetener with a mixer until stiff peaks form or put into a blender to whip (or put in a jar and shake vigorously for 1 to 2 minutes or until thickened). Spread on the pie and return it to the refrigerator (unless you just can't wait and need a piece right away).

NOTE: If your blender is not up to the task of pureeing the spinach, just leave it out. You can get a nice green color with a drop or two of liquid chlorophyll, or don't worry about turning your pie green.

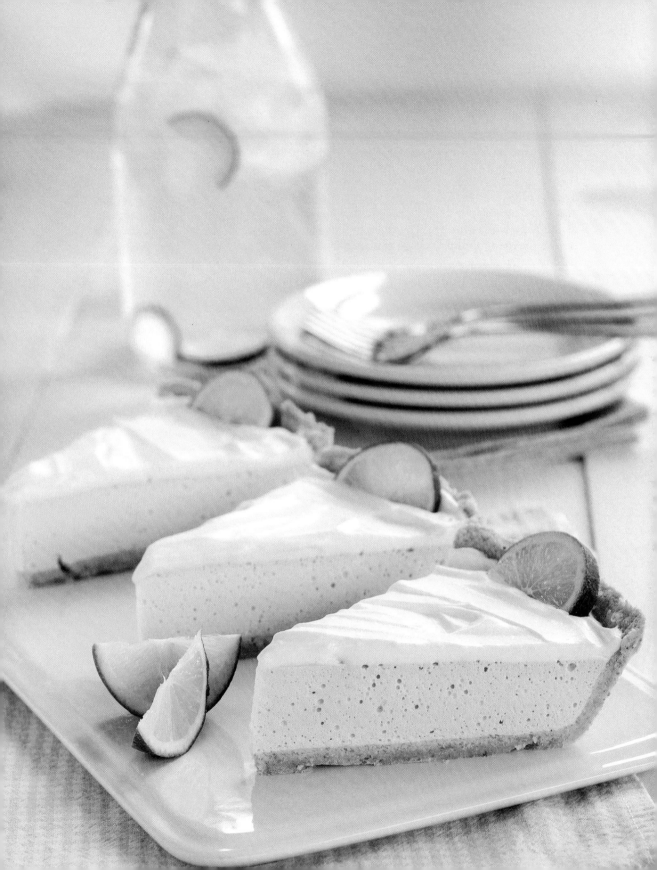

wigglemallow pies

Mmm . . . this pie is so marshmallowy, yet creamy with the cutest bit of a wiggle. We happened on this recipe by accident. We were working on perfecting our Skinny Chocolate Truffles (page 384) and had copious amounts of truffles that hadn't quite hit the bull's eye texture. It seemed horrific to waste them, so we went a bit "mad scientisty" in the kitchen. Lo and behold, this pie was born. It is truly the redheaded stepchild of another recipe, but we fell in love with it and the name just flowed. It was a true *Lion King* moment; we lifted the Wigglemallow cub into the air and proclaimed it heir to a page in the book. Below are our two favorite versions. Mocha would be a nice change, too. The collagen here is for extra protein and a balanced amino-acid profile. Allergen-free folks can use unsweetened almond milk or the cream from the top of a can of full-fat coconut milk instead of the whipped cream or use Whipped NoCream (page 490).

CHOCOLATE CHUNK WIGGLEMALLOW PIE

MULTIPLE SERVE

1¾ cups hot (not quite boiling) water

2 tablespoons Just Gelatin

1 cup extra-virgin coconut oil

1 cup frozen diced okra

¼ cup pastured raw cream or regular heavy cream

1 teaspoon Sunflower Lecithin (optional)

3 tablespoons unsweetened cocoa powder

½ cup Pristine Whey Protein

1 scoop Integral Collagen

4 pinches Mineral Salt

4 teaspoons Super Sweet Blend

3 to 4 teaspoons Gentle Sweet (optional for if you like more sweetness)

2 teaspoons vanilla extract

Piecrust of choice (see pages 323–325), prebaked

⅓ cup chunked Skinny Chocolate (page 377) or 85% dark chocolate or store-bought stevia-sweetened chocolate chips

This is a terrific pie, but an alternative is to layer parfait glasses with cubed Butterfly Wings Cake (page 301) or a cubed sweetened version of Swiss Bread (page 196) with this filling mix and whipped cream. Make two layers of these three tiers for a trifle effect, and let the party begin.

1. Place the hot water and gelatin in a blender and blend until the gelatin is dissolved. Add the coconut oil and blend again. Add the okra and blend until perfectly smooth. Now add all the other ingredients (except the piecrust of course) and chocolate chunks, and blend really super-duper well.

2. Pour the filling into the crust and sprinkle the chocolate chunks over the top. Some will settle into the filling and some will stay on the surface.

3. Transfer the pie to the refrigerator to set for a few hours.

SERVING IDEA: If desired, top the pie with whipped cream or Whipped NoCream (page 490) and shavings of grated Skinny Chocolate (page 377) or 85% dark chocolate.

MINT MATCHA WIGGLEMALLOW PIE

MULTIPLE SERVE

1¾ cups hot (not quite boiling) water

2 tablespoons Just Gelatin

1 cup extra-virgin coconut oil

1 cup frozen diced okra

3 tablespoons mild green powder
(such as barley grass), or handful of
baby spinach

¼ cup pastured raw cream or regular
store-bought heavy cream

1 teaspoon Sunflower Lecithin
(optional)

1 teaspoon matcha powder

½ cup Pristine Whey Protein

1 scoop Integral Collagen (optional)

4 pinches Mineral Salt

1½ teaspoons mint extract and/or
2 to 3 drops essential mint oil

3 to 4 teaspoons Super Sweet Blend

3 to 4 teaspoons Gentle Sweet
(optional for if you like more
sweetness)

2 teaspoons vanilla extract

Piecrust of choice (see pages 323–325)

1. Place the hot water and gelatin in a blender and blend until the gelatin is dissolved. Add the coconut oil and blend until perfectly smooth. Add the okra and spinach (if using), and blend until perfectly smooth. Now add all the other ingredients (even add the whey, as we actually want it to poof in this recipe) except the piecrust. Blend really super-duper well.

2. Pour the puree into the piecrust and place in the refrigerator until perfectly firm.

SERVING IDEA: Top the pie with whipped cream or Whipped NoCream (page 490) and grated Skinny Chocolate (page 377).

secret silk pie

FAMILY SERVE

1 cup hot (not quite boiling) water or coffee or espresso or chai tea

1½ tablespoons Just Gelatin

1 cup extra-virgin coconut oil

2 cups frozen diced okra

Generous 4 tablespoons unsweetened cocoa powder

3 tablespoons Super Sweet Blend, or 6 to 7 tablespoons Gentle Sweet

2 teaspoons vanilla extract

2 scoops Integral Collagen

Pinch of Mineral Salt

½ scoop Pristine Whey Protein (optional)

Simple Simon piecrust of choice (see pages 323–324)

This is an extremely rich pie and is completely dairy-free. It also has its origins in our Skinny Chocolate Truffles (page 384), but instead of being soft and marshmallowy, this is silky and will appeal to those who like intense richness in every bite. Trust us, with this pie just a small slice will suffice. It is so rich it comes with its own portion control. Try it out yourself if you wrestle with overeating issues; it satiates your body with an abundance of healing fats and your mind with that richness you crave, an effect you seldom get with "health food" desserts. It contains a whopping full 2 cups of that amazing secret ingredient we have banned your lips from uttering around other family members. Richness has never been so slimming! You might try adding other extracts or essential oils for unique twists on this recipe—orange and chocolate are wonderful together.

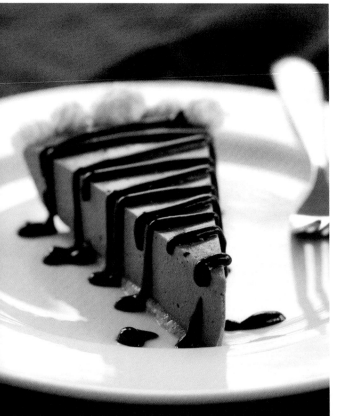

1. Put the hot liquid and gelatin in a blender and blend well. Add the coconut oil and blend again. Add the okra and blend until the okra is pureed. Add the remaining ingredients except the whey and piecrust and blend until well combined. Stir in the whey (if using) and blend for 10 more seconds (not seeking a poof effect here). Taste and adjust the flavors. Add more sweetening (use Gentle Sweet if you need it sweeter) or more vanilla or cocoa to your liking.

2. Pour into the piecrust and chill until firm and set before serving.

SERVING IDEA: This pie can be enjoyed as is or topped with whipped cream or Whipped NoCream (page 490).

DF (WITHOUT WHIPPED CREAM TOPPING)

crema la toppa squares

S

2 cups hot (not quite boiling) water

1½ tablespoons Just Gelatin

2½ teaspoons extra-virgin coconut oil

½ (15–ounce) can full-fat coconut milk, stirred

2 teaspoons vanilla extract

3 pinches Mineral Salt

1 scoop Integral Collagen

2 teaspoons Super Sweet Blend

2 to 3 drops pure essential lemon oil (optional)

Juice of 1 lemon (optional; add another ¼ teaspoon Just Gelatin if used)

Simple Simon piecrust of choice except peanut (see pages 323–324), pressed into an 8-inch square pan (see Note)

A great dessert, breakfast, or snack for our allergen-free Mamas—or for anyone who wants to get more health-promoting coconut and gelatin into their diet in a delicious way. The coconut fat naturally rises to the top while cooling and forms its own pretty layer.

1. Place the hot water, gelatin, and coconut oil in a blender and blend until smooth. Add the remaining ingredients except the piecrust and blend well. Put in the refrigerator to chill for several minutes.

2. Pour the filling into the piecrust and chill in the refrigerator until firm, then cut into squares.

NOTE: If you'd rather not bother with the crust, simply pour the mixture into 6 parfait glasses and chill.

DF

rich custard strawberry pie

S

4 tablespoons (½ stick) butter

⅓ cup Gentle Sweet

3 doonks Pure Stevia Extract

2½ teaspoons vanilla extract

¼ teaspoon grated nutmeg, plus more to sprinkle on top

2 cups unsweetened almond or cashew milk

6 large egg yolks, lightly beaten

1 tablespoon Just Gelatin dissolved in ¼ cup cool water

2 cups sliced fresh strawberries

Piecrust of choice (see pages 323–325), prebaked

This is a decadent way to use up those extra egg yolks you don't want to throw away.

1. Melt the butter in a large saucepan over medium-high heat. Add the sweeteners, vanilla, nutmeg, and ½ cup of the almond milk. Stir well. Add the egg yolks, turn the heat to medium-low, and whisk frequently while the mixture heats and soon begins to thicken. As you notice it thickening, do not stop whisking as you don't want any lumps. Allow the custard to come to a very gentle simmer (do not boil it), whisking the whole time, then remove from the heat.

2. Add the remaining 1½ cups almond milk and whisk well. Add the gelatin dissolved in the water. Whisk extremely well until smooth. (If it somehow gets lumpy, just blend in a blender and it will be fine.) Let the custard chill a bit in the fridge before filling the piecrust.

3. Layer the strawberries in the piecrust and add the filling. Sprinkle more nutmeg on top; refrigerate.

DF

chocolate berry wedding cheesecake ⓢ

FOR THE CHEESECAKE

Coconut oil cooking spray

3 (8-ounce) packages cream cheese
  (⅓ less fat works well)

3 large eggs

3½ tablespoons Super Sweet Blend, or
  ½ cup Gentle Sweet

Juice of 1 lemon

2 teaspoons vanilla extract

Piecrust of choice (see pages 323–325;
  optional), prebaked

FOR THE TOPPING

2 cups fresh or frozen berries

1 batch Skinny Chocolate (page 377),
  melted

Chocolate and berries are true soul mates; once combined, they live happily ever after together. This makes a large cheesecake, sure to impress. You can choose one of the pre-baked crusts here or go crustless.

1. Preheat the oven to 350°F. Lightly coat a 10-inch round springform (or other) pan with coconut oil spray.

2. Make the cheesecake. In a mixing bowl, beat the cream cheese with the eggs, Super Sweet Blend, lemon juice, and vanilla. (If you don't mind tasting batter with raw eggs, taste and adjust for sweetness.) Pour into the crust (if using), or directly into the prepared pan.

3. Bake for approximately 35 minutes. Allow the cheesecake to cool completely.

4. Make the topping. Top the cheesecake with the berries. Drizzle on the melted chocolate and then chill in the fridge so the chocolate sets.

NSI (IF YOU USE YOUR FAVORITE ON-PLAN SWEETENER)

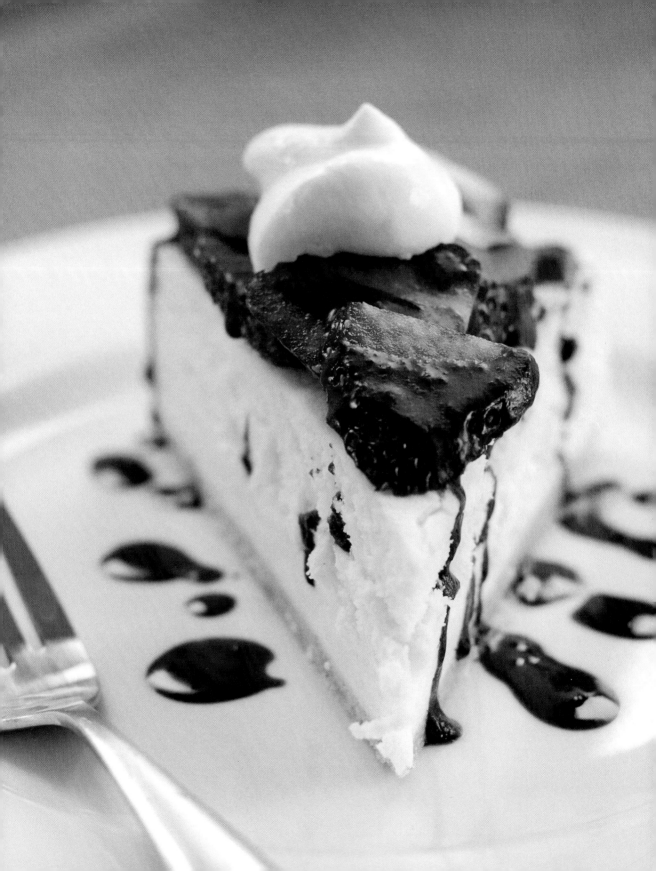

berry nocream cheesecake

FAMILY SERVE

2 cups very hot (but not boiling) water

1 tablespoon Whole-Husk Psyllium
Flakes

2 tablespoons Just Gelatin dissolved in
¼ cup cool water

2¼ teaspoons agar powder

½ teaspoon Sunflower Lecithin
(optional)

2 scoops Integral Collagen

3 tablespoons lemon juice

½ teaspoon lemon extract, or
4 to 6 drops essential lemon oil

2 tablespoons coconut oil

2 tablespoons plus 2 teaspoons MCT
oil (or if you don't have MCT oil, use
half amounts of ghee or additional
coconut oil)

2 teaspoons Super Sweet Blend

6 doonks Pure Stevia Extract

¼ teaspoon Mineral Salt

½ teaspoon vanilla extract

1½ cups frozen or fresh raspberries or
sliced strawberries

3,000 mg vitamin C powder (optional)

1 cup cold water

1 scoop Pristine Whey Protein
(optional)

Simple Simon piecrust of choice (see
pages 323–324), prebaked

SERENE CHATS: *We have no dairy intolerances in my home, but as a purist Freakzoid, my brain doesn't let me enjoy pasteurized cream cheese too often (don't worry, it's just me; Pearl eats it), so I seldom bake with it for myself. I really love the flavors and texture of cheesecake, though, so I enjoy this version regularly. I love it for an afternoon snack with whipped pastured raw cream or Whipped NoCream (page 490) on top. I feel like a spoiled princess when I sit down with my little girls, who love to play tea party with me, and we get to eat something so scrumptious and pretty.*

But I admit it: if you are used to eating real cheesecake on a regular basis, this may not taste exactly like what you are used to. But it is absolutely delicious in its own right, and I'm sure those of you who have had to say goodbye to real cream cheese because of food sensitivities will find it delightfully reminiscent of cheesecake. If you appreciate it for the creature it is (and don't compare), you will fall in love with this light, lovely, luscious, and lip-smacking dessert. (If you are dairy-free, let's hope you'll already have some of these special ingredients, like agar powder and Sunflower Lecithin on hand for, say, making the Hello Cheese (page 487) and Laughin' Mama Cheese (page 484) recipes.

1. Put the hot water, psyllium, dissolved gelatin, and agar powder in a small saucepan and whisk well while bringing to a boil over medium-high heat. Turn off the heat and stir well for 30 seconds.

2. Place this hot mixture in a blender with the remaining ingredients except the whey and blend well, until all the berry seeds are broken up and the mixture is a smooth puree. Add the whey protein and blend well again; you want the poof factor that whey gives, so let the blender go for at least 30 seconds.

3. Pour the filling into the piecrust and chill in the fridge. Do not serve until completely set.

DF (DAIRY-FREE OR THOSE SENSITIVE TO WHEY CAN LEAVE IT OUT AND STILL ENJOY THIS RECIPE, BUT IF YOU CAN TOLERATE IT, THE WHEY MAKES A BETTER, LIGHTER TEXTURE)

cobbler in a jar

S

1 cup Trim Healthy Mama Baking
   Blend

4 teaspoons Super Sweet Blend,
   plus 2 teaspoons for sprinkling over
   berries

3 cups frozen mixed berries

2½ tablespoons butter or coconut oil

4 tablespoons water

This is a wonderful prep-ahead trick you can use to help stay on plan if you work outside the home, or even if you don't! It's so easy. You'll end up with 4 cute jars of cobbler that you can take with you as a delicious snack or dessert, and that will help you resist other far less healthy and slimming temptations out there in the big wide world. This is so easy!

1. Assemble four 8-ounce jars (or ramekins that have lids) on a baking sheet. Preheat the oven to 375°F.

2. In a small bowl, combine the Baking Blend and 4 teaspoons Super Sweet Blend, and set aside.

3. Put ¾ cup frozen berries in each jar. Sprinkle ½ teaspoon each of the Super Sweet Blend over the berries. Then put 2 tablespoons of the sweetened baking mix in each jar and tap the jars so the blend goes down into the spaces around the fruit. Add 2 more tablespoons of that mix to each jar until you have used up all the mix. Tap the jars again.

4. Put 2 teaspoons of the butter onto the top of the baking blend in each jar divided, then add 1 tablespoon water to each jar. Bake for 35 minutes.

5. Allow the cobblers to cool, then screw on the lids and chill in the fridge.

DF (IF USING COCONUT OIL INSTEAD OF BUTTER)

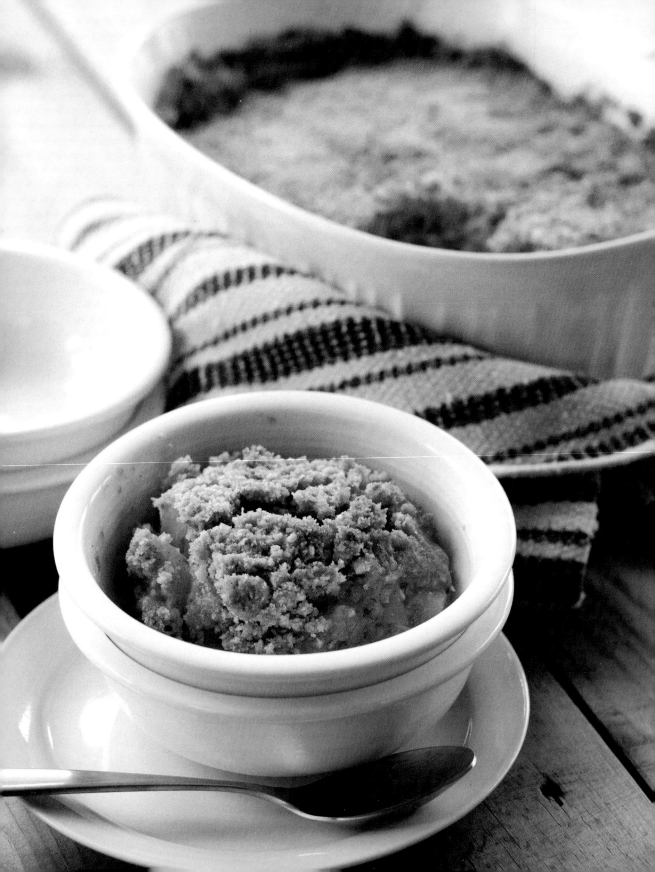

zapple crumble

FAMILY SERVE

FOR THE ZAPPLE

Coconut oil cooking spray

5 medium zucchini, peeled, seeded, and sliced

2½ cups water

Juice of 1 large lemon or 2 small lemons

½ teaspoon Gluccie

¼ teaspoon ground cinnamon

1½ teaspoons vanilla extract

2 tablespoons Gentle Sweet

FOR THE CRUMBLE TOPPING

1 cup Trim Healthy Mama Baking Blend (or ½ cup golden flax meal and ½ cup coconut flour)

3 tablespoons butter or coconut oil

2 pinches Mineral Salt

¾ teaspoon ground cinnamon

2½ tablespoons Gentle Sweet

Generous ½ cup unsweetened shredded coconut

¼ to ⅓ cup chopped walnuts or pecans

We talked about our friend Amelia in our first, self-published book. She was one of the first Mamas to start living the Trim Healthy Lifestyle. She learned the plan from us several years before the plan was ever written into a book, before there were products, before there was . . . well, before anything but our telling her about this food freedom we'd finally found!

Amelia is still going strong and has wrangled in so many new THM converts! She loves to tell new Mamas starting the plan not to complicate things. She did the plan without any special extras for years, and has been able to easily maintain her 30 pound initial weight loss to reach her goal weight all these years later. She has had two healthy pregnancies and births as a THM. She is now pregnant again—her third Trim Healthy Mama pregnancy! Congrats, Amelia, you fertile thing you! Amelia brought this treat over to us one recent afternoon, and we swooned over it. We could barely tell it wasn't made with apples—oh, so close to the real thing but made with zucchini! Hence the Zapple title. Since it is an S, we all indulged in some heavy cream poured over it—divine!

1. Preheat the oven to 375°F. Lightly coat an 8-inch square pan or a 7 × 9-inch baking pan with coconut oil spray.

2. Make the zapple. Put the zucchini, water, and lemon juice into a large saucepan and bring to a quick boil over high heat. Reduce the heat to low and simmer, bubbling gently, for 12 to 15 minutes.

3. Push the zucchini to the side of the saucepan and whisk like mad while sprinkling the Gluccie in slowly from a shaker so it does not clump. Whisk for another minute, then add the cinnamon, vanilla, and sweetener; stir well. Pour into the prepared pan.

4. Make the topping. Put the Baking Blend, butter, salt, cinnamon, and Gentle Sweet into a food processor and process for about 1 minute. Add the coconut and nuts, and pulse until they get chopped a bit more but not completely pulverized.

5. Sprinkle the crumble topping over the zapple and bake for 25 to 30 minutes, or until golden brown. Allow the baked dish to sit for at least 10 minutes before enjoying.

NSI (IF USING OTHER FLOURS) DF (IF USING COCONUT OIL)

apple crumble

FAMILY SERVE

FOR THE APPLE BASE

Coconut oil cooking spray

5 large apples, peeled, cored, and diced

½ cup unsweetened almond or cashew milk

1 teaspoon ground cinnamon

1 tablespoon Gentle Sweet

FOR THE CRUMBLE

1¼ cups old-fashioned rolled oats

1 tablespoon butter or coconut oil

1 teaspoon ground cinnamon

2 pinches Mineral Salt

2½ tablespoons Gentle Sweet

Coconut oil cooking spray

Nothing wrong with the real thing, right? Here's how to make an E-style apple crumble using regular old apples and regular old oats. This is a delish breakfast or afternoon snack with either unsweetened almond or unsweetened cashew milk poured on top. Drive Thru Sue's may want to use a squirt of fat-free Reddi-wip, and we'll just hide Serene's eyes. This crumble doesn't boast a lot of protein so if using alone as a meal or snack, pair it with a Collagen Tea (page 436), a Healing Trimmy (see pages 430–433), or some 0% Greek yogurt.

1. Preheat the oven to 350°F. Lightly coat an 8-inch square pan or 7 × 9-inch rectangular baking pan with coconut oil spray.

2. Make the apple base. Place the diced apples in the prepared pan. Pour the almond milk over the apples, then sprinkle on the cinnamon and Gentle Sweet. Stir together, then set aside.

3. Make the crumble. Place ½ cup of the oats in a food processor with the butter and process until the oats break down into small particles (not a smooth, finely ground flour but a very coarse flour). Add the rest of the oats, then add the cinnamon, salt, and Gentle Sweet, and pulse to combine. You can pulse enough so the rest of the oats get chopped just a little, but you still want them pretty chunky and almost whole.

4. Pour the crumble over the apples, then spray the top with a little coconut oil spray and bake for 30 to 35 minutes, or until the top is browned and a little crisp (you can broil at the end for a few minutes if desired for extra crispness, but watch out it doesn't burn).

NSI (IF YOU USE YOUR FAVORITE ON-PLAN SWEETENER) DF (IF USING COCONUT OIL)

SWEET BOWLS

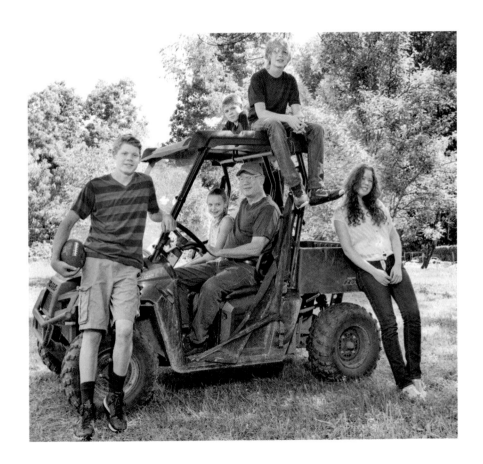

greekie swirl

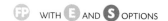

SINGLE SERVE – MAKES 1 TO 2 SERVINGS

2½ to 3 teaspoons Gentle Sweet

1 cup plain 0% Greek yogurt

Dash of extract of your choice

SWIRL OPTIONS

1 teaspoon natural-style, sugar-free peanut butter or 1 tablespoon Pressed Peanut Flour (use more peanut butter for **S** mode)

1 to 2 teaspoons unsweetened cocoa powder

2 tablespoons lemon juice

1 teaspoon all-fruit jelly

¼ to ½ cup berries

Cinnamon Crispy Addictions (page 458)

Diced apple, peach, or mango (for **E** mode)

Handy Chocolate Syrup (page 479)

1 tablespoon Sunflower Lecithin

Such a simple, fabulous, protein-rich snack or breakfast is Greek yogurt. (Don't worry, dairy-sensitive peeps; we have a solution for you coming up that will have you cheering!) The good news is that some yogurt companies are wising up and creating stevia-sweetened Greek yogurt options. Sweetening and flavoring your plain yogurt at home, though, is cheaper and you can make it exactly how sweet you like it (also, store-bought sweetened versions often include inulin (chicory root), which while on plan can make some of us gassy—oh no!). Enjoy up to 1 cup of Greek yogurt as a FP for a full breakfast or snack, and keep to ½ cup if eating it as a dessert after a meal or if you already have another protein source in your meal.

Since Gentle Sweet is already ground, it is a first choice for many of our Mamas when it comes to sweetening up their yogurt, so it is what we have listed here. You can just try a doonk or two of Pure Stevia Extract instead for an ultra-budget-friendly version (small amounts of ground Super Sweet Blend can work, too). The following recipe is the basic one, into which you can swirl any flavors or additions your heart desires. There's vanilla for sure, but try strawberry or raspberry extract if you are including berries.

1. Sweeten the yogurt, add the extract of choice, then add the desired swirl options, and enjoy.

NSI (IF YOU USE YOUR FAVORITE ON-PLAN SWEETENER AND IF YOU STICK TO COMMONLY FOUND SWIRL OPTIONS)

avo cream pudding

SINGLE SERVE

½ ripe avocado

1 scoop Integral Collagen

¾ cup berries (½ cup if using blueberries)

1 to 2 doonks Pure Stevia Extract

½ teaspoon vanilla extract

2 pinches Mineral Salt

OPTIONAL ADDITIONS (SEE NOTE)

4 teaspoons unsweetened cocoa powder (but then increase the sweetener)

2 tablespoons hemp protein powder

1 teaspoon maca powder

1 scoop favorite green powder

½ scoop Pristine Whey Protein (will make it more poofy)

1 tablespoon rehydrated rosehips

Chopped favorite nuts (added after processing)

SERENE CHATS: *Most afternoons during my current pregnancy, Pearl was over at my house because we were busy writing our two latest books. When the munchies hit and my brain and body got tired, I'd whip up this delicious treat. Each time I made it, I'd offer to make Pearl her own serving, but she always said she wasn't hungry. She'd say she just had a big snack before coming to my house, blah, blah. Every time, without fail, though she helped me eat my treat to the bottom of the bowl, always saying, "Just one more bite." She couldn't keep her spoon out of this pudding! I should have learned my lesson and just made extra for her! I guess stealing her preggo sister's portion was just way too much fun for her. She is going to try and delete this comment, but I plead freedom of speech!*

1. Combine all the main ingredients and optional ingredients of your choice in a food processor, and process until smooth.

NOTE: You don't have to put all of the optional ingredients into the one pudding, but you could use one or two or even three—the point is that their flavors don't all harmonize.

nogurts

Heads up, dairy-free Mamas! We spent hours doing science experiments in the kitchen because we felt your distress. Well, actually we didn't literally, physically, feel it, as we thrive on dairy, but we felt ya' in that, "Hey, if you're not happy, we're not happy" way. We know you long for the creamy, tart dairy sweetness yogurt brings. You want to top it with nuts, swirl your berries into it, top your pancakes with it, plop it next to your muffin, or just lick it straight off the spoon. Here is a heart-cheering recipe to lift your spirits. It might not be yogurt, but it might taste even better! We love this stuff and make it frequently, even though we do not have to be dairy-free.

You can find dairy-free yogurt alternatives in the store, but they are often drowned in blood sugar–spiking sweeteners and tapioca starches. You can also ferment canned coconut milk, but that takes a lot of time and is super-rich in calories. We love calories, but a whole can of full-fat coconut yogurt too many times a week is a bit much. This nummy NoGurt is rich in coconut's middle-chain fats, but not too dense that you can't dig into a whole cup (or more) guiltlessly.

NoGurt is healing to the digestive tract—the soothing mucilage in the okra, the healing and anti-inflammatory power of the glycine-rich collagen and gelatin, and the detoxing and constipation-relieving Gluccie all help. Add in the optional probiotics and this yogurt becomes a powerful treat that helps fight gut diseases. Whip it up in a few minutes, then let set in the fridge for yogurt consistency. There's no need to mess with thermometers, heating pads, or pilot lights—or 24 hours of worrying about whether the temperature is just right for inoculation of your starter. Just chill—literally—and relax and enjoy yogurt once again.

We have two versions for you. Give the S version a try first, but then don't forget about the FP version. It's great, too.

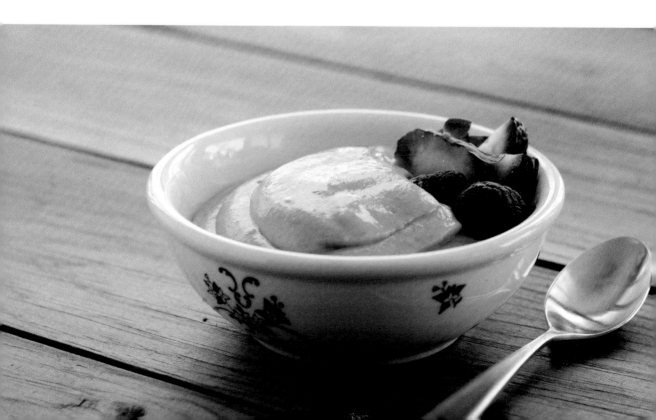

FRUITY NOGURT ⑤ WITH ⑰ OPTION

2 cups hot (not quite boiling) water

1½ tablespoons Just Gelatin

2½ teaspoons extra-virgin coconut oil, or 4 to 5 teaspoons MCT oil

½ (15-ounce) can full-fat coconut milk, stirred well

2 teaspoons vanilla extract

3½ pinches Mineral Salt

1 scoop Integral Collagen

2 teaspoons Super Sweet Blend

4 doonks Pure Stevia Extract

⅓ cup frozen diced okra

1 cup frozen strawberries or raspberries

½ teaspoon natural banana or strawberry extract, or a combination

½ teaspoon Gluccie

Juice of 1 large lemon or 2 small lemons

1 teaspoon dairy-free probiotic powder, or open 2 capsules of same (optional)

3,000 mg vitamin C powder (ascorbic acid, for more of a tart punch), or open capsules, or just blend tablets (optional)

1. Put the hot water, gelatin, and coconut oil in a blender and blend well. Add all the remaining ingredients and blend well until the okra is completely smooth. You won't know it's in there! Taste and adjust the flavors to "own it."

2. Chill in a quart jar with a lid in the refrigerator and allow to set before serving. The setting process takes about 4 hours, and best results are obtained when you stir or shake the jar about once or twice an hour.

FP VERSION — SAME AS ABOVE WITH THESE CHANGES: Add ¼ more teaspoon Gluccie, omit the coconut milk and use 1 extra cup hot water, and reduce the coconut oil to 2 teaspoons (or MCT oil to 3 teaspoons). Add ½ teaspoon Sunflower Lecithin (important for **FP** version) to the first blending process.

DF

NILLA NOGURT ⑤ WITH ⑰ OPTION

Use the same ingredients and preparation as in the master recipe, except omit the okra and the frozen berries. You can add ¼ teaspoon more of the Gluccie if desired for a thicker variety, but it's not necessary. The FP version is the same.

NOTE: Feel free to leave in the okra if you don't mind your yogurt looking green for no reason. Okra is supposed to be kept a secret from anyone you are eating this in front of and in this version there are no berries to disguise the color, but you could eat it in a hidden corner somewhere or use a camouflaged cup.

chia pud

SINGLE SERVE — MAKES 1 TO 2 SERVINGS DEPENDING UPON HOW HUNGRY YOU ARE

FOR THE FOUNDATION

1 cup unsweetened almond or cashew
   milk, or Foundation Milk (page 439),
   but use only water if adding avocado

1 teaspoon Super Sweet Blend

3 pinches Mineral Salt

½ teaspoon pure vanilla extract

½ to 1 scoop Integral Collagen

¼ to ½ scoop Pristine Whey Protein

3 tablespoons chia seeds

OPTIONAL ADDITIONS

½ cup berries (either blended in or
   stirred in after blending)

½ avocado, sliced

1 teaspoon cocoa powder (when using
   cocoa, up the sweetener by
   ½ teaspoon)

1 to 2 tablespoons pressed peanut
   powder

Cinnamon to taste

Ginger to taste

Pure extracts like mint, lemon,
   butterscotch, banana to taste

Pure essential oils like mint, orange,
   lime, chai spice blends to taste

2 teaspoons maca powder

2 teaspoons green superfood powder

2 to 3 tablespoons pastured raw cream
   (this little Pud is meant to be a
   superfood snack keeping in line with
   chia's superfoody status, so
   pasteurized regular cream can be
   used, but is not as optimal)

1 golden pastured egg yolk

Chopped raw nuts for garnish

Cinnamon Crispy Addictions for
   garnish (page 458)

SERENE CHATS: *Chia Pud, as opposed to chia pet—and it rhymes with "good"! It's short for pudding, but you can enjoy this for a breakfast or snack. Hydrating and blood-stabilizing chia provides energy stamina and slays the snacking monster at its ankles. This superfood of the ancient Aztecs has twice the potassium of bananas, three times the antioxidant levels of blueberries, and also triple the iron of spinach! Dig in, Mamas. It's all good!*

Build Your Own Chia Pud—use your imagination; we have listed some flavor ideas but the sky is the limit. At left are suggestions and of course all are not meant to go together in one Pud. Some can be combined but others will not harmonize together. My favorite way to eat this is to add the ½ avocado. Talk about a filling and hearty snack! When I am pregnant or nursing, which is most of the time, I throw in a golden pastured yolk and even some raw cream to boot. When I don't want Pearl eating any of mine and I am not in a sharing mood, I just make sure I put in a toddle of cod liver oil to scare her off. It always works like a charm . . . here she comes diving in with her spoon across the computer where we are working, and I just mention politely about the cod liver oil, and her hand snaps back with a disgusted jolt. Ha! Luv ya, Pearlie!

1. Make the foundation. Blend the milk or water with the basic foundational ingredients and any other additions, but leave out the whey and chia seeds at this point. After the initial blend, add the whey and blend on low for 3 seconds, or just until it combines. Don't let it froth!

2. Pour this blended mix into a refrigerator-safe container and stir in the chia seeds. Let set for at least 4 hours or overnight in the fridge and stir occasionally if you ever think about it. Just before eating, give it a final stir, garnish with whatever thrills you, or enjoy it simply as is, and dig in.

NOTE: If you become a chia pud addict, then we suggest making four batches of the same or different variations at the beginning of the week so you have it when the chia urge hits.

jigglegurt

2 teaspoons Just Gelatin

2 cups water

2 to 3 teaspoons Super Sweet Blend

1 to 3 tablespoons lemon juice, or 1 to 2 drops essential lemon, lime, or orange oil

2 teaspoons vanilla extract, or use 1 teaspoon vanilla and another of a natural flavor extract like butterscotch

1 to 2 teaspoons MCT oil (optional)

3,000 mg vitamin C powder or open capsules (optional)

1 to 2 scoops Integral Collagen (optional)

2 cups plain Greek yogurt

This is just plain yummy and super fun to eat. Even though we still enjoy regular Greek yogurt here and there, now that we have our fridges stocked with this delightful stuff, it's hard for us to go back. But the yumminess factor is not the reason we developed this recipe. There must be balance with all things, and even though Greek yogurt is welcome on plan and considered a Fuel Pull, it can be overdone. It can become such an effortless go-to snack that you may not realize you are eating it multiple times a day, and that can cause an imbalance of your very important amino acid levels. Cultured dairy like Greek yogurt is extremely healthy and, yes, slimming for those who tolerate it well, but we all need to vary our amino acid sources so our bodies can thrive.

There are certain Mamas who find that overconsuming dairy halts their weight-loss progress. They can handle a little, but too much makes that scale get stuck in limbo. Those who have thyroid antibodies may need to stay away from dairy totally (especially pasteurized), and you can try our NoGurts (see page 343), but others may simply need to eat less dairy and incorporate more glycine-rich foods that have balancing qualities before they can start seeing that scale move again (see "Note for Those with Stubborn Weight," page 347). We designed Jigglegurt so these Mamas can enjoy the benefits of yogurt without the problems that occur when it is eaten in excess.

This recipe stretches Greek yogurt to a larger volume so you feel like you are eating more but actually eating less. It also lowers the carbs and calories so it becomes a smarter late-night snack or dessert than Greek yogurt alone. Jigglegurt also saves a buck or two, since you are turning 2 cups of yogurt into 4 cups. So, this is not just for those with stubborn weight issues, it's for budget-minded Mamas, too.

1. Place the gelatin in a 1 cup measure. Add a little cool water, stir to dissolve the gelatin, then add a little hot (not quite boiling) water and give a good stir until you have no clumps. Top off the measuring cup with water to the brim.

2. Place the gelatin mixture in a blender. Add the remaining 1 cup water and all the remaining ingredients except the

(recipe continues)

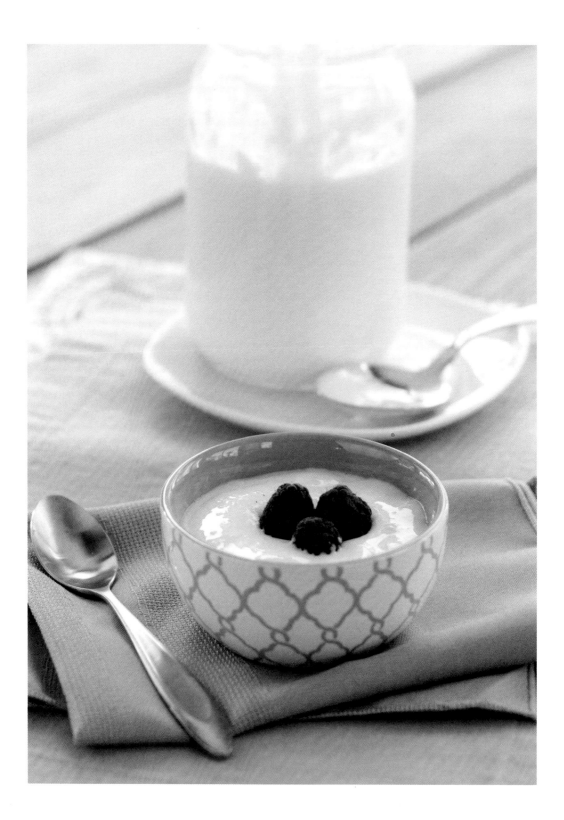

yogurt, and blend to a smooth mixture. Add the yogurt and gently pulse the blender just a few times to combine.

3. Place the yogurt mixture in a container with a lid in the fridge, and chill to set. It will take a good 24 hours to reach its peak, delicate jiggly curd, so be patient.

NOTE: If you would like your Jigglegurt to be more dense, add ½ teaspoon Gluccie to the first blending of ingredients or add another ¼ teaspoon Just Gelatin. And if you become a Jigglegurt lover, you can jigglify your whole tub of yogurt by doubling all the recipe's ingredients. That way, if you previously had to buy two containers of yogurt per week, now you'll get by with just one.

NOTE FOR THOSE WITH STUBBORN WEIGHT

This topic is explained in more detail in the "Heads Up: Turtle Losers!" chapter of *Trim Healthy Mama Plan,* but here's the information in a nutshell. If you find it harder to control your weight while nursing, or find you gain weight even in this season, then you might have hyper prolactin levels or be overly sensitive to this hormone, which is elevated during nursing. If you have PCOS or thyroid symptoms, but do not respond to most treatments for these, you might want to consider getting your prolactin levels tested and your pituitary gland checked. We've seen Mamas with benign cysts that can interfere with normal prolactin levels, and these can have a big effect on weight.

In both these cases, the way you tweak Trim Healthy Mama for your own challenges can make a huge difference. Dietary changes should include more generous supplementation of Just Gelatin and Integral Collagen (with less whey protein), as well as a diet rich in the bone cuts of meat and bone broth. Slightly reduce the amount of muscle meat (like steak and chicken breast) in your diet, as well as your dairy consumption. This should be easy when filling your other protein needs with glycine-rich collagen treats, drinks, bone broths, and soups. Jigglegurt can help reduce your dairy without cutting it out altogether.

glycine glory pudding

MULTIPLE SERVE – MAKES TWO 1-CUP SERVINGS OR FOUR ½-CUP SERVINGS

2 cups unsweetened almond or cashew milk, or Foundation Milk (page 439)

1 tablespoon plus ½ teaspoon Just Gelatin

1 to 2 teaspoons extra-virgin coconut oil or pastured butter, or 2 to 3 teaspoons MCT oil

3 pinches Mineral Salt

1 teaspoon vanilla extract

1 teaspoon butter extract or other (like butterscotch, maple, banana, or caramel) (optional)

2 scoops Integral Collagen (see Note)

2 to 2½ teaspoons Super Sweet Blend

This pudding smiles with all the benefits of the fat-releasing amino acid glycine in a smooth and sweet, perfect little snack or dessert. Glycine not only triggers your major fat-shredding hormone, but it also can help improve the elasticity of your skin, keeping it firm and youthful as you drop the pounds. Get that spoon ready and snack your way to Trim and Healthy.

1. Put ½ cup of the milk into a small saucepan over medium heat. As it warms, add the gelatin, whisking as the milk comes almost to a boil. Remove from the heat. (If you are using coconut oil or butter, add to the hot milk to soften; if using MCT oil, this is not necessary.)

2. Put the remaining 1½ cups milk and the remaining ingredients, including the MCT oil (if using), in a blender. Add the hot milk and blend well.

3. Pour the mixture into 2 snack-size jars or 4 very small containers, then refrigerate to chill and firm up. Give the puddings a little stir after 1 hour if you think about it; that will disperse any froth or bubbles that might be trying to set at the top.

NOTE: The ultra-budget-saving way to make this pudding is to leave out the Integral Collagen. It's not truly a pudding full of all glycine's glory that way, but, hey, it's got some there in the gelatin itself. The pudding will still be yummy and do your body plenty of good. If using the pudding as a snack or dessert instead of a breakfast, tight-budget Mamas might also use just 1 scoop of collagen instead of 2. You can "**S** it up" if desired with an added tablespoon of raw, pastured cream or heavy cream. Feel free to add 1 tablespoon unsweetened cocoa powder for a chocolate version; however, more sweetener will be needed.

DF

1 package Not Naughty Rice

½ cup 0% Greek yogurt or Jigglegurt (page 345), or the **FP** or **S** version of NoGurt (see page 343)

2½ to 3 teaspoons Gentle Sweet, or 1 teaspoon ground Super Sweet Blend, or 1 to 2 doonks Pure Stevia Extract

½ teaspoon vanilla extract, or ¼ teaspoon butter or caramel extract

½ scoop Pristine Whey Protein, or 1 scoop Integral Collagen (optional)

1 or 2 tablespoons heavy cream (for **S** version)

This makes a large bowl of goodness. You can enjoy it for breakfast or as a snack. A half-portion should be plenty if you are eating it as dessert, but if you are still super hungry, then feel free to eat the whole thing.

1. Drain and rinse the Not Naughty Rice in a colander, then press down with your hands to get rid of any excess water. Put the rice in a small bowl and add all the other ingredients.

2. Chill in the refrigerator until ready to enjoy.

DF (IF USING NOGURT)

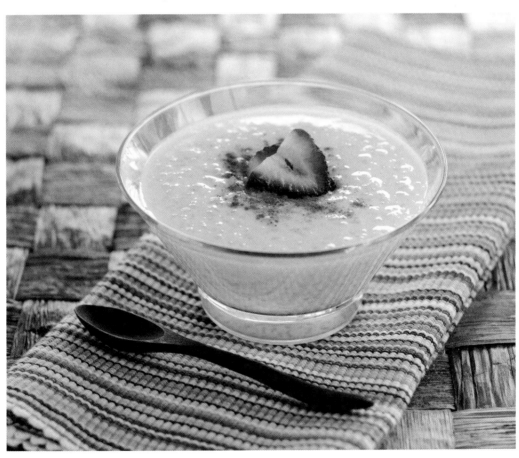

If you have stubborn insulin resistance, pre-diabetes, or full-blown diabetes, this pudding can help your blood sugar numbers. It's fantastic to eat at the end of an E meal if your body gets testy with carbs. If you have high morning blood sugar, try this is as a late-night snack. Even if you don't have blood sugar issues this is a delightful way to help you slim down. Glucomannan has powerful trimming abilities, it alkalizes your body, and it helps you stay full longer. Check out the "Specialty Food Stars" chapter in *Trim Healthy Mama Plan* for more in-depth information on the benefits of our friend Gluccie.

This pudding is great as a dessert after any meal because it has barely any fuel of carbs or fats, which is a nice change from heavy S desserts. We present the master recipe for Salted Caramel Gluccie Pudding and two variations.

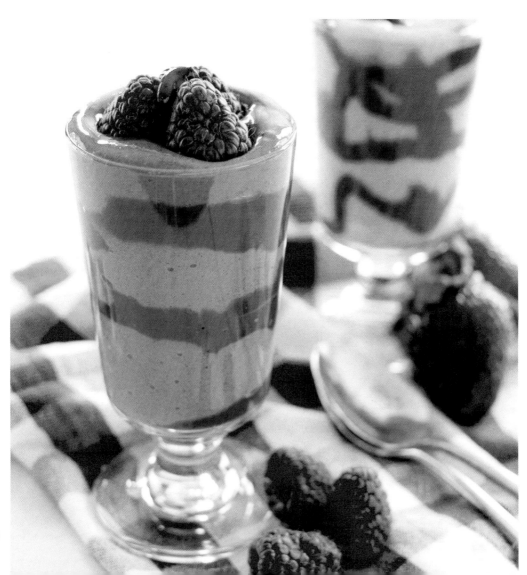

SALTED CARAMEL GLUCCIE PUDDING

MULTIPLE SERVE — MAKES 3 TO 4 SNACK OR DESSERT-SIZE PUDDINGS

2½ cups unsweetened almond or
    cashew milk
2 teaspoons Super Sweet Blend
2 doonks Pure Stevia Extract
Scant ½ teaspoon Mineral Salt
½ to ¾ teaspoon caramel extract
1½ teaspoons Gluccie (see Note)
1 scoop Pristine Whey Protein, or
    1½ scoops Integral Collagen
    (optional)

If you love the Salted Caramel Creamy Oolong (page 434), now you can get more of those scrumptious flavors in a pudding. Aleah Cronk (one of the admins for our social groups) tried that drink and loved it so much she had the brilliant idea of adding those flavors to our Gluccie pudding. We started making our pudding this way, and, oh, man—it's blazin'!

1. Put the almond milk in a blender with the two types of sweeteners, salt, and caramel extract. Start blending on low and then sprinkle in the Gluccie. Blend on high for 1 minute.

2. Let the blender rest for 30 seconds, then resume blending for another 1 to 2 minutes. Just before stopping, add the whey protein (if using) and blend for another 10 to 20 seconds on high. If it's not pudding texture yet, don't worry; the Gluccie will thicken up more after chilling in the fridge for a while.

3. Pour the pudding into a quart-size yogurt container or into four 1 cup containers with lids. Transfer to the refrigerator.

NOTE: This is a loose pudding; if you want it thicker, use another ¼ to ½ teaspoon Gluccie.

DF (IF USING COLLAGEN IN PLACE OF WHEY, BUT WHEY CREATES A LOVELY TEXTURE)

VANILLA GLUCCIE PUDDING

MULTIPLE SERVE — MAKES 3 TO 4 SNACK OR DESSERT-SIZE PUDDINGS

Same as in the master recipe, but reduce the salt to 2 to 3 pinches. Leave out the caramel extract and instead use 2 teaspoons vanilla extract.

MOCHA GLUCCIE PUDDING FP

MULTIPLE SERVE — MAKES 3 TO 4 SNACK OR DESSERT-SIZE PUDDINGS

Same as in the master recipe, but reduce the salt to 3 to 4 pinches. Leave out the caramel extract, and add 2 tablespoons unsweetened cocoa powder. Use 1 cup cooled strong brewed coffee in place of 1 cup almond milk. Increase the sweetener slightly to taste. It's fabulous drizzled with Handy Chocolate Syrup (page 479).

cheesecake berry crunch

SINGLE SERVE

1 generous handful frozen berries
  (about ¾ cup)
⅓ cup chopped dry-roasted nuts of
  choice
2 to 3 ounces cream cheese (⅓ less fat
  works well)
1 doonk Pure Stevia Extract, or
  ¾ teaspoon Super Sweet Blend
Squeeze of lemon juice
⅛ teaspoon vanilla extract
¼ teaspoon almond extract

If you love the taste of cheesecake, you will adore this super-simple but scrumptious treat. Here is a single-serving recipe, but feel free to multiply it by six or eight times, as it is a great dessert to take to parties.

1. Pulse all the ingredients in a food processor to combine and break down a little, but do not process to absolutely smooth.

NSI (IF YOU USE YOUR FAVORITE ON-PLAN SWEETENER)

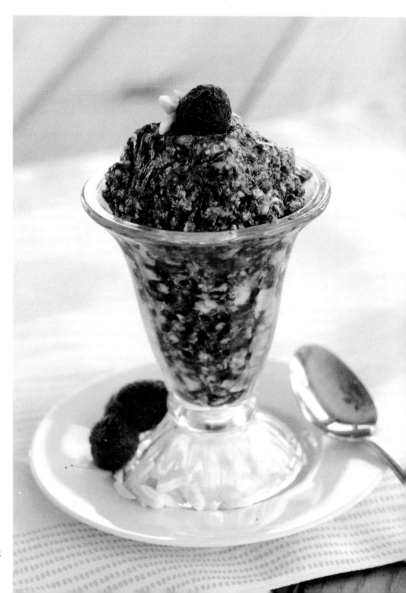

1 medium sweet potato, baked and
   with caramelized skin (see Note)
½ cup well-drained low-fat (1% or 2%)
   cottage cheese
½ scoop Pristine Whey Protein
1 scoop Integral Collagen (optional)
1 teaspoon Just Gelatin, softened in
   2 teaspoons cool water and then
   dissolved in 2 teaspoons hot water
   (optional)
2 doonks Pure Stevia Extract
3 pinches Mineral Salt
½ teaspoon ground cinnamon
½ teaspoon grated nutmeg
1 cup ice cubes

Srumptulicious and full of heartwarming spice, all served up in a cool treat. This is a lovely afternoon mini-meal that gets you through if you still have a few hours until dinner. Your metabolism will start revving for a hearty S meal later that night. This recipe is a wonderful thyroid stoker and adrenal aid, with its healthy dose of carbs cushioned with a large portion of protective protein.

1. Place all the ingredients except the ice in a blender. Blend on low speed for 30 seconds, then on high for 30 seconds.

2. Add the ice cubes ½ cup at a time, making sure the first cubes break down before adding the remainder. Blend until smooth and silky.

SERVING IDEA: If you wish to enjoy this as a smoothie instead, add a little unsweetened almond milk and a handful more ice. Taste and adjust the flavors to "own it". And if you live in the good ole South as we do and have wild persimmons falling from the trees in your backyard, then squeeze a few through some netting and harvest the nutritious sweet, deep orange pulp to use in this swirl. Oh, yeah, baby, the beta-carotene is soaring through the roof in this rendition of Sweetie Swirl.

NOTE: The caramelized skin of the sweet potato gives delicious warm and deep sweet notes. You could also quickly dice and simmer the potato in water until tender, if desired.

bread puddins'

The following five recipes make wonderful grab-n-go breakfasts. Make them the night before; grab them from the fridge the next morning, and you are good to go. They are filling, yummy, protein rich, and a perfect treat for anyone who has to do the THM plan dairy-free. You can also enjoy them as a delightful afternoon snack—or even a lunch. They are quite large, so a half-serving for dessert after a meal is about right. The "bread" part of this pudding is simply the Swiss Bread (page 196) with some sweetener and flavorings.

BANANA BREAD PUDDIN'

SINGLE SERVE

FOR THE BREAD
Coconut oil cooking spray
¼ cup Trim Healthy Mama Baking
  Blend
1 teaspoon Super Sweet Blend
Pinch of Mineral Salt
½ teaspoon aluminum-free baking
  powder
1 tablespoon water
¼ teaspoon vanilla extract
¼ teaspoon banana extract
¼ teaspoon grated nutmeg
2 large egg whites

FOR THE PUDDIN'
1 cup unsweetened almond or
  cashew milk, heated to just before
  boil in a saucepan
½ teaspoon extra-virgin coconut oil, or
  ¾ teaspoon MCT oil
½ teaspoon banana extract
3 pinches Mineral Salt
½ teaspoon vanilla extract
2 teaspoons Just Gelatin
½ to 1 scoop Integral Collagen
  (1 scoop as breakfast puddin')
2 teaspoons Super Sweet Blend

1 small (or ½ large) banana, sliced

1. Preheat the oven to 350°F. Lightly coat an 8-cup muffin tin with coconut oil spray.

2. Make the bread. Combine the ingredients in a small bowl, then divide the batter between 2 of the muffin holes and pour water into the other holes (for a nice steaming effect). Bake for 15 minutes.

3. Make the puddin'. Place all the ingredients except the banana in a blender and blend until smooth, then transfer to the refrigerator to chill.

4. Cut 1½ of the breads (see Note) into small cubes and put into a breakfast bowl (you can use the remaining half bread for another meal or snack). Add the banana, then top with the puddin', using a spatula to help. Stir together and put in the refrigerator to set. It takes roughly 2 to 3 hours for this pudding to set up completely. The longer it chills, the firmer it gets. If you like it less set and more gooey, then eat it sooner or warm it slightly before serving.

NOTE: If you are super hungry and using this as a full meal, go ahead and use both bread muffins in the pudding. However, even with 1½ muffins, this is a filling recipe. Drive Thru Sue's may want to use fat-free Reddi-wip on top for an extra treat.

DF

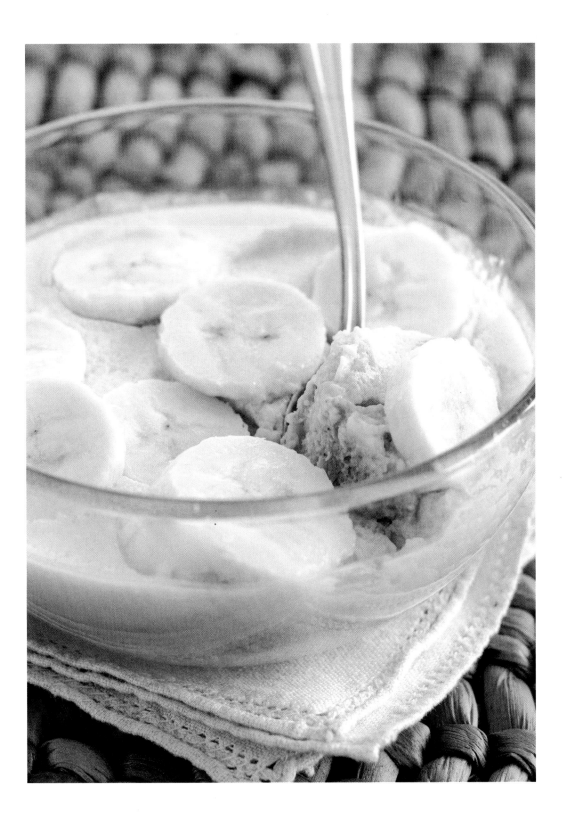

SPONGY PEACH PUDDIN'

SINGLE SERVE

Use the same ingredients for the bread and puddin' as in the master recipe, except substitute vanilla extract for the banana extract. Also, substitute 1 cup frozen or fresh diced peaches for the sliced banana. While the bread is cooking, put the diced peaches and 2 teaspoons water each in 2 or 3 of the empty muffin holes in the muffin tin. Then cook along with the 2 breads so those get a bit gooey and smooshy. Add the cooked peaches to the bowl with the cubed bread, then add the puddin' and stir well. Chill.

BERRY BREADY PUDDIN' OR

SINGLE SERVE

Use the same ingredients for the bread and puddin' as in the master recipe, except omit the banana extract and use only vanilla extract or strawberry extract. Instead of the sliced banana, use ¾ cup frozen or fresh berries and the juice of ½ lemon. Put the frozen or fresh berries in 2 or 3 of the empty muffin holes along with a squeeze of lemon in each hole, and cook along with the breads until gooey and smooshy. Add the cooked berries to the bowl with the cubed bread, then add the puddin' and combine well. Chill. If desired, top with real whipped cream for an S version or use Whipped NoCream (page 490) for a lactose-free version.

DF (WITHOUT THE OPTIONAL WHIPPED CREAM)

APPLE CAKE PUDDIN'

SINGLE SERVE

Use all the same ingredients as the master recipe for the bread and puddin', except omit the banana extract and substitute vanilla extract. Also add ½ teaspoon ground cinnamon or apple pie spice. Instead of the sliced banana, use 1 diced apple, the juice of ½ lemon, and a pinch of ground cinnamon. Put the diced apple pieces in 2 or 3 of the empty muffin holes in the tin along with a squeeze of lemon and the extra cinnamon in each hole, and cook along with the bread. Add the cooked apple to the bowl with the cubed bread, then add the puddin' and combine. Chill.

CRANBERRY NUT PUDDIN' WITH FP OPTION

SINGLE SERVE

Use all the same ingredients as in the master recipe for the bread and puddin', except omit the banana extract and replace with almond extract. Use ¼ cup chopped cranberries instead of the sliced bananas and add ⅛ to ¼ cup slithered almonds (use just a small amount of almonds for FP). Put the cranberries in 2 or 3 of the empty holes in the muffin tin along with a couple teaspoons of water in each hole, and cook along with the bread. Add the cooked cranberries to the bowl along with the cubed bread, then add the puddin' and combine. Chill.

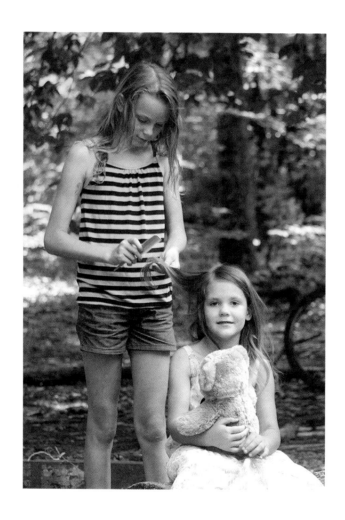

trim freezes

Welcome Trim Freeze into your life. This frozen treat makes a very large bowl of soft-serve ice cream all for you (unless you are nice enough to share with begging children or husbands), and it is super quick to whip up. If you prefer that sugar-sweet taste, try the Trim Freeze with double amounts of Gentle Sweet rather than using Super Sweet Blend.

ORANGE SHERBET TRIM FREEZE (FP) WITH (S) OPTION

SINGLE SERVE

¼ cup low-fat cottage cheese or
   reduced-fat ricotta

¼ cup unsweetened almond or
   cashew milk

¼ scoop Pristine Whey Protein

About 12 large ice cubes

4 baby carrots (for color and added
   health benefits)

1½ teaspoons orange extract, and/or
   1 to 2 drops pure essential orange oil

2 to 3 teaspoons Super Sweet Blend,
   or 2 to 3 doonks Pure Stevia Extract

Squeeze of lemon juice

1. Put a ceramic bowl in the freezer so your Trim Freeze won't melt while you eat it.

2. Put all the ingredients in a high-end blender and blend well (if your blender is supercheapo, use a food processor; however, it does not come out as smooth). Keep blending until the ice is completely broken down (this may take a few minutes). You may have to stop the blender and stir a few times, then blend again until perfectly smooth.

3. Scoop the Trim Freeze into the cold bowl and enjoy.

NOTE: For a creamy **S** version, add 1 tablespoon heavy cream.

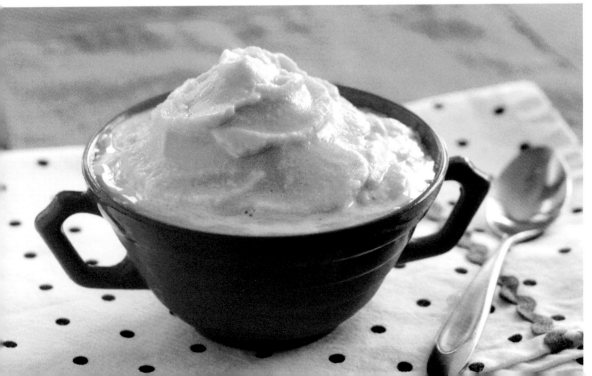

PEANUTTY TRIM FREEZE FP WITH S OPTION

SINGLE SERVE

2 heaping tablespoons Pressed Peanut
Flour

¼ cup low-fat cottage cheese or
reduced-fat ricotta

¼ cup unsweetened almond or
cashew milk

¼ scoop Pristine Whey Protein

About 12 large ice cubes

2 generous pinches Mineral Salt

4 to 5 teaspoons Gentle Sweet, or to
taste

Follow the same instructions as in the master recipe.

NOTE: For an indulgent **S**, add 1 tablespoon sugar-free, natural-style peanut butter.

CHOCOLATE-COVERED STRAWBERRY TRIM FREEZE FP WITH S OPTION

SINGLE SERVE

2 tablespoons unsweetened cocoa
powder

¼ cup low-fat cottage cheese or
reduced-fat ricotta

¼ cup unsweetened almond or
cashew milk

¼ scoop Pristine Whey Protein

¾ cup frozen strawberries

6 to 7 large ice cubes

4 to 5 teaspoons Gentle Sweet

Pinch of Mineral Salt

½ teaspoon strawberry extract
(optional)

Follow the same instructions as in the master recipe.

NOTE: For an indulgent **S**, add 1 to 2 tablespoons heavy cream.

tummy spa ice cream

 FP WITH S OPTION

MULTIPLE SERVE — MAKES 2 VERY LARGE OR 3 MEDIUM SERVINGS (HALVE INGREDIENTS FOR A SINGLE SERVE)

2 cups unsweetened almond or cashew milk, plus 1 to 2 tablespoons for blending

1 cup frozen diced okra

2 tablespoons unsweetened cocoa powder

1 tablespoon Super Sweet Blend, or 2 to 3 tablespoons Gentle Sweet

1 teaspoon vanilla extract

3 good pinches Mineral Salt

1 teaspoon MCT oil

1 to 2 drops pure essential oil (such as mint or orange), or ¼ teaspoon extract (optional)

If you love the Tummy Tucking Ice Cream (page 363), then you will definitely fall in love with the Tummy Spa. It tastes every bit as divine, but our "don't tell" ingredient in this version helps moisturize, soothe, and bring anti-inflammatory benefits to your tummy as an extra perk.

1. Place all the ingredients in a blender and blend until completely smooth. Pour into ice cube trays. Place in the freezer to harden.

2. When ready for your ice cream, put the bowl you want to eat it from in the freezer to chill.

3. Process the cubes in a food processor until powdery snow forms. (You can use a high-end blender, but if your blender gives you some trouble, let the cubes thaw for 5 minutes, then continue.) Turn off the processor and, with a spatula, push down any of the mixture that has risen up the sides. Add a little unsweetened almond milk for **FP** or heavy cream or canned coconut milk for **S**. Blend to incorporate into the icy mix and turn it creamy. Process until smooth, then taste and adjust the flavors to "own it."

NOTE: You have the option to add a scoop of collagen or ½ scoop of whey as you do the final blending. If you desire additional tummy spa therapy, and also to make this ice cream less icy, incorporate 1½ teaspoons gelatin dissolved in 1 tablespoon of the almond milk and 1 tablespoon hot water. Add this to the blender with all the other ingredients and proceed with the blending.

NSI (IF YOU USE YOUR FAVORITE ON-PLAN SWEETENER) DF

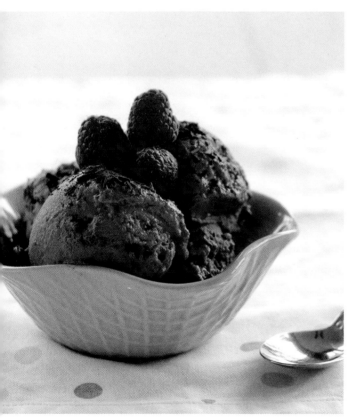

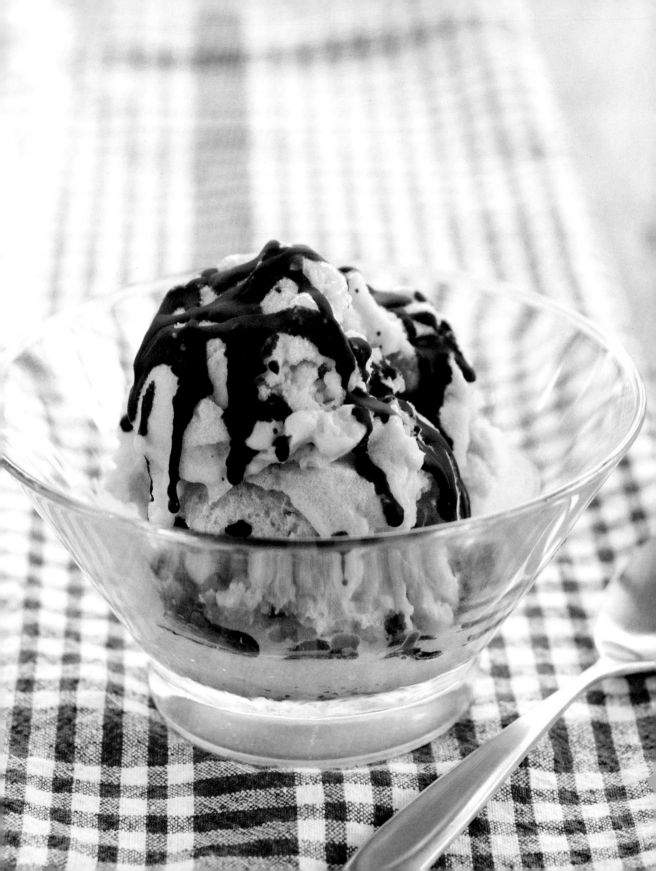

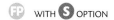
8 to 12 ounces unsweetened almond or cashew milk, plus 1 to 2 tablespoons for blending

1½ to 2 teaspoons Super Sweet Blend, or 3 to 4 teaspoons Gentle Sweet (or more to taste)

1 teaspoon vanilla extract

1 to 2 pinches Mineral Salt

¼ teaspoon Gluccie or xanthan gum

1 teaspoon heavy cream or tahini (or 2 to 3 full tablespoons for **S** option)

Not one special ingredient needed here. Xanthan gum can be found at most grocery stores, but this recipe will even work without Gluccie or xanthan. This makes a generous single-serve batch, but once you try it you may decide to quadruple the amounts next time. That will give you four large bowls of ice cream for your week, ready to be whizzed up in a jiffy. Variations are endless; the following is a basic vanilla recipe, but you can add cocoa for chocolate, or any other of your favorite flavors. Melted Skinny Chocolate (page 377) poured over the top of the basic vanilla version is an amazing S version—just like a chocolate shell.

1. Put the almond milk, sweetener, vanilla, and salt in a blender. Start blending, then add the Gluccie or xanthan. Blend for 20 seconds, then pour the mixture into a large ice cube tray or 1¼ trays (smaller cubes make it easier for less than stellar blenders or food processors). (If you want to use an electric ice cream maker, follow the manufacturer's directions.) Put the tray in the freezer to harden. (It's best to do this early in the day if you want to eat your ice cream in the evening after your dinner.)

2. Once the ingredients are frozen and you are ready for your ice cream, put the bowl you want to eat it from in the freezer to chill.

3. Put the frozen cubes in a high-end blender or food processor and blend or process on high until loose and grainy. If your machine is giving you any trouble, let the cubes thaw for a few minutes to blend more easily. Add the cream and remaining 1 or 2 tablespoons almond milk, and blend again on high or keep processing until mixture starts to be smooth and creamy. Add the other tablespoon of milk only if necessary. (In a high-end blender, like a Blend Tech, you'll get a lovely smooth ice cream texture in a few minutes; a food processor makes things quicker but gives perhaps not quite as smooth an end result.)

NSI (IF YOU USE XANTHAN GUM AND YOUR FAVORITE ON-PLAN SWEETENER) DF (IF USING TAHINI IN PLACE OF CREAM)

creamy indulgence ice cream Ⓢ

2 quarts pastured raw or regular heavy cream

8 large egg yolks

2 generous teaspoons Just Gelatin, softened in 4 teaspoons cool water and then dissolved in 4 teaspoons hot water

2 teaspoons glycerin (see Note)

4 teaspoons vanilla extract

6 pinches Mineral Salt

8 teaspoons Super Sweet Blend

1 teaspoon Sunflower Lecithin (see Note)

3 cups unsweetened almond or cashew milk, or water (see Note)

1 teaspoon Gluccie

SERENE CHATS: *This is a simple yet incredibly indulgent ice cream that my twelve-year-old son Cedar designed one night when he was in a desperate ice-cream mood after his mean mommy said she wasn't going to buy the sugary junk no mo'! As you can imagine, with nine children in my home (and one on the way), birthdays come around frequently. Our children get to eat real store-bought ice cream on their birthdays—yup, the stuff with sugar, but I make sure to buy brands without a whole lot of other junk. Well, my son started getting a taste for that stuff, and he'd been wearing me down and I'd been putting it in my grocery cart even without birthdays to celebrate. My children started digging into it every night. What was I thinking? I had to snap out of it and put my foot down. I told him to create his own healthier version with what we had at home. This ice cream blew me away. Pearl came over to visit and couldn't believe it, either. It is ultra-creamy and just-right sweet.*

This is a winner with children, but you're gonna love it, too, especially if you love rich desserts. My purist pals can even use their raw cream in this for a superfood kick. Yes, this is a very heavy S with all that cream, but for a now-and-then treat . . . oh, yum. Forget annoying ice-cream makers that only make a measly pint or quart of ice cream that usually gets all icy and stuck to the sides (and you have to freeze the bowl before you can even think of beginning). This is simple delightfulness made in the blender—a great way to use up leftover egg yolks, too.

1. Owing to the amounts here, blend the ingredients in 2 batches. For each batch, combine half the cream, egg yolks, gelatin mix, glycerin, vanilla, salt, sweetener, lecithin, and almond milk in the blender. Turn the blender on low and sprinkle in half the Gluccie, continuing to blend on low for several seconds, then blend on high for a full minute. Let it rest for a few seconds, then blend on high again for another full minute.

2. Pour the contents into a large plastic container with a lid. Repeat with the remaining ingredients for the second batch and combine in the container. Place in the freezer to harden.

3. Before serving, remove the ice cream and let it sit out for 10 to 15 minutes to soften a bit. Quick and simple delightfulness!

NOTE: The Sunflower Lecithin is very important in this recipe, as it makes the ice cream less icy and helps combine the cream with the other liquids. If you want to make this less rich and more budget friendly, dilute it with up to 2 more cups water per blending batch and add an additional 1 teaspoon Sunflower Lecithin per batch. Although it was not as creamy this way, our children very much enjoyed it and we thought it was successful for a lighter **S** version. It does take slightly more time to soften to spoonable, though. If your blender is too small to hold the additional 2 cups water per blending batch (making it 3½ cups water or milk to a batch), then you could consider blending in 4 batches.

You can try this without the glycerin. We heard that "real ice cream" needs glycerin to be spoonable. We don't know if this is true, since we have not tried making this without it. We know the Sunflower Lecithin makes a lot of difference, as mentioned above. We tried it without that, and it was not nearly as creamy. You could try a one-quarter version of this recipe to test whether or not it is needed, and let us know, okay?

My wiry children use raw whole milk in this recipe instead of the almond milk, and sometimes use some honey along with the sweetener listed, which then makes it a Crossover for them.

polar bear soft serve

6 cups water

2 scoops Pristine Whey Protein

3 tablespoons Super Sweet Blend, or
to taste

2 tablespoons vanilla extract

6 pinches Mineral Salt

1 teaspoon Gluccie

1½ tablespoons Just Gelatin

3 tablespoons cool water

3 tablespoons very hot (not quite
boiling) water

2 teaspoons coconut oil

2 tablespoons unsweetened almond or
cashew milk

Listen up, late-night snackers! This recipe can help you in times of trouble. It makes a batch of soft-serve ice cream to store in your freezer for whenever an ice cream fantasy hits. It is *ultra* Fuel Pull, and you won't believe how creamy it is. It's so gosh-darn perfect for evening snackies—a time when you shouldn't be taking in oodles of calories because all you'll be doing soon is sleeping. You can add mint extract or pure essential mint oil, or any other flavors you dream up that will harmonize with the whipped white clouds of this soft serve. Grated Skinny Chocolate (page 377) or shavings of 85% dark chocolate are gorgeously delicious sprinkled on top or stirred in. Of course, if you are a chocolate junky for real, you can make your Polar Bear slip into a puddle of tar, turning him into a chocolate brown bear by adding cocoa powder.

1. Place 2 cups of the water, the whey, sweetener, vanilla, and salt in a blender. Start blending, then slowly sprinkle in the Gluccie.

2. In a little cup, dissolve the gelatin first in the cool water and then add the hot water. Make sure there are no lumps. Then add the coconut oil so it melts into the warm mixture. Add to the blender and blend very well.

3. Pour the blended mixture into a large pitcher and add the remaining 4 cups water. Stir well, then pour into 6 ice cube trays. Fill each tray or container about three-fourths full. Put the trays in the freezer to harden. Once frozen, either leave them in the trays or transfer the cubes to zippies.

4. Once you are ready for your ice cream, put the bowl you want to eat it from in the freezer to chill.

5. Take out one serving's worth of cubes (one tray's worth) and put them in a food processor. Whiz until they make a grainy mixture. Add the milk, and process a good long time, until creamy and light. You might need to pulse the machine a few times, then turn it off and push some of the mixture down, then resume. You don't want it icy, so let it cream up well. (You could also use a high-end blender, letting it whir on low speed at first to break up the cubes, then slowly raise the speed and blend until whipped. The blender gives a lighter, cloudlike texture whereas the food processor yields a more regular soft-serve texture.)

mangosicles   Ⓔ

MULTIPLE SERVE — MAKES 4 TO 8 POPS

2 cups frozen mango chunks
1 cup water
4 doonks Pure Stevia Extract
1 to 2 teaspoons lemon juice

Enjoy these after any light E meal (if you still have room to reach 45 grams) or after a Fuel Pull meal—you'll be now heading into E territory, but that's fine. You could also have one as a mid-morning snack or evening treat (these do not have protein, so it's best not to have them alone as your important afternoon snack, which needs some protein to get you through to supper time). The number of pops made depends on the size of your molds.

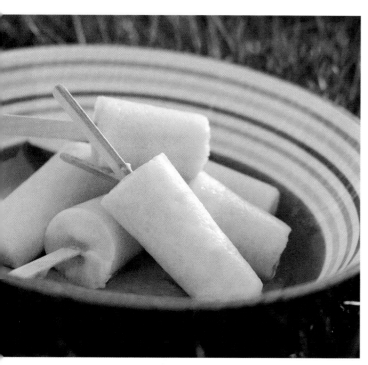

1. Place the mango, water, stevia, and lemon juice in a food processor. Process until smooth. Pour into ice pop molds and freeze until set.

2. To unmold the Mangosicles, run the molds under hot water or place in a bowl of hot water for 30 seconds, then twist gently to release.

NSI (IF YOU USE YOUR FAVORITE ON-PLAN SWEETENER) DF

STRAWBSICLES Ⓕ

Enjoy after any meal as a refreshing light treat. Use all the same ingredients as in the master recipe, except replace the mango chunks with 2 cups frozen strawberries.

mango creamsicles

2 cups frozen mango chunks
½ cup plain 0% Greek yogurt
6 doonks Pure Stevia Extract
1 teaspoon vanilla extract
1 teaspoon lemon juice
½ cup water
2 pinches Mineral Salt
½ teaspoon Gluccie

Sweet and creamy, these are a creamy version of the Mangosicles (page 367). They have a little protein, so now and then they can be a full snack alone.

1. Place all the ingredients (except the Gluccie) in a food processor and process until smooth. Sprinkle in the Gluccie, then process 20 more seconds to combine. Pour the mixture into ice-pop molds and freeze until set.

2. To unmold the ice pops, run the molds under hot water or place in a bowl of hot water for 30 seconds, then twist gently to release.

lemon creamsicles

1 cup unsweetened almond milk
½ cup plain 0% Greek yogurt
½ cup lemon Juice (fresh or from
   concentrate)
⅛ teaspoon grated lemon zest
   (optional)
4 tablespoons heavy cream
1 teaspoon vanilla extract
1 tablespoon Just Gelatin, dissolved in
   2 tablespoons of the coconut milk
   then whisked with 2 tablespoons hot
   (but not quite boiling) water until
   lumps disappear
⅛ to ¼ teaspoon Mineral Salt
2 tablespoons Gentle Sweet
3 to 4 doonks Pure Stevia Extract

1. Place all the ingredients in a blender and blend until smooth. Taste and adjust for desired sweetness. Pour into ice-pop molds. Freeze until set.

2. To unmold the ice pops, run the molds under hot water or place in a bowl of hot water for 30 seconds, then twist gently to release.

creamy fudge pops

MULTIPLE SERVE — MAKES 4 TO 8 POPS

1 (13½-ounce) can light coconut milk

2 tablespoons heavy cream

1 scoop Pristine Whey Protein

¼ cup unsweetened cocoa powder

¼ cup Gentle Sweet

2 to 3 doonks Pure Stevia Extract (optional)

1 tablespoon Just Gelatin, dissolved in 2 tablespoons of the coconut milk then whisked with 2 tablespoons hot (but not quite boiling) water until lumps disappear

1 teaspoon vanilla extract

2 to 3 pinches Mineral Salt

These are delish and reminiscent of pudding pops! They are perfect as a dessert or snack when you need to scratch that chocolately itch.

1. Put all the ingredients in a food processor or blender and whizz or blend until smooth. Pour the mixture into ice-pop molds and freeze.

2. To unmold the ice pops, run the molds under hot water or place in a bowl of hot water for 30 seconds, then twist gently to release.

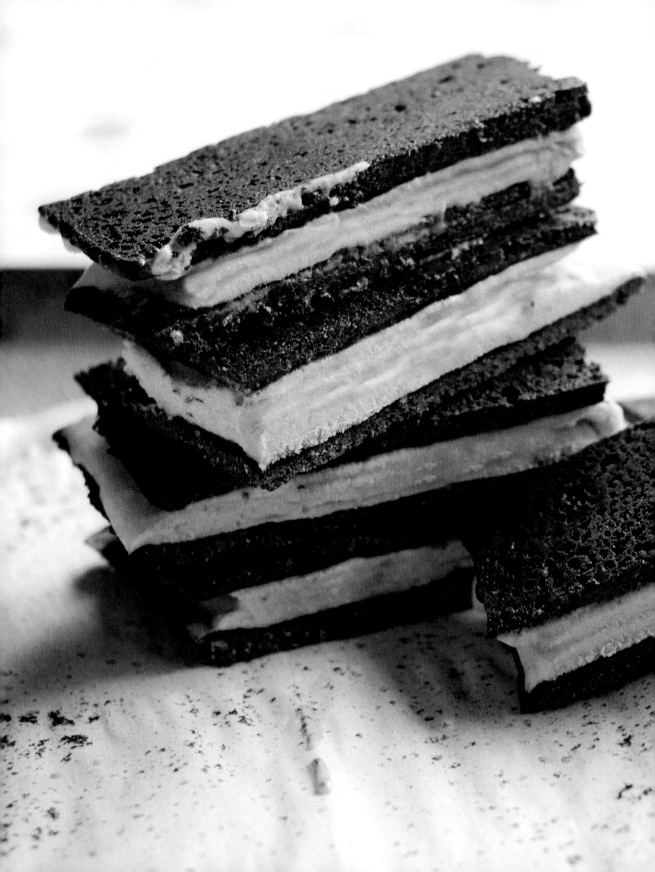

ice cream sandwiches

FOR THE BROWNIES

3 ounces unsweetened chocolate

½ cup (1 stick) softened butter

3 large eggs

¾ cup Gentle Sweet

¾ cup Trim Healthy Mama Baking Blend

1 teaspoon vanilla extract

½ teaspoon Mineral Salt

½ teaspoon baking soda

FOR THE STRAWBERRY FILLING

1 cup frozen strawberries

½ cup cottage cheese

2 scoops Pristine Whey Protein

3 to 4 teaspoons Super Sweet Blend

1 teaspoon vanilla extract

Pinch of Mineral Salt

PEARL CHATS: My daughter Meadow created these sandwich treats literally the night before we had to hand the book over to the publisher. The sandwiches are made from perfectly sweetened moist brownies while the filling here is a whipped strawberry ice cream (similar to Cottage Berry Whip, page 374) that harmonizes beautifully with the chocolate. I tasted it, flipped out, and made sure she gave me the recipe right away so I could pass it along to you.

1. Preheat the oven to 350°F. Line two 9 × 13-inch baking sheets with parchment.

2. Make the brownies. Melt the chocolate in a ceramic cereal bowl sitting atop a saucepan of simmering water over low heat (or melt in the microwave).

3. Place the melted chocolate in a large mixing bowl, add the butter, and beat until creamed. Add the remaining brownie ingredients and beat until smooth.

4. Divide the brownie batter between the prepared baking sheets and spread as thin as you can. The batter won't fill the sheets from end to end, but the point is to spread it thin enough to fill most of each sheet. Smooth the tops with a spatula.

5. Bake for 7 to 8 minutes. Allow to cool for several minutes, then put the sheets in the freezer.

6. Make the filling. Put all the filling ingredients in a food processor and process until smooth, then transfer to a container and put in the freezer to harden.

7. After about 1 hour of freezing, take the brownie sheets out and cut into uniform rectangles the size of ice cream sandwiches (smaller ones are more manageable). Carefully spoon a thick layer of ice cream onto half the pieces, then lightly place another brownie piece on top. The ice cream will not be set yet, so don't squeeze down with the top piece.

8. Put the sandwiches back in the freezer to freeze fully, for several hours.

slushies

Trim Healthy Mama slushies really shine when you want that something extra after a meal, but you know you already ate your full quota. These are a treat with lots of flavor but barely any fuel. They take a while to eat, so they are great to enjoy while watching a movie or relaxing in the shade on a hot Saturday afternoon.

LEMONADE SLUSHY (FP)

SINGLE SERVE

¼ cup lemon juice

½ cup water

12 to 14 large ice cubes

4 doonks Pure Stevia Extract

This lemon slushy can be enjoyed anytime. Think of it as your all-day sipper—it's truly free for whenever you want it.

1. Place the ingredients in a blender and blend very well until the ice is completely broken down. You may have to stop the blender, stir things around, then blend again a couple of times.

NSI (IF YOU USE YOUR FAVORITE ON-PLAN SWEETENER) DF

STRAWBERRY SLUSHY (FP)

SINGLE SERVE

¾ cup water

5 frozen strawberries

Juice of ½ lemon

1½ teaspoons strawberry extract

12 large ice cubes

3 to 4 doonks Pure Stevia Extract

1. Follow the directions in the master recipe.

GRAPEFRUIT SLUSHY (E)

SINGLE SERVE

½ grapefruit, halved and seeded

1 drop essential grapefruit oil
   (optional)

½ cup water

12 to 14 large ice cubes

3 to 4 doonks Pure Stevia Extract

1. Peel the grapefruit halves, leaving a lot of the white pith, which contains the health-promoting bioflavonoids. Place one half in the blender with the remaining ingredients. (Save the other half for a snack with 1% cottage cheese.) Follow the directions in the master recipe.

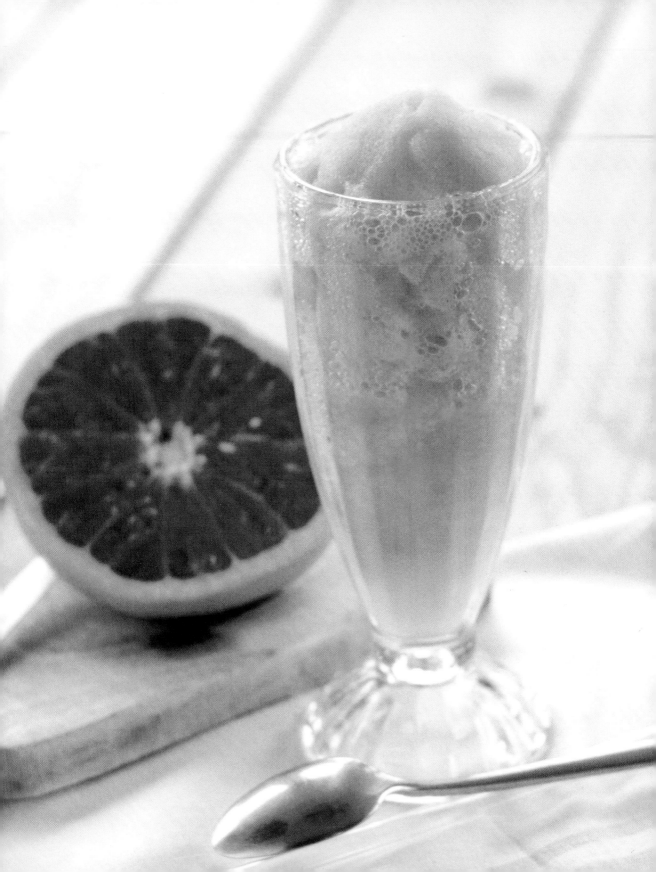

cottage berry whip

½ cup 1% cottage cheese
½ cup frozen berries
2 teaspoons Super Sweet Blend, or
   2 to 3 doonks Pure Stevia Extract

Don't overlook this simple frozen treat even if you detest the thought of cottage cheese. This recipe has won many a Mama over to the cottage-cheese-lovin' side. Whatcha waiting for? Be brave, give it a try, and you'll be surprised. Check out our Cottage Berry Whip video on YouTube, if you want us to take you through the easy steps on how to make this.

1. Place all the ingredients in a food processor and process until smooth.

NSI (IF YOU USE YOUR FAVORITE ON-PLAN SWEETENER)

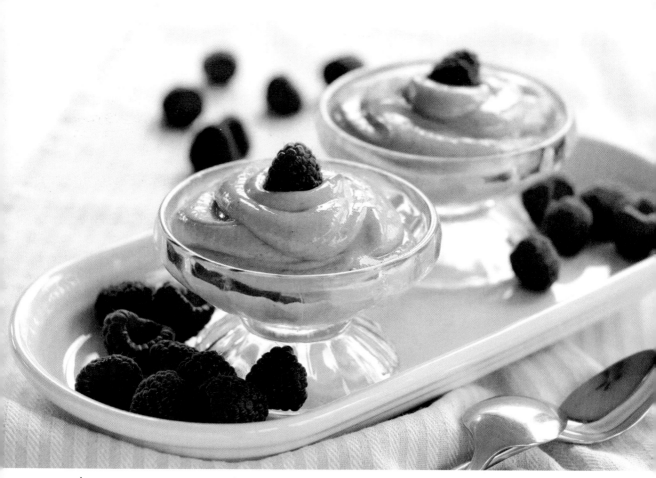

collagen berry whip

SINGLE SERVE

1 teaspoon Just Gelatin

2 tablespoons cool water

2 tablespoons very hot water

½ teaspoon Sunflower Lecithin

2 pinches Mineral Salt

1 to 1½ teaspoons Super Sweet Blend, or 2 doonks Pure Stevia Extract

1 scoop Integral Collagen

Juice of ½ lemon

1 cup frozen raspberries or mixed berries (if you use straight blueberries, you will be in **E** territory, and that's cool if you mean to)

1 teaspoon MCT oil (optional; use 2 teaspoons if full snack, not dessert)

Yay! A frozen berry whip that our dairy-free Mamas (or purists who don't eat pasteurized dairy) can dig into with glee! This is also a trophy recipe for those who have hyper-prolactemia (see the "Heads Up: Turtle Losers!" chapter in *Trim Healthy Mama Plan*) or who have thyroid antibodies and need to stay away from dairy but find that very hard to do. This could be the ticket that takes a plateaued Mama—stagnating because she is overdoing offending foods for her unique system—and puts her back on the road to healthy weight loss.

1. Put a ceramic bowl in the freezer to chill. Put the gelatin in a large cup and add the cool water. Stir, then add the hot water. Stir until completely dissolved.

2. Add all the other ingredients to the cup with the gelatin except the berries and MCT oil (if using). Stir well to combine.

3. Put the frozen berries in a food processor and process to break them down, but don't overdo it. Stop the processor, add the gelatin mixture, and quickly begin processing again so that the gelatin doesn't harden into a clump. Process and whip together until smooth. While the processor is running, add the oil (if using). Turn off, push any mixture that could have flung up the sides of the bowl back down close to the blades, and process for a tad bit more.

4. You are ready to serve. Don't worry if it looks a little thin and melty at first. By the time you put it into your chilled bowl and go get your spoon, it will have naturally started to thicken because of the gelatin.

NOTE: The first time we made this it didn't turn out quite right. We called it a "collagen berry wiggle" instead because it was more . . . Jell-O-ish. But it was awesome in its own right and it makes an even bigger serving of this yumminess so you can share it with a family member or just eat more. Originally we used 1 tablespoon gelatin and added ¼ cup water in the final processing; you can try it that way, too—it's all about preference.

DF

CANDIES AND BARS

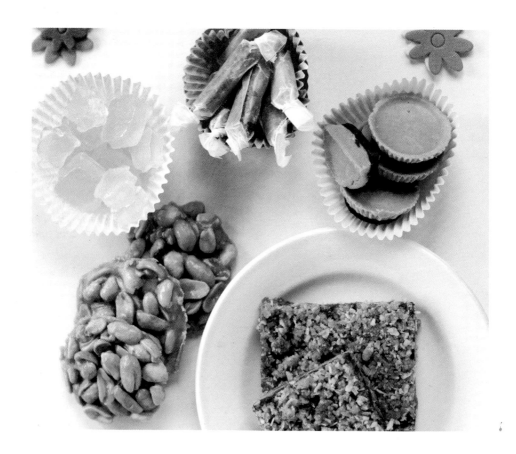

skinny chocolate

½ cup coconut oil, extra-virgin (or use cooking coconut oil for a neutral taste)

¼ cup unsweetened cocoa powder

2 teaspoons Super Sweet Blend, ground in a coffee grinder

Small pinch of Mineral Salt

24 packets truvia
1 C coconut oil
½ C cocoa powder

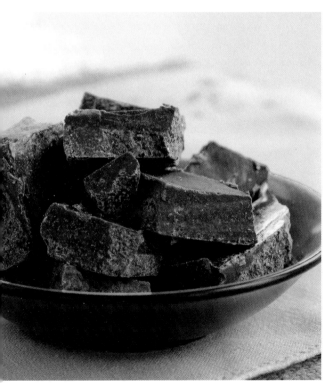

So long as you have some of this in your freezer, you will never have to feel chocolate deprived again. This is an easy recipe that has been the saving grace for many a Trim Healthy Mama when chocolate cravings hit. The coconut oil helps nourish your thyroid and rev your metabolism—that's why we call it "skinny."

Even though chocolate is usually hard to sweeten with stevia, the budget-friendly Super Sweet Blend works well in this recipe—just don't use too much. You'll get no bitter taste with the 2 teaspoons indicated. If you like much sweeter chocolate, or if you can't be bothered grinding your sweetener, use 3½ to 4 teaspoons of Gentle Sweet instead. Heads up: Skinny Chocolate is not a milk chocolate, so some people add heavy cream—that's fine, but don't go overboard with it, as it is still an S treat but not quite so skinnyfying.

The recipe makes about ¾ cup; we hate setting portion sizes, but up to one-third of this batch in a day is probably about right, but that is not a law.

1. If the coconut oil is solid, melt it by placing in a small bowl atop a small saucepan of water set over high heat.

2. Combine the melted coconut oil, cocoa, sweetener, and salt in a bowl and stir well. Pour into ice cube trays or chocolate or candy molds, or onto a plastic plate and put in the freezer to harden.

NOTE: You can make a delicious peanut version of this that is not quite as skinnyfying, but doesn't go overboard with the peanut butter. Add ¼ cup Pressed Peanut Flour plus an additional generous pinch of salt, then stir in 1 tablespoon natural-style peanut butter. Mmmmm.

NSI (IF YOU USE YOUR FAVORITE ON-PLAN SWEETENER) DF

treeces

Ⓢ

1 batch Skinny Chocolate (page 377)

½ cup coconut oil, extra-virgin or otherwise

¼ cup Pressed Peanut Flour

¼ cup natural-style, sugar-free peanut butter (see Note)

3 generous pinches Mineral Salt

2½ teaspoons Super Sweet Blend, ground in a coffee grinder

Get it? Trim Reeces . . . Treeces? Okay, we're batty, but who cares about the silly ol' name when you can eat these goodies? This is a layered tweak on the original Skinny Chocolate (page 377); it does include some peanut butter, but we're going for the yum factor here.

1. While still liquid, put 1 teaspoon of the Skinny Chocolate into the holes of a mini muffin tin (or you can just pour it in and eye the amounts). Place in the freezer to harden.

2. In another bowl, mix the remaining ingredients for the peanut butter layer.

3. When the chocolate layer has frozen, pour a little of the peanut mixture into each hole and freeze again.

4. Place the frozen Treeces in a zippy bag and store in the fridge for a softer version or keep in the freezer for the harder version.

NOTE: You can omit the peanut butter and use an additional ½ cup Pressed Peanut Flour instead for a bit more slimming effect, but the peanut butter does bring more rich creaminess to this candy—and let's not forget our "food freedom" approach. So enjoy these sometimes so long as you are also enjoying the original more "skinny" chocolate at other times.

DF

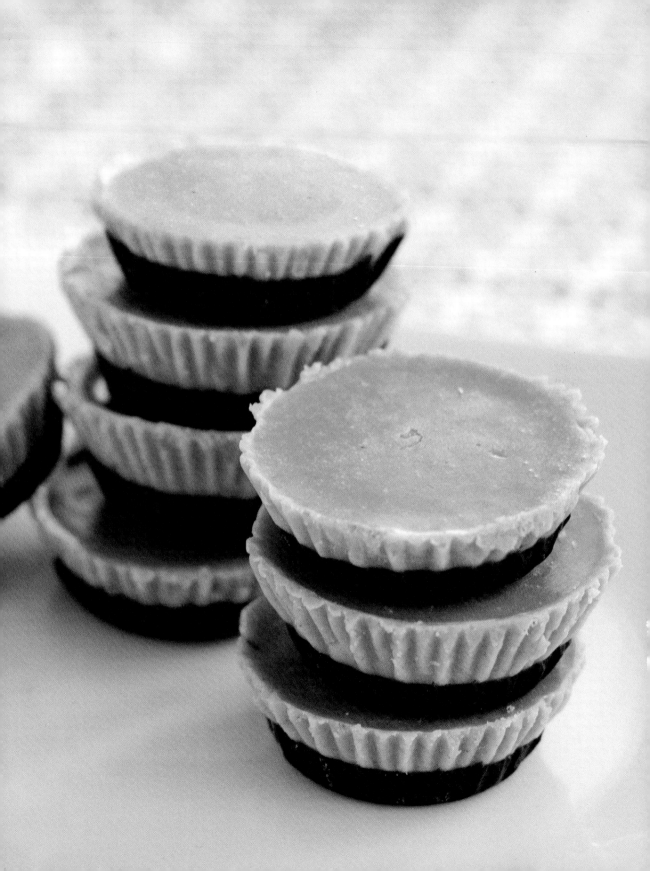

skinny peppermint patties ⓢ

Double batch of Skinny Chocolate (page 377)

3 ounces cream cheese (⅓ less fat works well)

1½ tablespoons coconut oil, extra-virgin or otherwise

1½ tablespoons softened butter

5 teaspoons Gentle Sweet

½ to 1 teaspoon peppermint extract, and/or 1 to 2 drops essential peppermint oil

½ teaspoon vanilla extract

1. While it's still liquid, drop teaspoonfuls of half of the double batch of the Skinny Chocolate into the bottoms of the holes of a mini muffin tin and put in the freezer to harden. Set the rest of the liquid chocolate aside.

2. While the mixture is freezing, in a small bowl, mix the cream cheese, coconut oil, butter, Gentle Sweet, peppermint extract, and vanilla.

3. When the chocolate layer is frozen, smear each one with some of the peppermint filling, then pour the rest of the Skinny Chocolate on top. Return the tin to the freezer to harden the chocolate.

NSI (IF YOU USE YOUR FAVORITE ON-PLAN SWEETENER)

pay off day candies

MULTIPLE SERVE – MAKES ABOUT 16 CANDIES

¼ cup Gentle Sweet

2 doonks Pure Stevia Extract (optional— for if you are a real sweetie)

2 tablespoons butter

2 tablespoons heavy cream

⅛ teaspoon caramel extract

2 teaspoons natural-style, sugar-free peanut butter

2 to 3 pinches Mineral Salt

¾ cup chopped peanuts

Your decision to stay on plan is paying off—reward yourself with this yummy creation by our friend Jennifer Morris. These are reminiscent of PayDay candy bars, but in this case they won't harm your health or your waistline.

1. Melt the Gentle Sweet, stevia (if using), and butter in a small saucepan. Add the cream and caramel extract and cook until the mixture reaches the desired caramel color, stirring often.

2. Take off the heat and add the peanut butter, salt, and peanuts. Stir well, then shape into mounds on parchment paper. Refrigerate until firm.

NSI (IF YOU USE YOUR FAVORITE ON-PLAN SWEETENER)

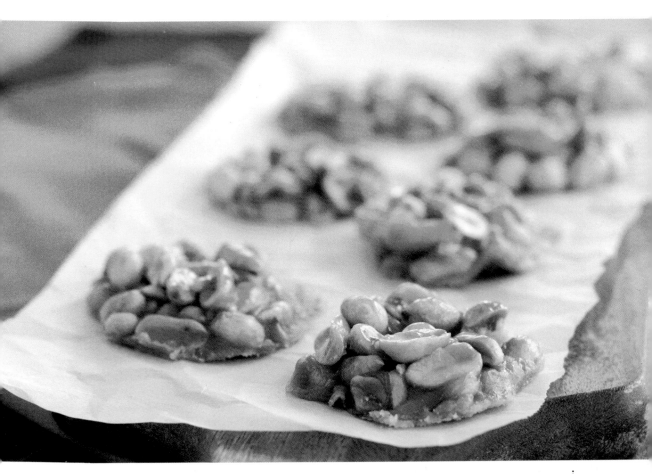

superfood chews

Others might scarf down sugar-laden candy, but we Trim Healthy Mamas don't deplete the health of our bodies like that. You don't have to miss out on chewy yumminess, though. Superfood Chocolate Chews are reminiscent of Tootsie Rolls—perhaps better, if we say so ourselves. They will give your taste buds a burst of rich chocolatiness, but they are also rich in protein, so feel free to have a few as part of any snack or dessert. All the following chew versions are high in glycine, which strengthens the immune system, promotes relaxation, detoxifies the body, beautifies the skin, repairs muscle, soothes digestion, promotes weight loss, gives luster to hair, is anti-inflammatory and anti-aging, and supports the maintenance of healthy bone and tissue. Deep breath—that was a long list of health benefits! But let's get real: Who cares about health benefits if something is not yummy? You've got both yummy and healthy here.

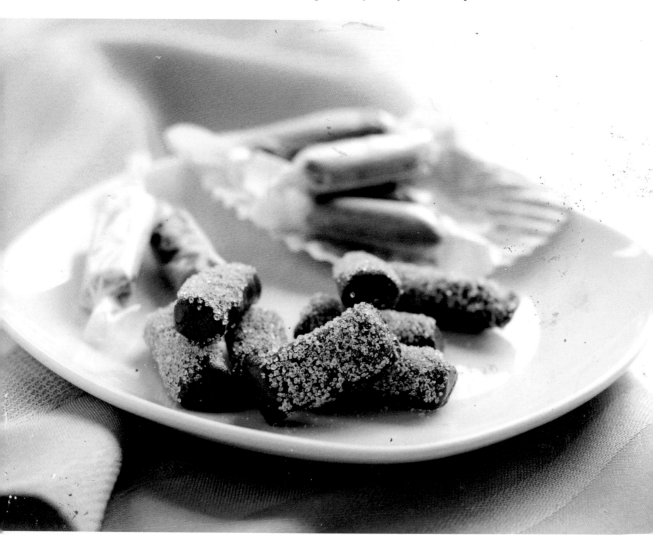

SUPERFOOD CHOCOLATE CHEWS (FP) WITH (S) OPTION

MULTIPLE SERVE – STICK TO NO MORE THAN $^1/_8$ OF THE RECIPE FOR FP
(GOING BEYOND THAT IS FINE FOR S)

2 scoops Pristine Whey Protein

½ cup Integral Collagen

¼ cup unsweetened cocoa powder

2 pinches Mineral Salt

2 tablespoons Super Sweet Blend,
   ground in a coffee grinder if desired,
   or 4 tablespoons Gentle Sweet

1 teaspoon vanilla extract

½ teaspoon mint or orange or other
   extracts, or 1 to 2 drops essential oil
   (optional)

1 to 2 doonks Pure Stevia Extract
   (optional)

4 generous teaspoons organic
   pastured butter or extra-virgin
   coconut oil

1 to 3 tablespoons water, as needed

1. Place the whey, collagen, cocoa, salt, and sweetener in a food processor. Begin processing and add the vanilla and other extracts (if using). Add the butter or oil and process a bit more. Drop in 1 tablespoon of water to moisten the mixture. After a minute or two of processing, stop and press some of the mixture between your fingers to see if it holds together. (It might still be a little crumbly but should hold together when pinched.) If it's too dry, add 1 teaspoon of water at a time and process until you can get a nougat texture when pressed together. Taste to see if you would like more sweetness.

2. Pull off little bits of the mixture and form into small squares, pressing between your fingers as you shape them. Or roll the mixture into a long thin roll and cut the roll into bite-size pieces. (If you like a crunchy coating, roll the pieces in erythritol; it makes them look pretty but is not necessary.)

3. Refrigerate the chews. (If you take them with you on errands for a couple of hours, they should be just fine.) Wrap the individual pieces in wax paper or plastic, if desired.

DF (IF USING COCONUT OIL INSTEAD OF BUTTER)

SUPERFOOD LEMON COCONUT CHEWS (FP) WITH (S) OPTION

If you like eating cookie dough, this recipe can help, and it has the bonus of tangy lemony flavor. Replace the cocoa in the master recipe with 2 tablespoons coconut flour. Leave out the vanilla, and use 2 tablespoons lemon juice and no water. Process as directed in the master recipe.

SUPERFOOD CHOCOLATE-COVERED PEANUT CHEWS (S)

Replace the cocoa in the master recipe with Pressed Peanut Flour and process as directed. Make a batch of Skinny Chocolate (page 377). While it is still liquid, pour half of it into chocolate molds or ice cube trays. Add some peanut batter to each mold, then pour the rest of the chocolate on top. Freeze to harden; transfer to the refrigerator.

skinny chocolate truffles

(S)

1 cup hot (not quite boiling) water (see Note)

2¼ to 2½ teaspoons Just Gelatin, as needed

1 cup extra-virgin coconut oil

6 tablespoons unsweetened cocoa powder

1 tablespoon Super Sweet Blend

2 to 3 teaspoons Gentle Sweet (optional for real sweet lovers)

2 teaspoons vanilla extract or other extract of choice (see Note)

OPTIONAL COATINGS

Ground espresso beans, finely chopped nuts, unsweetened coconut flakes, Gentle Sweet, or erythritol, mixed with ground cinnamon or other nummy spice (optional; see Alternative Method)

We brought you Skinny Chocolate (page 377), but now let's kick it up a notch and indulge in the truffle form. Guilt? What is that? These truffles make that word obsolete for chocolate lovers. The best thing about these truffles is that you can eat them with breakfast, as medicine for a healthier body, or with lunch or dinner just because you want to, or you can shove one in your mouth before a workout for some immediate middle-chain triglyceride energy. Here is the basic recipe. Creative ideas on how to dress them up follow.

1. Place the hot water in a blender, add the gelatin, and blend for a few seconds to dissolve. Add the coconut oil and blend well; this should happen very easily as the warm water should liquefy the coconut oil. Stop the blender and add the remaining ingredients except the optional coatings, and blend until smooth. Taste and adjust the flavors to "own it."

2. Pour the mixture into ice cube trays and freeze until solid. When frozen, turn one tray at a time upside down and twist to release the truffles. Place the desired amount that you wish to eat during the week into a zippy bag and put in the fridge. They are not ready to sample yet—don't even try a weeny bit. Wait until they melt from their frozen state into a perfect fridge temperature. They will not taste like truffles until they reach that new, unfrozen refrigerated temp.

ALTERNATIVE METHOD: Place the blended mixture into a gallon zippy and lay it flat in the freezer until the mixture is just hard enough to spoon out. Put your chosen coatings on a plate and roll the truffles in them to cover. Divide into zippered bags and refrigerate.

CREATIVE IDEAS: The hot water can be replaced with hot espresso, regular or decaf strong coffee, chai tea, oolong tea, fragrant jasmine tea, mint tea, and so on. You can also drop in some internal-grade essential oils, natural extracts, and spices. The extra nutritional and energy benefits, as well as weight-loss-boosting effects, of these additions can catapult the truffles into a super-duper superfood category. Our personal favorite truffle creations are made with jasmine green tea, or oolong tea/ginger tea, or ginger powder/mint, or essential orange oil, or natural raspberry extract—the list goes on and on.

DF

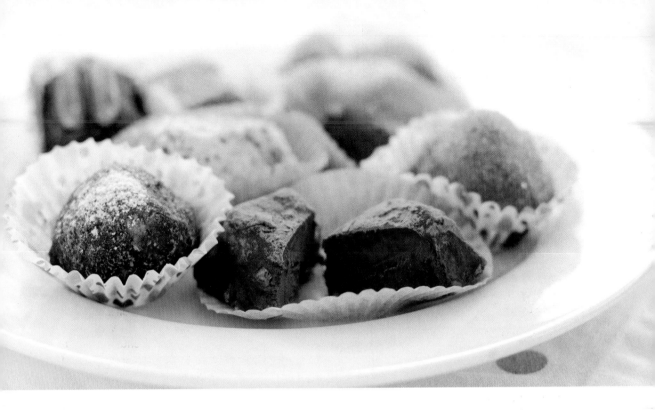

MINT CHOCOLATE CHUNK SKINNY TRUFFLES

MULTIPLE SERVE

These are gorgeous green truffles with chocolate featured only as chunks. This recipe will reveal the endless possibilities to be had with this basic truffle idea.

Use all the same ingredients as the master recipe except omit the cocoa and replace with 3 tablespoons Pristine Whey Protein (or Integral Collagen) and 3 tablespoons green powder (not the kind with bitter herbs or additions that make the flavor too strong; just regular barley grass powder or similar grass powders). (Alternatively, you could use a large handful of baby spinach and a few drops of liquid chlorophyll for extra color.) Reduce the vanilla to 1 teaspoon and add 1 to 1½ teaspoons mint extract and/or a few drops essential mint oil or to taste. Include the desired amount of chopped Skinny Chocolate or store-bought stevia-sweetened chocolate chips, or chopped 85% dark chocolate. Do not blend in the whey protein until the last 10 seconds, then stir in the chocolate chunks at the end.

DF (IF USING INTEGRAL COLLAGEN OVER WHEY PROTEIN)

meadow's lemon coconut truffles

3 ounces cream cheese (⅓ less fat
  works well)
Juice of ½ to 1 large lemon
2 tablespoons coconut flour
2½ to 3 tablespoons Super Sweet
  Blend, ground in a coffee grinder or
  use double amounts Gentle Sweet
2 tablespoons butter
1 tablespoon extra-virgin coconut oil
Dash of vanilla extract
Pinch of Mineral Salt
Unsweetened shredded coconut, for
  rolling

PEARL CHATS: My nineteen-year-old daughter Meadow has a way with Trim Healthy Mama desserts. She constantly comes up with scrumptious (and kind-to-the-waistline) sweet treats. Our whole family is only too happy to sample. This is one of my favorite recipes of hers.

1. In a medium bowl, mix all the ingredients except the coconut. Roll the mixture into little balls, then roll the balls in the coconut.
2. Place the truffles on a nonstick surface, store in the freezer until serving, then allow to sit out for 10 minutes or so for the best texture.

NSI (IF YOU USE YOUR FAVORITE ON-PLAN SWEETENER)

lemon pucker gummies ⓕⓟ

⅔ to 1 cup fresh lemon juice or from
concentrate (use a full cup for
punch-in-your-mouth lemon flavor)

1 to 1⅓ cups water (use only 1 cup if
you used a full cup of lemon juice)

3 to 5 teaspoons Super Sweet Blend,
or 3 to 6 doonks Pure Stevia Extract

3,000 mg vitamin C powder (optional)

6 tablespoons Just Gelatin (see Note)

Gummies made the Trim Healthy Mama way are not just sweet little treats—they are also protein-rich superfood blessers for your body! The degree of sweetness is an individual preference. Serene likes her gummies incredibly sour without much sweetness, so she uses only 2 teaspoons Super Sweet Blend. Pearl likes 3 to 4 teaspoons in this, and our friend Rohnda, who has been our photographer and food tester for this book, likes even more—a whopping 5 to 6 teaspoons! So taste as you go and "own it," or try these with Gentle Sweet instead for a more sugarlike taste.

1. Put all the ingredients except the gelatin in a medium saucepan over medium-low heat. Slowly sprinkle in the gelatin as the mixture warms, and whisk until dissolved. Bring to a "good 'n hot" point but not boiling, then pour into molds or a baking dish.

2. Place in the freezer to harden for 10 minutes, then store in the refrigerator until fully set. Cut into squares or slice into worms.

NOTE: This amount of gelatin will give a melt-in-the-mouth gummy texture; if you want a chewier gummy, add 1 to 2 more tablespoons gelatin.

DF

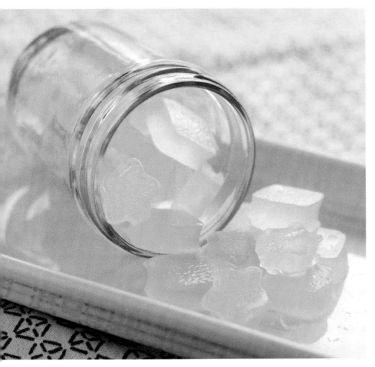

berry yummy gummies

MULTIPLE SERVE

¾ cup fresh or frozen strawberries or
    blueberries
1¼ cups water
3 to 5 teaspoons Super Sweet Blend,
    or 3 to 6 doonks Pure Stevia Extract
3 tablespoons lemon juice
6 tablespoons Just Gelatin

**See the headnote for Lemon Pucker Gummies (page 387)
regarding the amounts of sweetness and gelatin for these
gummies as well.**

1. Place all the ingredients except the gelatin in a blender
   and blend until smooth. Turn the blender off and add the
   gelatin. Blend for 3 seconds on low, until combined but not
   aerated too much.

2. Place the mixture in a medium saucepan and slowly heat
   over medium-low heat while stirring, until it reaches a
   "good 'n hot" point but not boiling.

3. Pour the mixture into molds or into a baking dish. Chill in
   the freezer for 10 minutes, then store in the refrigerator
   until fully set. Cut into squares or worms.

DF

peanutty fudge

MULTIPLE SERVE

½ cup (1 stick) butter or ghee (clarified
    butter) or coconut oil
5 teaspoons Super Sweet Blend (or
    use double amounts of Gentle
    Sweet)
¾ cup Pressed Peanut Flour
3 ounces cream cheese (⅓ less fat
    works well)
2 to 3 pinches Mineral Salt (extra pinch
    if using coconut oil or ghee)

**Rich and fabulous, this fudge is perfect around the holidays
or anytime when you are seeking sweet, peanutty indulgence. You can replace half the peanut flour with cocoa if
you desire a chocolate version.**

1. Melt the butter in a medium saucepan or skillet over
   medium-low heat. Add the sweetener and allow it to dissolve. Turn the heat to low and add all the other ingredients.
   Combine well.

2. Spread the mixture onto a parchment-lined baking sheet
   and shape into a block. Score the block into squares, then
   place in the freezer to harden and store.

3. Cut off pieces of fudge whenever desired.

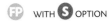
2 tablespoons Just Gelatin

1½ cups water

7 tablespoons Gentle Sweet

¼ teaspoon xanthan gum

1½ teaspoons vanilla extract

¼ teaspoon Mineral Salt

1 scoop Pristine Whey Protein

PEARL CHATS: I was determined to come up with a Trim-healthymamafied marshmallow because—what is not to love about a Fuel Pull candy that you can eat plenty of? Sadly, I kept failing miserably in this quest. All my attempts turned out very non-marshamallowish and nowhere near cookbook worthy. My daughter Meadow said I should let her give it a try. Her first attempt delivered this "'mazing" result. What!!???? Well, I might be bested by my teenage daughter, but I now have yummy marshmallows so I'm happy.

1. Combine the gelatin with ½ cup of the water in a small bowl and stir a little, not a lot. Allow to sit so the gelatin dissolves.

2. Place the remaining 1 cup water in a small saucepan over high heat and bring to a rapid boil.

3. In a large bowl, combine the sweetener, xanthan, vanilla, and salt. Add the gelatin mixture, then slowly pour in the boiling water. Start beating on high speed until the mixture gets thick and marshmallow-like. Be patient; it takes a while. After beating for the first 5 minutes, add the whey protein a little at a time, then beat for another few minutes.

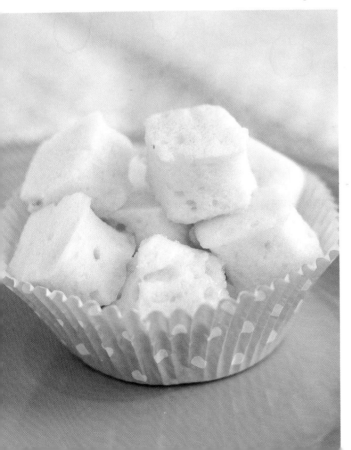

4. Pour the mixture into a parchment-lined 9 × 13-inch pan and spread it out with a spatula. Place in the refrigerator and chill for at least 2 hours. Cut into squares.

NOTE: For an **S** version, dip the squares in melted Skinny Chocolate (page 377) and then top with unsweetened shredded coconut. Return to the refrigerator to set the chocolate.

BARS

quicky-quick protein power balls ⓢ

MULTIPLE SERVE — MAKES 20 TO 25 BALLS, DEPENDING ON SIZE

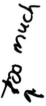
too much

1 cup unsweetened shredded coconut
2½ scoops Integral Collagen
1 scoop Pristine Whey Protein
½ cup extra-virgin coconut oil
2 teaspoons vanilla extract
2 pinches Mineral Salt
2 teaspoons Super Sweet Blend
1 tablespoon unsweetened almond or
  cashew milk

A super-quick, well-balanced high-protein treat that soothes and tranquillizes the snacking monster.

1. Place all the ingredients in a food processor and process until well blended. When it begins to take shape as a nice dough ball, remove and roll into small balls.

2. Freeze the balls on a parchment-lined tray for 10 minutes, until firm. Store in the fridge for use in the next week, or keep in the freezer for an extended period.

DF

chewy chotein logs ⓢ

MULTIPLE SERVE — MAKES 10 TO 20 SMALL LOGS, DEPENDING ON HOW BIG YOU MAKE THEM

½ cup Pristine Whey Protein
½ cup Integral Collagen
5 tablespoons chia seeds, ground in a
  coffee grinder
3 tablespoons plus 2 teaspoons water
4 tablespoons Pressed Peanut Flour
4 tablespoons unsweetened cocoa
  powder
2 tablespoons extra-virgin coconut oil
2 generous pinches Mineral Salt
½ to 1 teaspoon Super Sweet Blend
4 doonks Pure Stevia Extract
Unsweetened shredded coconut
  (optional)

SERENE CHATS: *These are great for on-the-go snacks made with our superhero friend, chia. My toddler loves them and calls them "chewies." Whenever she gets snacky in the car, she yells out for a "CHEEEEWWWWWYYYYY!!!!! MAAMMMA!!!"*

1. Place all the ingredients except the shredded coconut in a food processor and process until it forms a pressable dough ball that holds its shape. This may not happen at first. You will need to stop the machine and press the crumbles together to see if you can form balls that won't crumble and are moist but not gooey. You may need to add a tiny bit more water and process some more. If you need your mix to be drier, then add additional cocoa.

2. Roll pieces of the dough ball into logs using a little water- or oil-moistened fingers. You can choose to roll them in coconut or leave as is. Freeze most of the batch in little throw-in-your-purse baggies but put some in the fridge for snackies for the next few days. Wait until they are chilled and firm before enjoying.

DF

390 trim healthy mama cookbook

praline protein bars

MULTIPLE SERVE — MAKES 5 BARS

1 cup Pristine Whey Protein

⅓ cup Pressed Peanut Flour

¼ cup Integral Collagen

¼ cup Gentle Sweet, or 1½ to
2 tablespoons Super Sweet Blend

¼ teaspoon Mineral Salt

1 teaspoon MCT oil, butter, or
coconut oil

¼ to ½ teaspoon caramel or maple
extract

4 tablespoons water

¼ cup chopped pecans

These are a spinoff from the **Superfood Chocolate Chews** (page 383), an amazing protein bar with close to 25 grams of protein (part of it coming from the glycine-rich collagen). They're perfect for a slimming, on-the-run afternoon snack. Each bar contains 5 grams of fat (mostly from the nuts) and negligible carbs, so they just fit into FP mode; add any more fat to your snack and you are in S mode, which is perfectly okay.

1. Place the whey, peanut flour, collagen, sweetener, and salt in a food processor and blend well. Add the oil and extract and blend again. With the processor still on, add the water, 1 tablespoon at a time, adding just until the mixture is sticky enough to press together. Add the chopped pecans and pulse just a few times to mix.

2. Scoop out the mixture onto a piece of parchment and form into a flat rectangle. Cut into 5 bars.

3. Place in the refrigerator to firm up. You may wrap the bars individually in wax paper.

DF (IF USING MCT OR COCONUT OIL INSTEAD OF BUTTER)

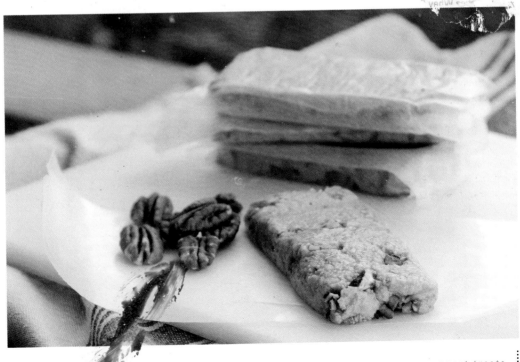

berry crunch bars

MULTIPLE SERVE – MAKES 12 BARS

1½ cups Trim Healthy Mama Baking Blend

3 tablespoons Super Sweet Blend

1 teaspoon aluminum-free baking powder

¼ teaspoon Mineral Salt

½ cup (1 stick) cold butter, plus 3 tablespoons melted butter

2 tablespoons extra-virgin coconut oil

¼ teaspoon blackstrap molasses (optional)

1 teaspoon vanilla extract

¼ cup old-fashioned rolled oats (see Note)

½ cup finely chopped pecans or walnuts

¼ cup unsweetened shredded coconut

1½ cups Slim Belly Jelly made with full amount of Gluccie (page 478)

A couple of these buttery, berrylicious bars make a fabulous grab-and-run-out-the-door breakfast or snack. The original idea was inspired by thirteen-year-old Katie Myers. Katie's mom, Jessica, is the awesome Mama who oversees all our Trim Healthy Mama social media chat groups. Her nature of grace and encouragement set the tone for the positive atmosphere in the groups.

We usually make this recipe with budget-friendly Super Sweet Blend. It works well because these bars are not supposed to be ultra sweet. If you desire a sweeter bar, simply sprinkle Gentle Sweet over the tops once they are set. They will look pretty that way, you'll save money by not having to use a lot of Gentle Sweet in the recipe, and you'll get that extra-sweet pop you're looking for.

1. Preheat the oven to 350°F.

2. Place the Baking Blend, sweetener, baking powder, and salt in a food processor. Add the cold butter, coconut oil, molasses (if using), and vanilla, and pulse until the mixture resembles coarse crumbs.

3. Press approximately two thirds of the mixture into a parchment-lined 9 × 13-inch baking pan. Bake the layer for 10 minutes and then remove from the oven to slightly cool. Leave the oven on.

4. Put the oats, nuts, and coconut in the food processor with the remaining dough and pulse a couple times; you don't want to break this mixture down too much but just get it combined and a little more chopped. This will be your crunch topping.

5. Spoon the jelly over the cooled bottom layer, then carefully use the back of a spoon to spread it evenly. Sprinkle the crunch topping over the top and drizzle on the melted butter as evenly as you can. Gently pat everything down and bake for another 30 to 40 minutes, or until golden brown.

6. Remove from the oven and let cool in the pan. It might still look and act a little gooey for a while; that is okay. When cooled somewhat, transfer the pan to the freezer and freeze until firm. Cut into bars and refrigerate.

NOTE: The small amount of oats here should not pose any major mixing of fuels in this recipe.

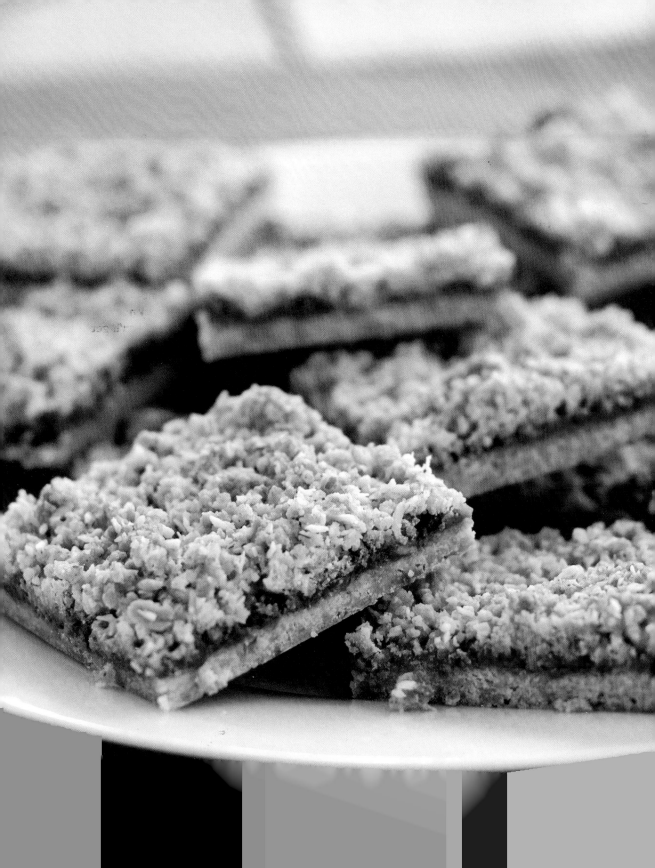

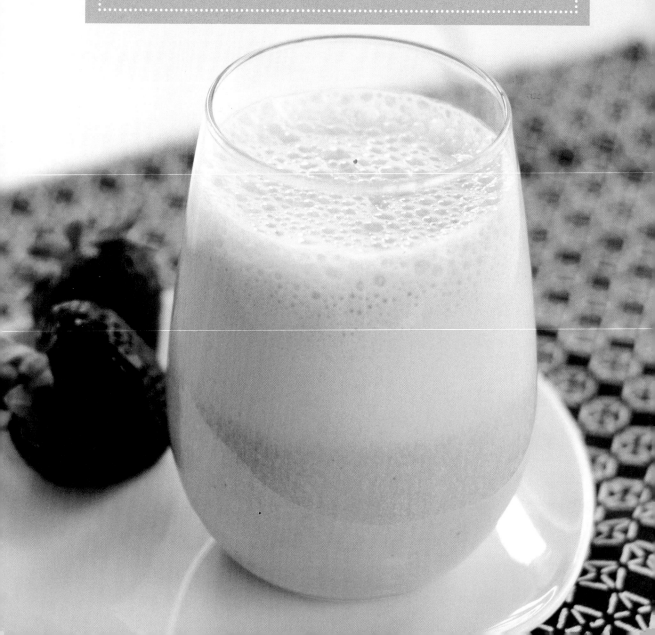

beverages

● = S   ● = E   ○ = FP   MORE THAN ONE DOT INDICATES OPTIONS

ALL-DAY SIPPERS

These drinks help heal your body, curb the snackies, shrink fat cells, and hydrate you all day. The spices in the following sippers are incredible health tonics. Learn more about their super powers in the "Specialty Food Stars" chapter of *Trim Healthy Mama Plan*. Budgeting Mamas, don't waste money using Stevia blends in your sippers. The pure extract works great and saves you money.

good girl moonshine

1 to 2 tablespoons apple cider vinegar (preferably one with mother)

1 teaspoon ground ginger (see Note)

2 to 4 doonks Pure Stevia Extract, or 2 to 3 teaspoons Super Sweet Blend, or to taste

Extracts of choice (optional; for different flavors)

Water and ice cubes

Stay hydrated with this slimming, health-promoting drink. It's your Baptist-friendly buzz toddy—no alcohol involved, yet it just might make you say "Eeee Ahhh!" and do a wild karate kick after you take your first sip. It is refreshing, zingy, and tantalizing; many Mamas doing the THM plan have found it helps them kick the soda habit. Ginger and apple cider vinegar, the superfood stars of this drink, are both powerful digestive aids. GGMS (this recipe's affectionately abbreviated name) detoxifies, clarifies, alkalizes your body, and aids in weight loss. It can also be made with sparkling water for a fizz effect or with any fruit-flavored herb tea.

1. Put the vinegar, ginger, sweetener, and extract of choice (if using) into a quart-size jar. Add a little bit of water so you are able to stir the ingredients.

2. Fill the jar with ice cubes, then add more water (or cooled tea of choice) until the liquid reaches the top of the jar. Stir well, then taste and adjust the flavors to "own it!"

NOTE: If you'd rather use fresh ginger, blend a good-size nob of the root (about 5 ounces) with ¾ cup water until it is completely broken down. Now add 1¼ cups more water (for a total of 2 cups) and blend well again. Pour into ice-cube trays and place in freezer. When frozen, put the cubes in zippies and store in the freezer. Use 1 or 2 of these ginger cubes in place of the powder in your Good Girl Moonshine.

NSI (IF YOU USE YOUR FAVORITE ON-PLAN SWEETENER) DF

singing canary

2 lemons

1½ cups water, plus more for the jar

½ to 1 teaspoon turmeric, as needed

1 teaspoon MCT oil, or ½ teaspoon extra-virgin coconut oil

1 teaspoon Pristine Whey Protein or Integral Collagen, or both

2 generous pinches Mineral Salt

1 to 2 splashes vanilla extract

2 to 4 doonks Pure Stevia Extract, or 2 to 3 teaspoons Super Sweet Blend, or to taste

3 to 4 drops pure essential lemon oil (optional)

2,000 mg vitamin C powder (optional)

Ice cubes

Are you exhausted? Living under chronic stress? If you've been diagnosed with adrenal fatigue, you'll want to make this drink frequently. But all of us can benefit. If you've had too many late nights or simply need a battery recharge, then drink the Singing Canary. It detoxes the body, beautifies the skin (super-high vitamin C content), has cancer-fighting power (thanks to curcumin), and has weight-loss benefits to boot! It has been especially formulated for tired, inflamed bodies, with each ingredient carefully chosen to be a powerful adrenal healer. There is no caffeine. It contains only deeply nourishing, soothing, hydrating, healing, tenderly awakening ingredients that create a delicious adrenal reviver! And despite the fact that it contains 1 full teaspoon of adrenal-rebuilding, inflammation-fighting turmeric powder, it's remarkably delicious—think *Sunny D meets Orange Creamsicle*. If you'd rather gulp it in one go, check out the Singing Canary Shot option next.

1. Peel the yellow rind off the lemons using a sharp paring knife, leaving as much of the white pith as possible (bioflavonoids in the pith are a healing component). Slice each lemon into 4 chunks, remove the seeds, and throw the lemon pieces into your blender along with the water. Blend well. Strain the mixture through a fine sieve or nylon mesh bag into a bowl or pitcher. (You can purchase these bags at a paint store inexpensively.) If you are pressed for time, just use the juice of the lemons and don't worry about the straining.

2. Pour the strained juice into the blender. Add all the other ingredients except the ice cubes, and blend really well.

3. Fill a quart jar with ice to the tippy top and then pour the blended lemon mixture over the ice. If it doesn't reach the top, add remaining water until it does. Put a tight lid on the jar and shake it like you are a professional drink mixer. Uncap and adjust the flavor to "own it." (Quite a bit of stevia is required to offset the strong tart effect of the lemon pith and turmeric and to balance the salt. If your Canary has too much bite, add more sweetener and/or vanilla and scale back on the turmeric next time.)

DF (IF USING INTEGRAL COLLAGEN)

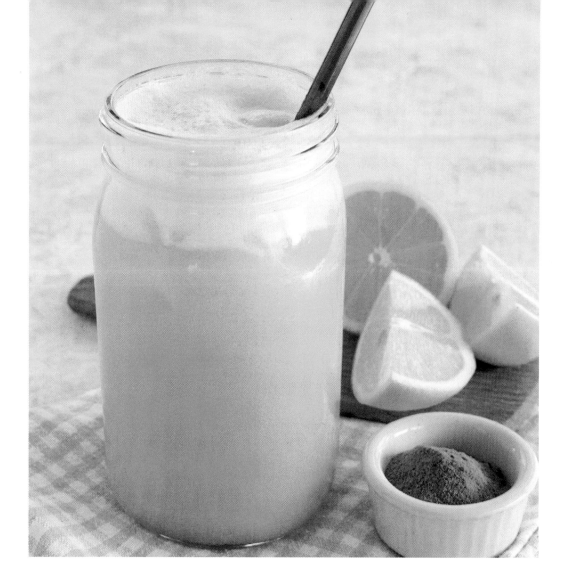

SINGING CANARY SHOT (FP)

SINGLE SERVE – MAKES 1 SMALL CUPFUL

Juice of 1 lemon
½ to 1 scoop Integral Collagen
½ to 1 teaspoon turmeric
1 teaspoon MCT oil (or ½ teaspoon, if having with an **E** meal that includes other fat)
2 doonks Pure Stevia Extract
½ to 1 teaspoon Pristine Whey Protein
2 pinches Mineral Salt
¾ cup water

Gulping this version of Singing Canary is the fastest way to get a good daily dose of turmeric and the other healing goodies. You can chug it as part of a mid-morning or mid-afternoon snack, or have it right before your meal as it helps to suppress the appetite.

1. Place all the ingredients in a blender and blend well, then throw down the hatch!

SINGLE SERVE – MAKES 1 FULL QUART TO BE SIPPED ON ALL DAY (CAN BE DOUBLED FOR A 2-QUART SIPPER)

2 oolong tea bags

1 mug boiling water

¼ cup unsweetened almond or cashew milk (see Note)

1 to 2 generous pinches Mineral Salt

1 to 2 teaspoons vanilla extract

2 to 4 doonks Pure Stevia Extract, or 2 to 3 teaspoons Super Sweet Blend, or sweeten to your own taste

½ to 1 teaspoon ground cinnamon

1 to 2 pinches cayenne pepper (or enough to make you feel like a feisty tiger)

Ice cubes and cold water

As its name suggests, this drink helps shrink your fat cells! Its combined thermogenic-boosting ingredients promote energy and help speed your metabolism. But you'll want to drink this simply because it tastes good! The Shrinker is not a meal replacement, so keep up your regular THM meals and snacks. It is designed to be sipped between set times of eating. It helps resist the urge to graze, scarf, or over-snack. You can find organic oolong tea at www.trimhealthymama.com, but some stores have it and you can also check online.

1. Steep the tea bags in a mug of boiled water. Allow to cool somewhat and discard the tea bags.

2. Pour the tea into a blender and add the almond milk, salt, vanilla, sweetener, cinnamon, and cayenne. This is your Shrinker concentrate. Blend well.

3. Place the concentrate in a quart jar and fill to the top with ice cubes. Add enough cold water so the liquid reaches the top of the jar. Put a lid on the jar, shake well, then taste and adjust flavors. "Own it!!!!"

NOTE: You can make this a healing shrinker by omitting the milk and replacing with ½ teaspoon of Just Gelatin, 1 teaspoon Integral Collagen, 1 teaspoon MCT oil, and an optional ¼ teaspoon Sunflower Lecithin. You will dissolve the gelatin into the mug of hot brewed tea, stir very well, then add to the blender along with the collagen, oil, lecithin, and ½ cup cold water. This makes an ultra-creamy shrinker.

NSI (IF YOU USE YOUR FAVORITE ON-PLAN SWEETENER) DF

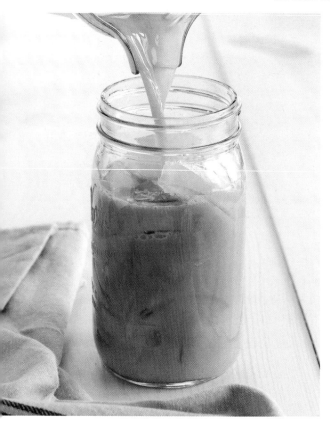

pumpkin pie sip

2 rooibos tea bags

1 mug boiling water, plus more for the jar

1 tablespoon pumpkin puree (not pie filling)

¼ teaspoon pumpkin pie spice

1 to 2 dashes vanilla extract

1 to 2 generous pinches Mineral Salt

2 to 4 doonks Pure Stevia Extract, or 2 to 3 teaspoons Super Sweet blend, or to taste

½ teaspoon coconut oil, or 1 teaspoon MCT oil (see Note)

1 teaspoon Pristine Whey Protein (see Note)

Ice cubes and cold water (optional)

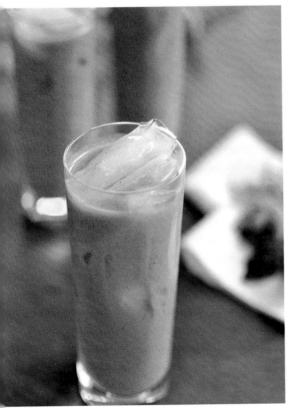

You *can* get your trim on while satisfying your holiday taste buds—never denying them one mouthful of "festive flavor" indulgence. This was the first drink in our Holiday Life Line series of all-day sippers. It is enriched with the flavors of the festive seasons, fall and winter. You can win the holiday head games because this sipper makes you feel blessed with a giant "can have" while it weakens the naughty "shouldn't have's." Of course, this can be enjoyed all year long if you are a diehard pumpkin pie lover. Choose whether you want to drink it refreshingly chilled or soothingly hot.

1. Steep the rooibos tea bags in a mug of boiled water for several minutes. Discard the tea bags and pour the tea into a blender with all the remaining ingredients except the ice (if using). Blend until smooth and frothy. This is your sipper concentrate.

2. For a chilled sip, pour the concentrate into a quart jar. Fill to the brim with ice cubes, then pour in the concentrate and top off with cold water. Stir, taste, and adjust the flavors until it rocks your holiday world. For a hot sip, pour the concentrate into a quart jar and add enough boiling water to reach the top. Taste and adjust as necessary.

NOTE: You can put this yummy mixture in a large stay-warm carafe and use an insulated cup when you are on the go. Sip your pumpkin pie all day, but please don't forget to enjoy it at night by the fire. If you do not have the Pristine Whey Protein or MCT or coconut oil, you can substitute ¼ cup unsweetened almond or cashew milk.

NSI (IF SUBBING WHEY PROTEIN AND OIL FOR UNSWEETENED ALMOND OR CASHEW MILK) DF

earth milk sip

1 cup boiling water

2 oolong or green tea bags, or 1 teaspoon matcha powder (if caffeine sensitive, leave tea out or use rooibos tea) (see Note)

1 tightly packed cup of soft baby greens

3 doonks Pure Stevia Extract

4 pinches Mineral Salt

¼ teaspoon ground cinnamon (optional)

1 teaspoon MCT oil, or ½ teaspoon extra-virgin coconut oil

½ teaspoon Sunflower Lecithin (optional, but makes a creamier drink that won't separate)

1 teaspoon Pristine Whey Protein or Integral Collagen

½ teaspoon Just Gelatin

1 cup ice cubes for blending and 2 cups ice cubes for serving

Here's a way of enjoying the benefits and nutrition of a salad without having to chew one leaf. It is also a great cleansing detox aid, and is a lot gentler on blood sugar levels than typical juice cleansing drinks that remove fiber or rely on carrots, beets, or apples, which in juice form can spike your blood sugar. The weight-loss and energy merits of oolong or green tea, combined with the blood sugar–busting power of cinnamon and the blood-stabilizing properties of gelatin and collagen, make this sipper a winner for your health journey.

1. Pour the boiling water into a quart jar and steep the tea bags in it for several minutes.

2. Put the greens, stevia, salt, cinnamon (if using), MCT oil, lecithin (if using), whey or collagen and salt in a blender. Don't add the coconut oil (if using instead of MCT oil).

3. Remove the tea bags and discard. Stir the gelatin and coconut oil (if using) into the hot tea. When the gelatin is dissolved, add the 1 cup ice and let cool for 10 seconds.

4. Add the tea mixture to the blender and blend everything together for 1 full minute. Let the blender rest for a few seconds, then run it again for 1 minute, until the greens have been pureed and there is no sign of leaf sediment.

5. Fill a quart jar a little over halfway with the remaining 2 cups ice cubes, pour the earth milk concentrate over the ice, and add water to the top of the jar, if necessary. Taste and adjust the flavors to "own it."

NOTE: If using matcha powder instead of tea bags, you will still have to use hot water to soften the gelatin before continuing with the recipe. You just won't have to wait for the tea to steep. If you love everything chocolaty, add 1 to 2 teaspoons unsweetened cocoa powder to the mix when blending.

DF

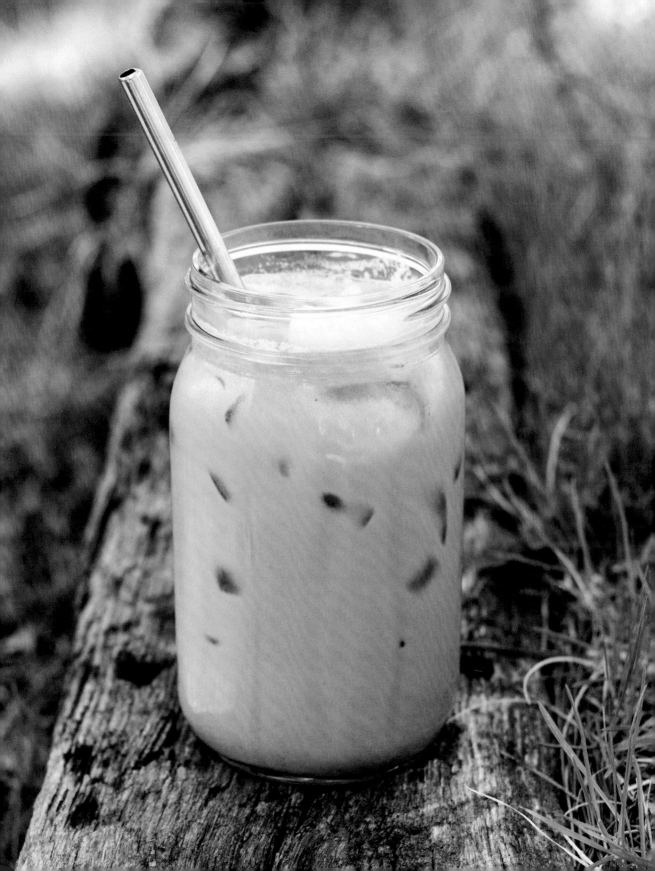

apple pie sip

2 chamomile tea bags

1 mug boiling water, plus more for the jar as needed

¼ teaspoon apple pie spice

Juice of 1 lemon

½ teaspoon coconut oil, or 1 teaspoon MCT oil (see Note)

1 teaspoon Pristine Whey Protein (see Note)

2 doonks Gluccie or xanthan gum

1 to 2 pinches Mineral Salt

1 teaspoon vanilla extract

¼ teaspoon butterscotch extract, or ½ teaspoon additional vanilla extract

2 to 4 doonks Pure Stevia Extract, or 2 to 3 teaspoons Super Sweet Blend, or to taste

1,000 mg vitamin C powder (optional)

Ice cubes and cold water (optional)

If apple pie is what gets you going, then you are about to dive headfirst into the deep end of that scrumptious flavor. Apple pie and vanilla ice cream were the inspiration for this recipe, and it delivers. You can roll your tongue around the flavors of good ole American apple pie at your whim on crisp fall days, while still making great strides toward reaching your goal weight. Like our Pumpkin Pie Sip (page 401), this is here to save you from feeling holiday deprived and "Grinchified" (if that could pass for a word). It is also here to help defend you from the onslaught of holiday pounds and common holiday illnesses. Your choice—enjoy this drink hot or cold.

1. Steep the chamomile tea bags in a mug of boiled water for several minutes. Remove the tea bags and discard.

2. Pour the tea into a blender and add all the remaining ingredients except the ice (if using). Blend until whipped and frothy. This is your pie concentrate.

3. Choose whether you want your sip soul-warming hot or chilled over ice. For a chilled sip, pour the concentrate into a quart jar. Fill to the brim with ice cubes, then pour in the concentrate, and top off with cold water. Stir, taste, and adjust the flavors until it rocks your holiday world. For a hot sip, pour the concentrate into a quart jar and add enough boiling water to reach the top. Taste and adjust as desired.

NOTE: If you do not have Pristine Whey Protein or MCT or coconut oil, you can substitute ¼ cup unsweetened almond or cashew milk.

NSI (IF SUBBING WHEY PROTEIN AND OIL FOR UNSWEETENED ALMOND OR CASHEW MILK) DF

winter wonderland sip

2 peppermint tea bags

1 mug boiling water, plus more for the jar as needed

½ teaspoon butter, or 1 teaspoon MCT oil

1 rounded teaspoon Pristine Whey Protein

2 to 4 doonks Pure Stevia Extract, or 2 to 3 teaspoons Super Sweet Blend, or to taste

Pinch of Mineral Salt

½ teaspoon vanilla extract

½ to 1 teaspoon peppermint extract, and/or 1 to 2 drops essential peppermint oil

2 doonks Gluccie or xanthan gum

Ice cubes and cold water (optional)

This drink has a wintry peppermint snap with a sugar-cookie hint. Use it to curb your winter cravings and as something to look forward to instead of second helpings! This sip will tantalize your taste buds while halting abuse of "over the top" holiday grazing. If you are a peppermint lover, feel free to make this any time of the year.

1. Steep the peppermint tea bags in a mug of boiled water for several minutes. Discard the tea bags.

2. Pour the tea into a blender along with all the other ingredients except the ice (if using). Blend until whipped and frothy. This is your pie concentrate.

3. Choose whether you want your sip soul-warming hot or chilled over ice. For a chilled sip, pour the concentrate into a quart jar. Fill to the brim with ice cubes, then pour in the concentrate, and top off with cold water. Stir, taste, and adjust the flavors until it rocks your holiday world. For a hot sip, pour the concentrate into a quart jar and add enough boiling water to reach the top. Taste and adjust as desired.

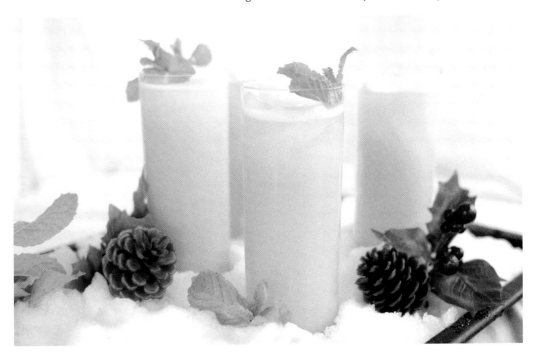

cranberry wassail

2 cups fresh or frozen cranberries

3 cinnamon sticks

1 teaspoon whole cloves (use only ½ teaspoon if you prefer a less "spiced" toddy)

3 star anise (optional)

Generous ¼ teaspoon Pure Stevia Extract, or to taste

2 teaspoons orange extract, and/or a few drops pure essential orange oil

SERENE CHATS: *The aroma that festively leaps from the holiday "wassail pot" as it brews is so inviting. It asks you to sip Christmas's spiced, warming fruity goodness without any hint of hidden pudge. My children smell it, and come running from every corner of the house, thinking I must have morphed into some kind of "Betty Crocker meets Mama Claus." But it's just plain ole me, feeling oh so clever! Cranberries are high in vitamin C, so get this drink brewing once the cold and flu season starts!*

1. Put the cranberries, cinnamon sticks, cloves, and star anise (if using) into a large pot and cover with about 1½ quarts of water. Place a lid on the pot and bring to a rolling boil over medium-high heat. Turn the heat down to a gentle simmer and brew for 1 hour while you become completely intoxicated with the "heart and home"–warming aroma.

2. Fit a 2-quart jar or large jug with a circle of fine cheesecloth, tying it over the mouth of the jar, or insert a funnel-type coffee filter into the mouth of the jar (I use the permanent filter from my coffee maker for this). Using a ladle, scoop the spicy mixture into your filter to strain it into the jar. Occasionally you might need to swish things around in the filter and maybe even remove some of the mush to allow the liquid to flow through.

3. Remove the filter and add very hot water to top off the jar. Add the stevia and orange extract, stir very well, and taste. Adjust the flavorings accordingly to "own it."

SERVING IDEA: Pour your wassail mixture into a warmed crockpot, leave it on a warm setting, and enjoy the wassail at your leisure to delight your senses on Thanksgiving Day, Christmas, and beyond.

NSI (IF YOU USE YOUR FAVORITE ON-PLAN SWEETENER) DF

SHAKES, SMOOTHIES, FRAPPAS, AND THIN THICKS

Sweet, creamy drinks are a big part of a Trim Healthy Mama's life. We've got you well covered here, with lots of different flavors and varieties, so there's no chance of your getting bored. Instead of piling on the pounds, these thick and creamy drinks will help strip the weight off of you—woo hoo! Unless otherwise noted, they can be used as a breakfast, a snack, or even as a quick lunch for on-the-go days.

If you are a Mama on a very tight budget and cannot afford the whey protein or any of the other special ingredients, try 1% cottage cheese or plain 0% Greek yogurt in your creamy drinks. Those two options cream the drinks up nicely and offer protein, which is a must for all our shakes, smoothies, and frappas. You can always add a tablespoon or two of heavy cream for more **S**-style indulgence. And please don't fret about the collagen, gelatin, or lecithin, either. In most of the recipes (Thin Thicks excluded) they are optional, and if you can't afford them, you're still fine. Remember, you will do THM your own way, and for some that means limiting the use of special ingredients.

Those with elevated prolactin levels can omit the whey protein and use 1 to 2 scoops Integral Collagen instead. (Read the "Heads Up: Turtle Losers!" chapter in *Trim Healthy Mama Plan* for more about why elevated prolactin levels and whey protein are sometimes not compatible.) Allergen-free Mamas who cannot even tolerate whey protein (it is lactose-free, so many do fine with it) can stick to the collagen and leave out any cottage cheese.

creamy key lime shake

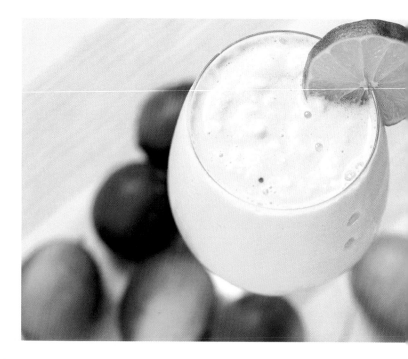

SINGLE SERVE — MAKES 2 TO 3 CUPS

Juice from 1 lime (about 2 tablespoons); can be a key lime, but they are smaller, so you may need juice from 2 of those—or use any old lime

7 fresh spinach leaves (you won't taste them), or 1 tablespoon frozen chopped spinach

½ cup unsweetened almond or cashew milk

¼ cup water

½ cup 1% cottage cheese

1 rounded tablespoon ⅓ less fat cream cheese

1 tablespoon heavy cream

2 to 3 teaspoons Super Sweet Blend, or to taste

1½ to 2 cups ice cubes

½ scoop Pristine Whey Protein

¼ teaspoon Gluccie (optional)

2 drops pure essential lime oil, or ½ teaspoon lime extract (really makes this drink more amazing to include the lime oil)

1. Place the lime juice, spinach, almond milk, and water in a blender and spin until a smooth puree with no spinach bits floating around. Add all the other ingredients and blend very well.

NSI (IF YOU USE YOUR FAVORITE ON-PLAN SWEETENER, OMIT WHEY PROTEIN, AND USE XANTHAN IN PLACE OF GLUCCIE)

orange creamsicle shake

SINGLE SERVE — MAKES 2 TO 3 CUPS

1 orange, peeled and seeded
½ cup unsweetened almond or
    cashew milk
¼ cup water
½ cup 1% cottage cheese
½ scoop Pristine Whey Protein
¾ teaspoon orange extract, or 2 drops
    pure essential orange oil
3 teaspoons Super Sweet Blend
1½ to 2 cups ice cubes
¼ teaspoon Gluccie (optional)

This shake makes a nice large breakfast or snack just for you or to share with a friend or family member as a refreshing E dessert.

1. Place the orange sections in a blender with the almond milk and water, and blend to a smooth puree. Add all the other ingredients and blend well.

NSI (IF YOU USE YOUR FAVORITE ON-PLAN SWEETENER, OMIT WHEY PROTEIN, AND USE XANTHAN IN PLACE OF GLUCCIE)

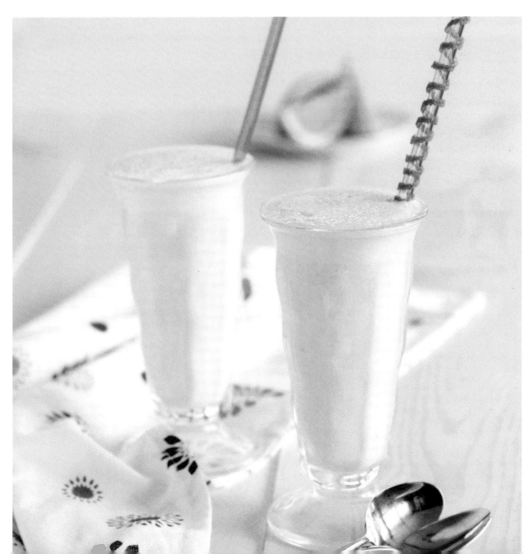

thin mint chocolate chip shake

(S)

½ ounce 85% dark chocolate, or ½ to 1 ounce stevia-sweetened chocolate or Skinny Chocolate (page 377)

½ cup low-fat cottage cheese (1% works fine but 2% Daisy is Gwen's favorite)

1½ to 2 cups ice cubes

1 cup unsweetened almond or cashew milk

2 tablespoons heavy cream or half-and-half (see Note)

1½ teaspoons vanilla extract

¼ teaspoon peppermint extract, or 1 to 2 drops pure essential mint oil (see Note)

2 to 3 teaspoons Super Sweet Blend, or 4 to 5 teaspoons Gentle Sweet Pure Stevia Extract to taste

⅛ teaspoon Gluccie or xanthan gum (optional)

Gwen Brown was the Mama who started the first Trim Healthy Mama Facebook group with us (which grew to over 100,000 members), and she is the one we have to thank for this recipe, which literally went viral in the THM community from the moment she shared it. Gwen has many incredible THM recipes on her blog, and you can read about her journey to goal weight with Trim Healthy Mama at www.gwensnest.com.

1. Chop the chocolate into smallish chunks and set aside.

2. Put all the remaining ingredients into a blender, and blend until well combined and smooth. Add the chocolate and blend or pulse to chop small enough to fit through a straw.

SERVING IDEA: Pour the mixture into a tall glass and top with whipped cream and chocolate curls, if you're feeling fancy.

NOTE: Want to add a superfood boost and a lovely soft green color to your mint shake? Add mint-flavored chlorophyll instead of the mint extract. You can go all the way to using ¼ cup cream now and then, but don't use the full ¼ cup if this is a dessert rather than a snack.

NSI (IF YOU USE YOUR FAVORITE ON-PLAN SWEETENER AND XANTHAN IN PLACE OF GLUCCIE)

shake gone nuts

SINGLE SERVE — MAKES ABOUT 1 QUART

1 cup water

2 tablespoons Pressed Peanut Flour

6 pinches Mineral Salt

2 teaspoons Super Sweet Blend

3 doonks Pure Stevia Extract

1 scoop Integral Collagen

¼ teaspoon Gluccie

1 teaspoon vanilla extract

1 teaspoon ghee (clarified butter) or
butter, or 2 teaspoons MCT oil

½ teaspoon butter extract (or
1 teaspoon if using MCT oil; optional)

¼ teaspoon Sunflower Lecithin
(optional but adds extra creaminess)

2 cups ice cubes

½ scoop Pristine Whey Protein, or
additional ½ scoop Integral Collagen
(optional)

Are you crazy for peanuts? Do you find yourself with a peanut butter jar and a spoon when times get tough? If you go nuts for nuts, then this recipe is a sane approach to soothing your addiction. Unlike most high-caloric peanut treats, which carry obscene amounts of calories and the guilt that goes with them, this scrumptious nutty indulgence is decadently rich in taste, but not in abuse to your body, and it is completely lactose-free.

1. Put all the ingredients in a blender except the ice and whey protein, and blend well. Add the ice cubes and blend until smooth. Add the whey and blend for 10 seconds more.

NOTE: You can easily convert this to an **S** treat by adding 1 tablespoon natural-style peanut butter and sprinkling some chopped roasted peanuts on top. Delish—and you're still not going overboard on peanut butter, just enjoying it wisely.

DF (IF USING ALL COLLAGEN IN PLACE OF THE WHEY PROTEIN)

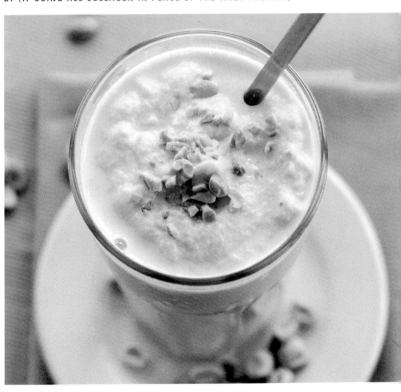

strawberry cheesecake shake

½ to ¾ cup frozen strawberries (or raspberries)

½ cup 1% cottage cheese

½ cup unsweetened almond or cashew milk

¼ cup water

½ scoop Pristine Whey Protein

2 to 3 teaspoons Super Sweet Blend

1 rounded tablespoon ⅓ less fat cream cheese

1½ to 2 cups ice cubes

¼ teaspoon Gluccie (optional)

1. Place all the ingredients in a blender and blend until smooth.

NSI (IF YOU USE YOUR FAVORITE ON-PLAN SWEETENER, OMIT WHEY PROTEIN, AND USE XANTHAN IN PLACE OF GLUCCIE)

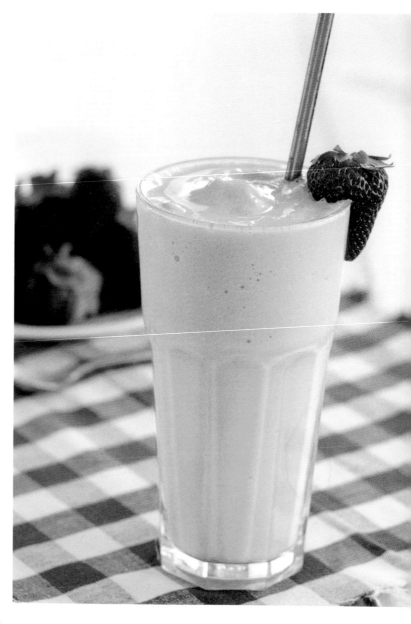

banana oat shake

(E)

SINGLE SERVE — MAKES 3 CUPS

½ large banana (or 1 small banana)

½ cup cooked old-fashioned rolled oats

¾ cup unsweetened almond or
   cashew milk

½ cup 1% cottage cheese

1½ to 2 cups ice cubes

½ scoop Pristine Whey Protein

1¾ teaspoons Super Sweet Blend, or
   4 teaspoons Gentle Sweet

⅓ to ½ teaspoon banana extract

⅛ teaspoon ground cinnamon or
   nutmeg, plus extra for sprinkling

Pinch of Mineral Salt

¼ teaspoon Gluccie (optional)

Here's a great way to fuel your morning with protein and healthy carbs. It's helpful for a nursing Mama's milk supply, too!

1. Put the banana, cooked oats, and almond milk in a blender and blend well. Add all the other ingredients and blend until a smooth puree. Pour into a glass and top with an extra sprinkling of nutmeg.

NOTE: Nursing and pregnant women who need more Crossovers can include 1 tablespoon sugar-free, natural-style peanut butter or 1 tablespoon heavy cream, if desired.

NSI (IF YOU USE YOUR FAVORITE ON-PLAN SWEETENER, OMIT WHEY PROTEIN, AND USE XANTHAN IN PLACE OF GLUCCIE)

german chocolate shake

(S)

SINGLE SERVE — MAKES 2 TO 3 CUPS

1 cup unsweetened almond or
   cashew milk

½ cup water

1 scoop Pristine Whey Protein

1 tablespoon unsweetened cocoa
   powder

4 teaspoons Gentle Sweet, or 2 to
   3 teaspoons Super Sweet Blend

½ teaspoon Gluccie or xanthan gum

¼ cup 1% cottage cheese

2 tablespoons heavy cream

½ teaspoon coconut extract (optional)

½ teaspoon vanilla extract

1 tablespoon coconut oil

12 large ice cubes

1 tablespoon unsweetened shredded
   coconut

1 ounce store-bought stevia-
   sweetened chocolate or 85% dark
   chocolate, roughly chopped

This shake was created by Jennifer Griffin, who dropped 75 pounds on plan. It has made many other Trim Healthy Mamas happy as clams since she shared it. Check out her other great THM recipes at www.ahomewithpurpose.com.

1. Place all the ingredients except the shredded coconut and chocolate in a blender. Blend well until it's a smooth shake consistency. Add the coconut and chocolate, and blend again until the coconut is almost but not quite pureed (small enough to fit through a straw).

NSI (IF YOU USE YOUR FAVORITE ON-PLAN SWEETENER, OMIT WHEY PROTEIN, AND USE XANTHAN IN PLACE OF GLUCCIE)

strawberry big boy

SINGLE SERVE — MAKES ABOUT 1 QUART

1 cup unsweetened almond or
   cashew milk

1 cup frozen strawberries

12 to 16 large ice cubes

2½ to 3 teaspoons Super Sweet Blend

2 pinches Mineral Salt

Dash of vanilla extract

Squeeze of lemon juice

1 scoop Integral Collagen (optional)

¼ teaspoon Sunflower Lecithin
   (optional)

1 scoop Pristine Whey Protein (or
   ½ scoop if using Integral Collagen)

This is the original Big Boy Smoothie that has helped keep thousands of Mamas happily on plan. It makes a huge weight-stripping smoothie that is all yours! Enjoy it for breakfast, lunch, or as a snack. Be sure to check out the following new "secret" variations of this that we have recently come up with.

1. Place all the ingredients except the whey protein in a blender. Blend until the ice and strawberries have pureed. Add the whey and blend for another 10 to 20 seconds. Taste and adjust the flavors to "own it"!

secret big boys

The following are our new takes on the Big Boy Smoothie. They are large and satisfying protein drinks that soothe digestion, moisturize your insides, and help shed stubborn pounds. The "secret" comes from the fact that you would never guess all that creamy goodness contains a full cup of okra—unless somebody spills the beans. Don't spill the beans! Even your children will enjoy this unless they find out about the okra—and then, and only then, will they turn up their noses. Hide the okra bag, Mamas!

CHOCO SECRET BIG BOY

1 cup water

1 cup frozen diced okra

2 tablespoons unsweetened cocoa powder

1 teaspoon extra-virgin coconut oil, or 2 teaspoons MCT oil

½ teaspoon vanilla extract

3 generous pinches Mineral Salt

3 teaspoons Super Sweet Blend

1 scoop Integral Collagen (optional)

¼ teaspoon Sunflower Lecithin (optional)

12 to 16 large ice cubes

1 scoop Pristine Whey Protein (or ½ scoop if using Integral Collagen)

1. Place all the ingredients except the ice cubes and whey in a blender and blend until very smooth. It is very important not to blend the ice and whey yet. You want all the okra completely broken down first. Add the ice and blend well again. You may have to stop the blender and stir a couple times or add the ice slowly.

2. Add the whey and blend for 10 to 15 seconds more. (If you blend too long, the whey causes this smoothie to get super poofy. You might like this, but we like a balanced poof. Experiment for fun, if you want.) Taste and adjust the flavors if needed to "own it"!

CHOCO NUT SECRET BIG BOY FP

Use all the same ingredients as the master recipe except add 4 teaspoons Pressed Peanut Flour to the blend.

BERRY SECRETIVE BIG BOY

Use all the same ingredients as in the master recipe, except omit the cocoa and add ½ cup frozen berries and 2 table-spoons lemon juice. Reduce the salt to 1 to 2 pinches, use only 8 to 10 ice cubes, and reduce the Super Sweet Blend to 2 to 2½ teaspoons. Add the berries at the same time as you add the ice.

GREEN SECRET BIG BOY

Use all the same ingredients as in the master recipe, except omit the cocoa and add 1 handful of soft-fiber greens like young lettuce or spinach, or a serving of your favorite green powder (barley grass, wheat grass, spirulina, or kamut grass). Reduce the Super Sweet Blend to 2 teaspoons. Blend the greens with the okra—you want them to become a smooth puree—before adding the ice cubes and whey protein.

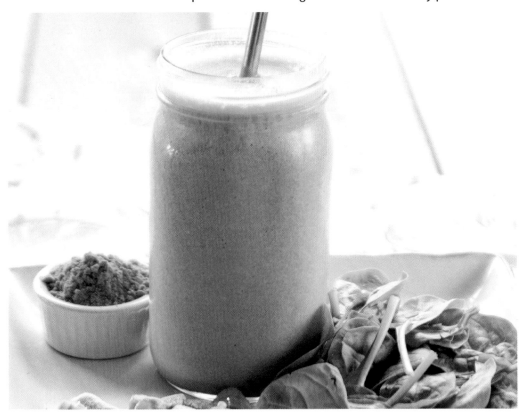

2 teaspoons Just Gelatin

1 tablespoon cool water

1 tablespoon very hot (not quite boiling) water

1 cup water

1 cup frozen diced okra

8 cardamom seeds (not pods; use the little seeds that come from inside the pod)

1 teaspoon vanilla extract

3 pinches Mineral Salt

3 to 4 doonks Pure Stevia Extract, or to taste

1 scoop Integral Collagen

½ teaspoon Sunflower Lecithin (helps to fluff the smoothie in place of whey protein)

Handful of soft lettuce greens (butter lettuce, baby romaine), stems removed

1 teaspoon ghee (clarified butter) or coconut oil (1 tablespoon for an **S** option)

12 to 16 large ice cubes

Have a sensitive tummy that reacts and bloats with many foods? Perhaps you don't tolerate whey protein very well and plan-approved sweeteners other than Pure Stevia Extract leave you bloated. Make good friends with this creamy drink. We created it for our allergen-free Mamas and those who need a soothing tonic in a smoothie.

This smoothie has all the tummy-soothing and healing power of okra, just like the other Secret styles but it has the addition of gelatin, which moisturizers and protects the mucosal lining of your intestinal tract and brings healing to an irritated bowel. The gelatin and collagen in this drink will supply your protein needs, so you can leave out the whey and still get a protein boost. You will also get a nutritional punch from the greens, but not the greens that are too high in roughage to digest easily. We have purposefully kept this drink gentle on fiber and sweeteners. No sugar alcohols are used, and there is plenty of fiber in here, but mostly the soft, soothing type from okra.

The cardamom is not only delicious (especially when paired with vanilla) but was specifically chosen for its ability to soothe a cranky digestive system. This aromatic medicinal spice helps combat nausea, constipation, or the other extreme, diarrhea, as well as acidity, heartburn, bloating, and a bad case of what we call "fluffs," which is a bunch of tooting. Another great perk is it is an effective breath freshener. Ever get a bad case of the hiccups? Cardamom is an antispasmodic—the perfect natural answer. Other involuntary muscle spasms, like stomach and intestinal cramps, are relaxed by cardamom, too. This talented spice makes the smoothie taste like you need to sit crosslegged in an exotic Bedouin tent as you sip. It is also a powerful antioxidant that helps prevent major disease dragons like cancer.

Go ahead—now even with a tender tummy, you can eat like a Big ole Boy.

1. Dissolve the gelatin in a cup by adding the cool water and stirring to soften, then adding the hot water to dissolve it.

2. Put all the remaining ingredients except the ice cubes into a blender and blend until very smooth. Make sure the okra and greens are fully blended, then add the dissolved gelatin and blend again. Add the ice cubes a little at a time, and keep blending until smooth.

DF

fat-stripping frappas

PEARL CHATS: I'll never forget the day I tasted this drink. It was the Fourth of July, we were at our annual community picnic by the creek, and Serene kept disappearing behind a tree. I got glimpses of a big jar of something yummy and chocolaty coming out of a tote bag she was hiding there. She'd take a secretive sip or two, then come back to join the party. I followed her during one of her disappearing acts and cajoled her into giving me a taste. I couldn't believe it! She was drinking a full quart of thick creamy chocolate amazingness. It tasted incredible! She had to rip the jar out of my hands as I began to guzzle it. As usual, she was nursing and hungry, and wasn't willing to part with it! When she assured me it was a Fuel Pull, I could barely believe it. Yep, I have to admit: my little sister is a genius for inventing this drink. But I'm only saying that once. She won't hear it cross my lips again.

These Fat-Stripping Frappas have now become a staple in kitchens all over the globe, with so many new varieties invented by our Mamas. It can be a super-large afternoon snack or perhaps a breakfast or lunch on the run now and then (but don't replace too many meals with it, as it is a Fuel Pull and you don't want to overdo those as meals); having a couple a few times a week is probably fine if you are not nursing or pregnant. Here are some of our personal favorite versions.

CHOCOLATE FAT-STRIPPING FRAPPA (FP)

SINGLE SERVE – MAKES 1 FULL QUART

2 tablespoons unsweetened cocoa powder

½ cup unsweetened almond or cashew milk

½ cup water

3 to 3½ teaspoons Super Sweet Blend, or 5 to 6 teaspoons Gentle Sweet, or more to taste (newbie THM's may want to start with Gentle Sweet)

2 to 3 pinches Mineral Salt

½ teaspoon Gluccie

18 to 20 large ice cubes (or 1¼ trays of large ice cubes)

1 scoop Pristine Whey Protein

1. Put all the ingredients except the ice cubes and whey protein in a blender and blend for 10 to 15 seconds. Add the ice a little at a time, and blend until smooth.

2. Add the whey protein at the end while the blender is still running. Continue to blend until the mixture is thick and fluffy.

3. Taste, and adjust the flavors to "own it," then pour into a quart jar.

NOTE: A fun trick! Once the ice has broken down in the blender, transfer frappa to a food processor and add the whey protein. Process for a minute or two. This creates a much poofier frappa. It literally grows in volume and creaminess, so you have even more to enjoy!

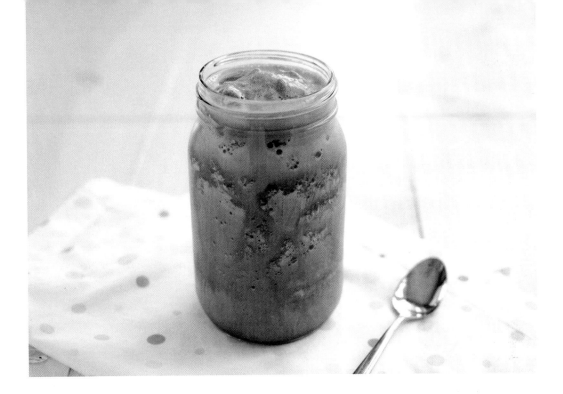

MOCHA FAT-STRIPPING FRAPPA 🅕🅟

Use all the same ingredients as in the master recipe, except use 1¼ trays of coffee-flavored ice cubes (coffee frozen into ice cubes) in place of regular ice. You may want to increase the sweetener just a tad.

SALTED CARAMEL FAT-STRIPPING FRAPPA 🅕🅟

Use all the same ingredients as in the master recipe, except omit the cocoa and add ½ to ¾ teaspoon caramel extract. Up the salt to 3 to 4 generous pinches and reduce the Super Sweet Blend to 2½ to 3 teaspoons.

LEMON FAT-STRIPPING FRAPPA 🅕🅟

Use all the same ingredients as in the master recipe, except omit the cocoa and add the juice of 1 to 1½ lemons, depending on how lemony you like things. Reduce the salt to 1 to 2 pinches and add a dash of vanilla extract.

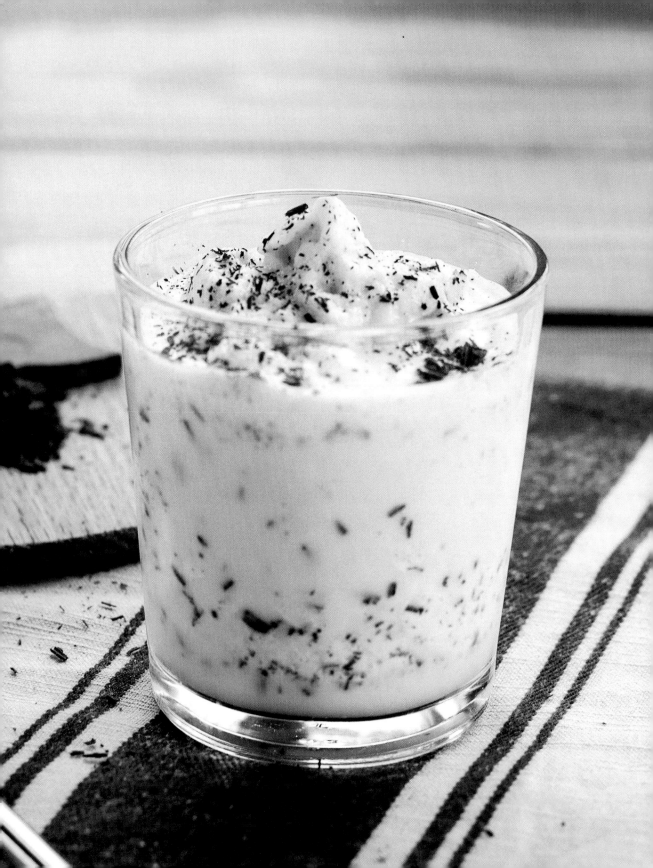

choco chip baby frap (FP)

¼ cup unsweetened almond or
  cashew milk

¼ cup water

1 to 2 pinches Mineral Salt

⅓ teaspoon vanilla extract

1 to 1½ teaspoons Super Sweet Blend,
  or to taste

⅛ to ¼ teaspoon Gluccie

7 to 8 large ice cubes

1 heaping tablespoon Pristine Whey
  Protein

¼ ounce Skinny Chocolate (page 377)
  or store-bought stevia-sweetened
  chocolate or 85% dark chocolate,
  chopped (this small amount still
  keeps you in FP mode)

Get to know the Baby Frap. It does not make a full meal, but it is an excellent dessert, small snack, or part of a snack. The huge Fat-Stripping Frappas can sometimes stand alone as a breakfast or lunch, but they are really too much to pair with other food unless you are ravenously hungry, and then there is no law against it.

You've finished your meal and are not filled up yet? This is where the Baby Frap can shine. Add it on to the end of your meal or snack. It's ultra Fuel Pull, very low in calories, yet it is gonna do the filling trick in a sweet way. You can make any variety of Baby Frap you want. This recipe is a yummy chocolate chip version, but you can easily omit the chocolate chips and make it straight chocolate by adding cocoa, or you can use any of your favorite flavors for the original large frappa and just halve the flavor amounts.

1. Put all the ingredients except the ice cubes, whey, and chocolate in a blender and blend for 10 to 15 seconds. Add the ice and blend until smooth. Add the whey while the blender is still running and blend for 10 to 15 seconds more.

2. Turn the blender off and add the chocolate. Pulse briefly, until the chocolate is broken into tiny pieces small enough to suck through a straw (don't overblend). Taste, and adjust the flavors to "own it."

thin thicks

We're introducing our latest trimming drinks! We've been enjoying these for several months now, and we want you to join in on the fun. These "thickies" will thin you down and nourish you up, with their key fat-kicking and health-promoting ingredients. We have a new mantra: "Let your shake be thick, not your waistline!"

Thin Thicks are not as large as the Fat-Stripping Frappas or the Big Boys (they make a manageable pint), but, man, oh man, are they thick! Like turn-your-glass-upside-down thick! These thickies make an awesome snack, but they're not large enough for a meal replacement unless you're in the mood for a very light meal. Have them alongside a sandwich or salad for lunch. Or enjoy as a filling dessert after dinner. You won't come away hungry until it is wisely time to eat again, and your body will be flooded with superfood nutrition.

Yes, these drinks do use a few special ingredients that are not optional, so you don't have to try them right out of the gate if you are a newbie THM, but many of our seasoned Trim Healthy Mamas will want to dive deep into these babies! Okra and Gluccie are like quicksand to rising blood sugar. Putting them together as a dynamic duo in one recipe is a double whammy-kabammy to out-of-control blood sugar levels. They also satiate hunger pangs and cleanse your digestive system. Whey is a fat stripper and the glycine in the collagen is one of the most intense glucagon triggers, which is the hormone that releases fat from storage.

The whey and collagen are a crime-fighting pair, providing you with 20 grams of protein in a very balanced amino acid profile. *SO PLEASE TAKE NOTE OF THE FOLLOWING:* if you are pairing this shake with a meal that already contains protein, reduce the collagen and whey by half. Sorry we had to yell, but we don't want you wasting money. If you already have sufficient protein, there's no need throwing tons more into your meal and ruining your budget or overdoing your protein counts. Collagen is not optional in these Thin Thicks, and it is not exactly cheap, so go easy.

The high antioxidant levels in cocoa used in the Chocolicious Thin Thick help your body use its insulin more efficiently to control blood sugar. Cocoa consumption has been shown to lower diabetes risk by 31 percent. The mint used in the Mintylicious Thin Thick also helps lower elevated blood sugar levels and soothes gas and bloating, which makes you feel thinner—woot! The addition of spinach in that version is not just for color; it also aids weight loss through its green leaf membranes called thylakoids, which have been shown in research to boost the production of satiety hormones. Foods rich in antioxidants, like the raspberries in the Berrylicious Thin Thick, are linked with weight loss, while the ketones in raspberries help rid the body of deep abdominal fat, called visceral fat, along with overall adipose tissue. The Matchalicious Thin Thick is a weight-kicking powerhouse. One serving of matcha powder is 137 times more potent in metabolism and disease-fighting polyphenols, called epigallocatechin gallate (EGCG), than a regular brewed cup of green tea! New studies reveal EGCG's promising ability to help prevent the growth of new fat cells. Don't miss the reasons we want you to drink the BBBB Thin Thick at the end of this section. They needed their own space.

CHOCOLICIOUS THIN THICK

SINGLE SERVE —MAKES 1 PINT

½ cup water

⅓ cup frozen diced okra

¼ teaspoon Sunflower Lecithin

1 teaspoon Just Gelatin

2 teaspoons cool water

1 tablespoon hot (not quite boiling) water

¼ teaspoon Gluccie

1½ tablespoons unsweetened cocoa powder

1 scoop Integral Collagen

½ teaspoon vanilla extract

¼ teaspoon butter extract

1 teaspoon MCT oil, or ½ teaspoon extra-virgin coconut oil

2½ teaspoons Super Sweet blend

2 pinches Mineral Salt

1½ cups ice cubes

½ scoop Pristine Whey Protein

1. Place the water, okra, and lecithin in a blender.

2. Soften the gelatin in the cool water in a cup. Stir, then add the hot water and stir well again to dissolve the gelatin.

3. Add the dissolved gelatin to the blender, followed by the Gluccie. Blend very well, until the okra is pureed. Add all the remaining ingredients except the ice and whey protein, and blend some more. Stop blending, then add the ice gradually and blend until smooth.

4. Add the whey protein and blend for 10 seconds only.

5. Put the mixture into a pint jar with a straw, and slurp this thick creaminess to the last satisfying drop. Cheers to your health!

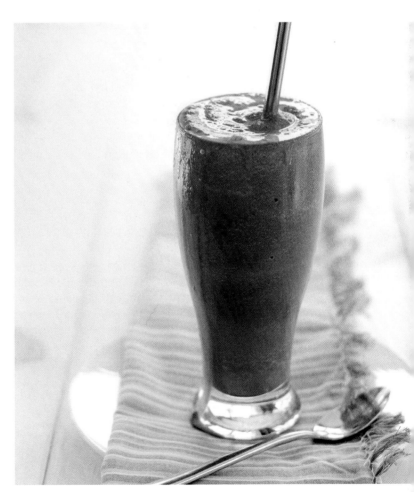

BERRYLICIOUS THIN THICK (FP)

SINGLE SERVE – MAKES 1 PINT

1. Use all the same ingredients as in the master recipe, but omit the cocoa and butter extract, and reduce the ice to 1 cup. Add ½ cup frozen raspberries, 2 tablespoons lemon juice, and an optional drop or two of essential lemon oil. You can also add 1,000 mg vitamin C powder, if desired, for a tart burst and for helping adrenal function. Reduce the Super Sweet Blend to 2 teaspoons. Add the raspberries with the first batch of ice so they get pureed. Then add the remaining ice and blend until fully smooth. Add the whey at the end and blend for 10 seconds on high.

MINTYLICIOUS THIN THICK (FP)

SINGLE SERVE – MAKES 1 PINT

1. Use all the same ingredients as in the master recipe, except omit the cocoa and add a handful of fresh spinach, or 5 to 6 drops liquid chlorophyll, ¼ teaspoon mint extract, and/or a couple drops of essential mint oil. Reduce the sweetener to 1½ to 2 teaspoons. Add the spinach with the ingredients that are blended first.

MATCHALICIOUS THIN THICK (FP)

SINGLE SERVE – MAKES 1 PINT

1. Use all the same ingredients as in the master recipe except omit the cocoa and add 1 teaspoon matcha powder.

BBBB THIN THICK Ⓢ

(BABY, BRAIN, AND BOOBY BUILDER)

SINGLE SERVE – MAKES 1 PINT

SERENE CHATS: *This rich and creamy drink is so filled with hormone-healing, brain-boosting, pregnancy-nurturing, nerve-calming goodies that it will catapult your health into a new state of flourishing. I devoured this smoothie during my recent pregnancy, but it benefits any woman, pregnant or not. I have chickens who run around my backyard, and I love to use the raw yolks because they are so golden and spectacular.*

Okra is a super veggie to support pregnancy, as it is ultra-rich in folic acid and vitamin C. Sunflower Lecithin supports brain health (including the brain health of a baby in utero), is nerve healing, prevents dementia, and treats depression. It is also a suggested supplement for nursing Mamas to prevent breast infections, and is a studied breast-cancer fighter—in short, a booby helper! MCT oil is the brain's "super unleaded fuel" and raw vitamin D–rich egg yolks support hormone health. Collagen and gelatin help build healthy babies, support perky boobies, and help a blossoming pregnant Mama's skin as it stretches and grows so it will snap back firmly. And the high-antioxidant cocoa is a true beauty food, helping with healthy blood oxygenation and circulation. Cheers! Whatever you're drinking to, whether it be a healthy baby, a more focused brain, or flourishing curves, enjoy every yummy sip along the way!

1. Use all the same ingredients as in the master recipe, except reduce the cocoa to 2 teaspoons, and use 1 teaspoon of MCT oil as the fat and 1 to 2 tablespoons of Sunflower Lecithin. Add 1 teaspoon of ghee (clarified butter) for a rich buttery flavor, if desired, or use 1 teaspoon butter extract. Add 1 raw pastured egg yolk (or the healthiest store-bought egg yolk you can find), and increase the salt to 3 to 4 pinches. Put the egg yolk in the blender at the beginning of blending your ingredients.

HOT DRINKS

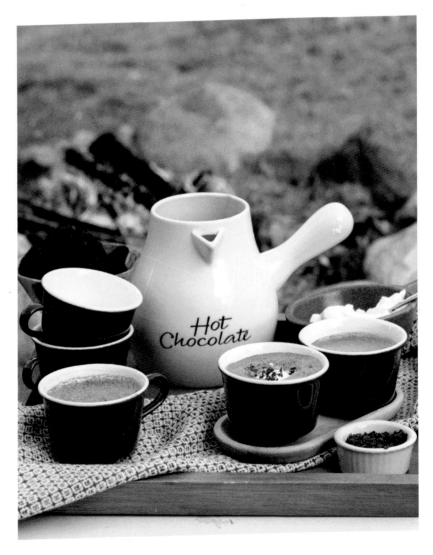

Cuddle Family Hot Chocolate (page 435)

trimmies

Welcome the Trimmaccino into your life! It's fondly known as the "Trimmy" in THM land. Start your day the Trimmy way, and your health and weight-loss goals will be reset every morning. If you're addicted to chemical-laden coffee creamers, oust them from your life with the help of the Trimmy. Coffee with heavy cream or half-and-half is on plan, so there's no need to demonize that yummy stuff. And if you are determined to do the plan without special ingredients, that's perfectly fine, too. Trimmies are not mandatory on plan; you'll be doing Trim Healthy Mama your way by sticking only to your cream or half-and-half, and we are fiercely proud of you for how far you have come. But some of us can sabotage our health and weight-loss goals by overdoing the cream. You don't have to raise your hand. And let's be honest; store-bought ultrapasteurized cream is not necessarily a superfood. Let's enjoy it when we want to, but let's have another go-to creamer option that shoots our health forward. The Trimmy fits that role perfectly.

Trimmaccinos are designed to raise the thermogenic temperature of your body, which means they heat you up and help you burn fat more efficiently. They boost and protect your brain function, offer your body some super protein, and even beautify your skin and hair—all in a delicious cup of creamy, steaming goodness! They allow you to harness the energizing power of coffee, but not overdo the fuel amounts in one simple cuppa. You can also "Trimmy" up any creamy drink you could want. Don't stop with the Joe—keep the Trimmies coming.

The Trimmy recipe has evolved over the last couple of years since we first shared it on our Facebook fan page. We have continued to tweak it to have a better mouth feel and to stay creamy looking with no separation or evaporation of milkiness to the last drop. There are two types of Trimmies you can make: the budget-friendly basic Trimmy or the super-duper Healing Trimmy. In the basic version, you use only 1 teaspoon of Integral Collagen, whereas in the healing version you use ½ to 1 scoop of this glycine-rich, body-renewing superfood. Your choice will depend on how protein rich your meal may already be, or you may choose the basic Trimmy because of budget concerns. If your meal contains lots of protein, you won't need the Healing Trimmy with its full scoop of collagen; you can do half a scoop or just a teaspoon.

Just as there are two types of Trimmies, there are two ways to fuel your Trimmy. The Trimmy Light uses just 1 to 2 teaspoons of MCT oil and can pair with an FP or an E meal (if the FP or E meal includes 1 teaspoon fat, then stick to 1 teaspoon MCT oil). The Trimmy Rich uses 1 tablespoon of oil and needs to pair with S meals unless you are seeking a Crossover. If you don't mind the taste of coconut oil or butter (from grass-fed is best for this recipe) in your coffee, you can substitute the MCT oil with ½ to 1 teaspoon of either of those for the Trimmy Light and 2 to 3 teaspoons for the Trimmy Rich.

But coconut flavor in coffee is not for everybody. People either love it or loathe it. We list MCT oil as the first option, not only for its neutral taste but also for its incredibly decadent silky mouthfeel that comes from a very small amount. We also like to use it in our Trimmies because it has such powerful brain-charging and fat-stripping abilities. Feel free to use the other fats if MCT oil is unavailable, however.

You will be using just a small amount of Sunflower Lecithin in each Trimmy. Yes, it is another special ingredient, but buy just one bag and it will last you many months. This incredible brain-protecting, nerve-calming substance keeps your Trimmy creamy looking to the last drop, and

HAPPIFY YOUR CREAMY DRINKS!

To any of the drinks in this chapter that would suit a creamy, chocolaty flavor and aroma, you can add 1 to 2 teaspoons of cocoa butter (which of course will make your drink an **S**; don't add it to **E** drinks unless you're choosing a Crossover). This richly nutritious and chocolaty scented superfood is one of the happiest foods God ever invented. It deliciously raises endorphins and serotonin levels in the brain and imparts feelings of giddy glee. The very reason chocolate is known to make us happy is due to the abilities of cocoa butter! It is known to raise levels of dopamine (the "wellbeing" hormone) and oxytocin (the "attachment" hormone) in the body. High in oleic fatty acids, this delicious food medicine is protective against heart disease, and its high magnesium content helps prevent headaches and drops in progesterone, which are linked to PMS. We all know PMS *ain't* a happy feelin'. Cocoa butter sure is not a mandatory ingredient on this plan, but if you suffer from severe PMS symptoms, go find some online (it's more expensive in health food stores, but you can usually find it there, too).

There are many other reasons to get happy about cocoa butter. It is loaded with vitamins, flavonoids, antioxidants, and minerals that replenish sluggish health, protect against damaging free radicals, and fight disease. You will also be elated to know that cocoa butter is packed with cocoa mass polyphenol (CMP), which is a powerful anti-cancer weapon. It also has a talent for soothing arthritis symptoms and preventing cardiovascular disease. CMP has been shown in studies to help control excessive T-cell activity, which is the known trigger of dysfunctional immune disorders like psoriasis, fibromyalgia, and chronic fatigue syndrome. Cocoa butter wields a double attack against cancer with its rich quantities of a preventative substance known as Pentamer.

When adding cocoa butter to cold, creamy drinks, you might want to let it sit in a lid on top of a cup of hot water to let it soften just a bit. If you want to add it to any hot drinks, like the Trimmies (see pages 430–433), just stick it straight into the blender.

has oodles of health benefits of its own, which you can read about in the "Specialty Food Stars" chapter of *Trim Healthy Mama Plan.*

Following are the two main Trimmies recipes—Light and Rich; a comparison reveals the differences between what we call the "healing" version and the "basic" version. Then we offer lots of fun varieties.

NOTE: An Iced Trimmy is simply the chilled version of any of the Trimmies recipes that follow. You use half the liquid (cooled to room temperature) instead of the 1½ cups called for in the hot drink recipes, and blend with a heaping cup of ice cubes.

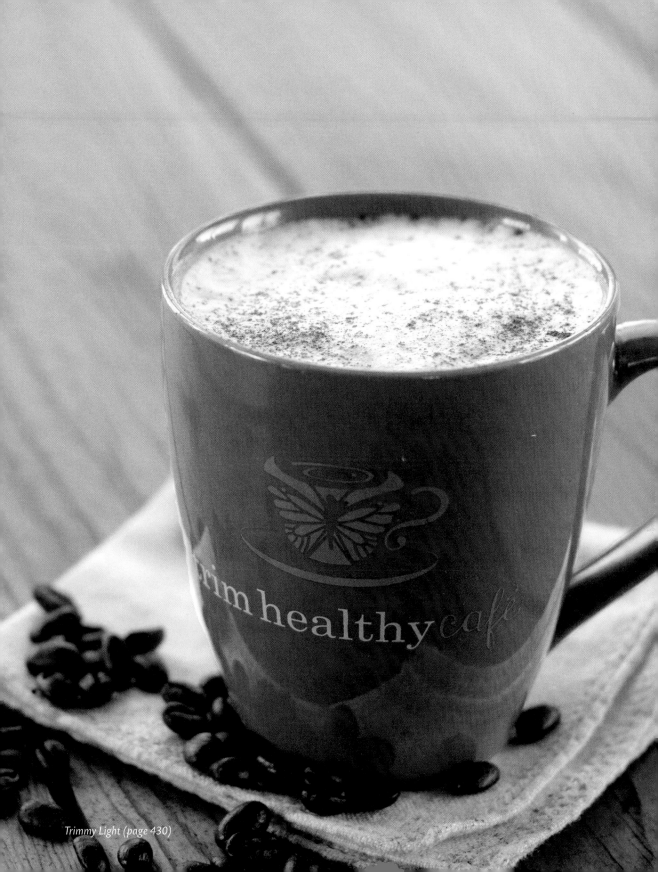

Trimmy Light (page 430)

TRIMMY LIGHT

SINGLE SERVE

12 ounces (1½ cups) your favorite hot
  brewed coffee
1 to 2 teaspoons MCT oil, or ½ to
  1 teaspoon pastured butter or
  coconut oil
½ to 1 scoop Integral Collagen (Healing
  Trimmy), or 1 teaspoon (basic
  Trimmy)
⅛ teaspoon Sunflower Lecithin
Super Sweet blend, Gentle Sweet, or
  Pure Stevia Extract to taste (optional;
  we personally prefer our coffee
  unsweetened)
1 teaspoon Pristine Whey Protein
  (optional but makes an even frothier
  Trimmy)

1. Place all the ingredients in a blender. Hold the lid on tightly
   and blend for 10 seconds, until frothy and deliciously creamy
   (or use a stick blender).

DF

TRIMMY RICH

SINGLE SERVE

12 ounces (1½ cups) your favorite hot
  brewed coffee
1 tablespoon MCT oil, or half pastured
  butter and half MCT oil (see Note)
½ to 1 scoop Integral Collagen (Healing
  Trimmy), or 1 teaspoon (basic
  Trimmy)
⅛ teaspoon Sunflower Lecithin
Super Sweet Blend, Gentle Sweet, or
  Pure Stevia Extract to taste (optional)
1 teaspoon Pristine Whey Protein
  (optional but makes an even frothier
  Trimmy)

1. Place all the ingredients in a blender. Hold the lid on tightly
   and blend for 10 seconds, until frothy and deliciously creamy
   (or use a stick blender).

NOTE: Those with sensitive tummies might need to get used to
MCT oil slowly, and at first will want to halve this rich variety
with unsalted butter. You can "happyize" this Trimmy by replacing the 1 tablespoon MCT oil with 1 teaspoon cocoa butter and
2 teaspoons MCT oil.

DF

hot chocolate trimmy (FP) WITH (S) OPTION FOR RICH VERSION

SINGLE SERVE

12 ounces (1½ cups) just-off-the-
    boil water
2 teaspoons unsweetened cocoa
    powder
1 teaspoon Super Sweet Blend, or
    more to taste
¼ teaspoon Sunflower Lecithin
1 to 2 teaspoons MCT oil or 1 full
    tablespoon for rich version (or
    use 1½ teaspoons butter and
    1½ teaspoons MCT oil for rich
    version)
½ to 1 scoop Integral Collagen (Healing
    Trimmy), or 1 teaspoon (basic
    Trimmy)
3 pinches Mineral Salt
½ teaspoon vanilla extract
1 to 2 drops essential peppermint or
    orange oil
1 teaspoon Pristine Whey Protein
    (optional but makes an even frothier
    Trimmy)

Here is an awesome Trimmy take on hot chocolate, followed by other variations on the Trimmy idea.

1. Place all the ingredients in a blender. Hold the lid on tightly and blend for 10 seconds, until frothy and deliciously creamy (or use an immersion blender).

NOTE: You can "happyize" this hot chocolate (or other drinks here except coffee) by replacing one of the teaspoons of MCT oil with 1 teaspoon of cocoa butter as part of the full table-spoon for the rich version (see "Happify Your Creamy Drinks!" page 428).

DF

MATCHA MARVEL TRIMMY (FP) WITH (S) OPTION FOR RICH VERSION

SINGLE SERVING

1. Use the same ingredients as in the master recipe, except omit the cocoa and replace with 1 teaspoon matcha powder.

MIGHTY MACA TRIMMY (FP) WITH (S) OPTION FOR RICH VERSION

SINGLE SERVING

1. Use the same ingredients as in the master recipe, except omit the cocoa and replace with 1 teaspoon gelatinized maca powder.

GINGER CREAM TRIMMY **FP** WITH **S** OPTION FOR RICH VERSION

SINGLE SERVE

1. Use the same ingredients as in the master recipe, except omit the cocoa and replace with ¼ to ½ teaspoon ground ginger.

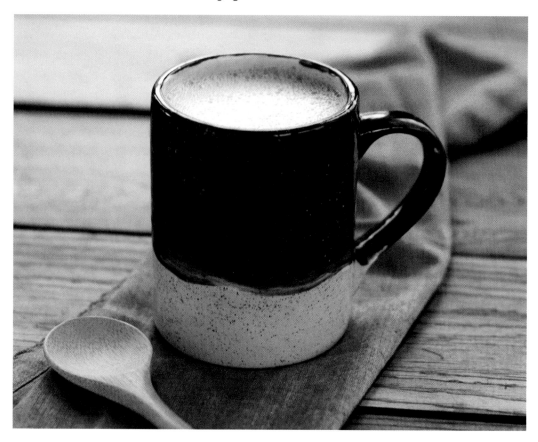

CHAI TRIMMY **FP** WITH **S** OPTION FOR RICH VERSION

SINGLE SERVE

1. Use the same ingredients as in the master recipe, except omit the cocoa and brew your favorite chai tea in a large mug of just-off-the-boil water; cover while brewing to retain heat. Add all the other ingredients to the blender before adding the tea. Blend for a few seconds or use an immersion blender.

VANILLA ROOIBOS TRIMMY WITH **S** OPTION FOR RICH VERSION

SINGLE SERVE

1. Use the same ingredients as in the master recipe, except omit cocoa and brew the rooibos tea in a large mug; cover while brewing to retain heat. Add all the other ingredients to the blender before adding the tea. Blend for a few seconds or use an immersion blender.

TURMERIC TODDY TRIMMY **FP** WITH **S** OPTION FOR RICH VERSION

SINGLE SERVE

1. Gorgeously golden, this unique drink is a spin on an Ayurvedic curative remedy from India. It is an acquired taste, but if you are not afraid of turmeric it can be an incredibly healthy toddy to restore exhausted adrenals, cleanse the liver, beautify the skin, and jump-start the cardiovascular system. Perfect for a late-evening soothing balm for your adrenals before bed. Use the same ingredients as the master recipe, except omit the cocoa and replace with ½ teaspoon turmeric (but soon scale up to ¾ or 1 teaspoon). You may need to increase the sweetener a bit if you go higher on the turmeric.

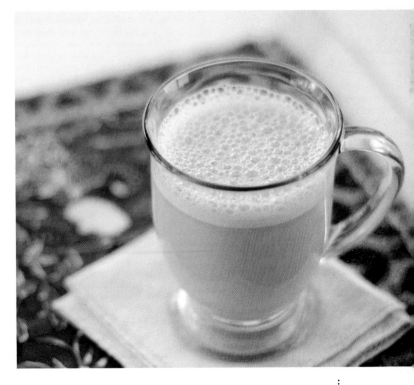

Now on to some hot drinks that are not Trimmies . . .

salted caramel creamy oolong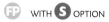

SINGLE SERVE

12 ounces (1½ cups) just-off-the-
    boil water
1 oolong tea bag (or regular tea)
⅛ teaspoon Mineral Salt
¼ teaspoon caramel extract
1 tablespoon half-and-half, or
    1 teaspoon cream (or 1 to
    2 tablespoons heavy cream for
    an indulgent **S**)
1 teaspoon Super Sweet Blend
Scant 1 tablespoon Pristine Whey
    Protein
Squirt of fat-free Reddi-wip (optional;
    for Drive Thru Sue's)

You really need to try this deliciousness. Here's a great way to enjoy a creamy hot drink without any special ingredients except the whey protein. Cindy Young shared this recipe with us. She uses 2 tablespoons low-fat half-and-half for a Fuel Pull version to be on the safe FP side, but 1 tablespoon of regular half-and-half easily fits into FP. If you want to create a really indulgent version of this drink, use heavy cream for an S version. These ingredients can be used with a variety of flavored teas, or even try it with coffee or cocoa. It's super yummy.

1. Place the hot water in a large mug and add the tea bag; cover while brewing.

2. Place all the remaining ingredients except the whey protein and Reddi-wip in a blender. Add the tea and blend for a few seconds.

3. Add the whey and blend for 5 to 10 seconds more. Serve with a squirt of Reddi-wip on top, if desired.

cuddle family hot chocolate

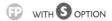

FAMILY SERVE — MAKES 6 TO 8 GENEROUS CUPS (HALVE INGREDIENTS IF YOUR FAMILY IS SMALLER OR DOUBLE FOR LARGER FAMILIES)

8 cups just-off-the-boil water

5½ tablespoons unsweetened cocoa powder

2 teaspoons vanilla extract

⅛ teaspoon Mineral Salt

6 to 8 teaspoons Super Sweet Blend or use double amounts of Gentle Sweet

5½ teaspoons Just Gelatin

1½ to 2 tablespoons butter, coconut oil, or ghee (clarified butter) (see Note)

½ to 1½ teaspoons Sunflower Lecithin (this really makes it, but you can get away with ½ teaspoon if you are budgeting all your ingredients)

1 cup frozen diced okra (optional but recommended)

SERENE CHATS: *This drink brings the family together. We make it on family movie nights, or on any evening when we are all just hanging together. It helps my little ones settle down, and it seems to make our family experience somehow cozier and cuddlier. This recipe is completely milk free, even free of milk substitutes, which is great for us purists, because if we have a raw milk source, then why heat that and destroy its rawness, right? This hot chocolate has key ingredients, like glycine-rich gelatin that acts as a soothing dietary lullaby to settle down wired little (or adult) bodies and ready them for sleep. The tiny bit of healthy fat and tummy settling and satiating okra will help quiet nighttime, post-dinner hunger. Cocoa may be thought of as stimulating, but this high-antioxidant ingredient is also rich in magnesium, which calms the nervous system; when tempered with healthy fat and the smooth viscosity of okra, its effect is not awakening but relaxing. Remember, if you choose to use the okra, keep the secret to yourself if you think it will dampen your children's acceptance of this yummy drink. We promise if they don't know it's in there, they will never taste it! This is a great way for veggie-hating children to get a daily or (nightly) health dose.*

Mix up the batch in the evening, keep it on a warming element, and then ladle out the hot chocolate throughout the evening to your eager sippers.

1. Place 4 cups of the hot water in a blender. Add all the remaining ingredients except the okra (if using) and blend until very smooth.

2. Pour the puree into a saucepan. Add the remaining 4 cups hot water to the blender, add the okra (if using), and blend until completely broken down and creamified.

3. Pour into the saucepan and whisk briskly while heating the mixture over medium heat. Taste and adjust to "own it."

NOTE: You can **S** this drink by adding more butter or coconut oil or ghee, if desired.

DF (IF USING COCONUT OIL OR GHEE; THE GHEE IS TOLERATED WELL BY MANY WHO ARE DAIRY SENSITIVE)

collagen tea

SINGLE SERVE

12 ounces (1½ cups) just-off-the-
   boil water
Tea bag of choice
½ to 1 scoop Integral Collagen (see
   Note)

Any hot tea (or iced tea, for that matter) can become a superfood protein booster for your meal or snack. Let's say you want some fruit for a snack, but don't want to go to the bother of having cottage cheese or Greek yogurt with it—you're in a hurry. Simply add 1 scoop of Integral Collagen to your hot tea. It dissolves fully and you will never taste it. This is also a great way to end your meal if it did not include a lot of protein. Perhaps you only had 3 to 4 ounces of meat on your salad or a bean or lentil soup—you could do with a bit more protein. Collagen Tea to the rescue, baby!

1. Place the hot water in a large mug and add the tea bag; cover while brewing. Remove the tea bag, then stir the collagen into the hot tea with a fork. Keep stirring until completely dissolved. At first the tea will appear cloudy, but after 30 seconds to 1 minute, it will be clear. Enjoy!

NOTE: If you want Collagen Iced Tea, dissolve the collagen in the tea while it is hot, then chill.

DF

MORE DRINKS

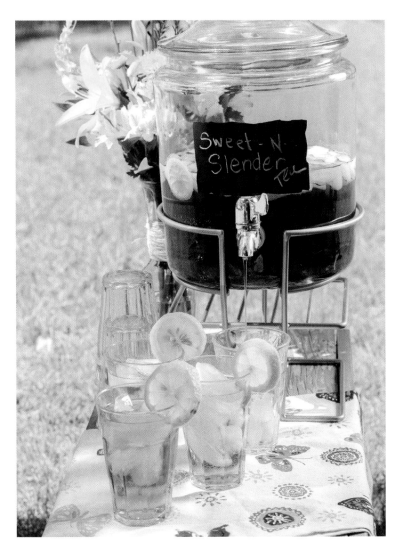

Sweet 'n' Slender Iced Tea (page 438)

sweet 'n' slender iced tea

1 gallon chilled brewed black tea
½ teaspoon Pure Stevia Extract

Heads up, sweet tea drinkers! This is the most economical way to sweeten a full gallon of iced tea. While coffee can be a little tricky when it comes to using stevia, the flavors of tea lend themselves perfectly to stevia. Don't waste your Super Sweet Blend or Gentle Sweet on tea when the pure extract will do the trick nicely and save your budget!

1. Pour 1 cup of the tea into a jar and add the stevia. Whisk until the stevia is dissolved (don't taste; it will be way too strong). Pour the cup of tea back into the gallon. Close tightly and shake well to combine, or stir well. Return the tea to the refrigerator for anytime use.

DF

strawberry milk

SINGLE SERVE

1 cup chilled unsweetened almond or
   cashew milk
3 whole frozen strawberries
1½ teaspoons Super Sweet Blend
1 to 2 tablespoons Pristine Whey
   Protein or ½ scoop Integral Collagen
Dash of vanilla extract

A wonderful way to end any meal if you are not quite filled up yet—or enjoy it anytime.

1. Put all the ingredients in a blender and blend until smooth.

DF (IF USING COLLAGEN INSTEAD OF WHEY PROTEIN)

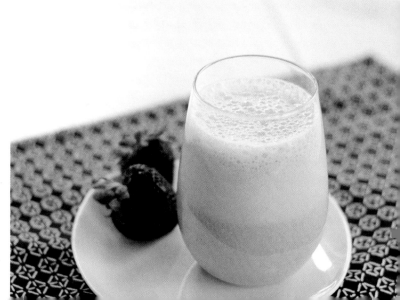

easy chocolate milk

SINGLE SERVE

1 cup chilled unsweetened almond or cashew milk

1 rounded teaspoon unsweetened cocoa powder

1½ teaspoons Super Sweet Blend (or use double amount of Gentle Sweet)

1 to 2 tablespoons Pristine Whey Protein or ½ scoop Integral Collagen

1. Place all the ingredients in a blender and blend until smooth.

NOTE: In place of the cocoa, sweetener, and whey protein, you can use 2 to 3 tablespoons TrimQuik (page 494).

DF (IF USING COLLAGEN INSTEAD OF WHEY PROTEIN)

foundation milk

SINGLE SERVE

1½ cups water

½ to 1 teaspoon extra-virgin coconut oil, or 1 to 2 teaspoons MCT oil (see Note)

¼ teaspoon Sunflower Lecithin

¼ scoop Integral Collagen (optional)

Pinch of Mineral Salt

1 doonk Pure Stevia Extract (optional)

SERENE CHATS: *This is a simple milk substitute for when you don't have any unsweetened nut, seed, or coconut milk on hand. I frequently use it for my smoothie or drink-milk purposes, and no longer have to rely on store-bought unsweetened almond or cashew milk all the time. If you have nut or dairy allergies, this milk can be your new BFF. Or, if you're a purist and don't like the thought of fillers in the carton stuff, worry no longer. Foundation Milk whips up in a jiffy and is a superfoodie, simply delicious option. If you're using the milk in a recipe that already has collagen, then leave it out here. Similarly, if using the milk in a savory preparation, omit the stevia. The recipe can be doubled, tripled, or even quadrupled, but all results should be stored in the fridge for use within a few days.*

1. Place all the ingredients in a blender and blend until very smooth. Pour into a glass jar and store in the refrigerator until ready to use.

NOTE: If you are concerned about fuel stacking (as described in the "Higher Learning" chapter of *Trim Healthy Mama Plan*), and are adding this to other ingredients with oils or fats, then decrease the oil to ½ teaspoon coconut oil or ¾ to 1 teaspoon MCT oil.

DF

beauty milks

Sip your way to more youthful and resilient skin. Raise your glass to lustrous hair, skin, nails, and stronger muscles and joints. Beauty Milk is a simple daily regimen for repair and preservation that works from the inside out. Don't just drink this milk because it's absolutely yumsers; drink it also because you are being responsible, kind, and nurturing to yourself.

VANILLA BEAUTY MILK

SINGLE SERVE

1 cup water
1 teaspoon MCT oil
½ to 1 scoop Integral Collagen
1 to 2 doonks Pure Stevia Extract, or
  ½ to ¾ teaspoon Super Sweet Blend
2 pinches Mineral Salt
½ teaspoon vanilla extract
4 to 5 large ice cubes

1. Place all the ingredients in a blender and blend until completely smooth.

NOTE: If you also add ⅛ teaspoon Sunflower Lecithin, it will make your milk creamy white and stay that way for future enjoyment. It does make this vanilla version a tiny bit bitter and slightly malty tasting, so if you are drinking it immediately and don't care about the perfect creamy color, you needn't bother with it. (Serene likes the flavor added by the lecithin.)

DF

CHOCOLATE BEAUTY MILK

SINGLE SERVE

1. Use all the same ingredients as in the master recipe, except use 2 to 3 doonks Pure Stevia Extract, add another pinch of salt, and add 1 teaspoon unsweetened cocoa powder. Adding the Sunflower Lecithin works well here because the chocolate masks any malt flavor.

GREEN VIBRANCE BEAUTY MILK

SINGLE SERVE

1. Use all the same ingredients as in the master recipe, but add 1 teaspoon green powder of choice (like barley grass).

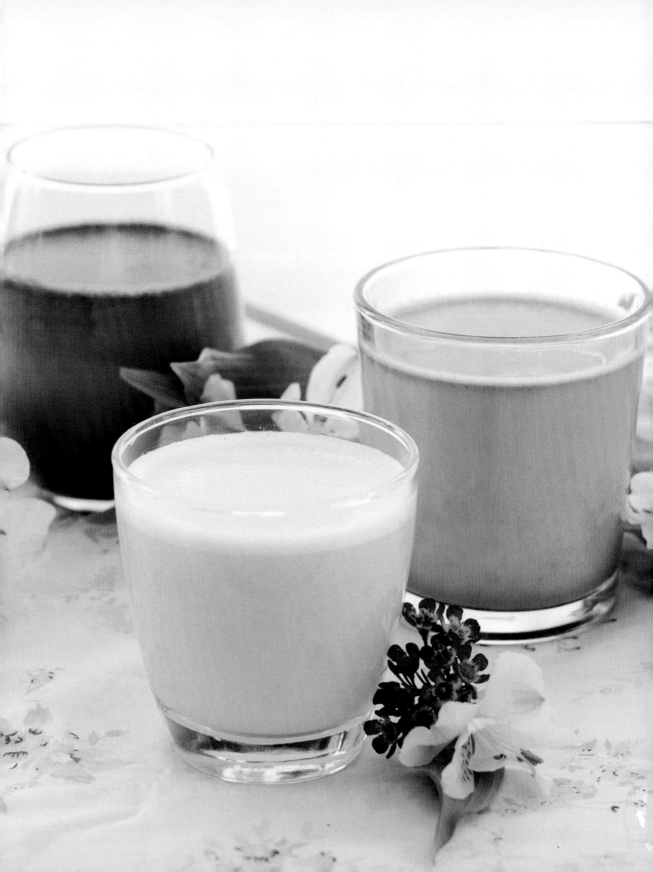

iced coffee

SINGLE SERVE – ENJOY ALL FOR YOURSELF OR SHARE WITH A FAMILY MEMBER

1 cup unsweetened almond or
　cashew milk
½ scoop Pristine Whey Protein or
　1 scoop Integral Collagen
10 to 12 large ice cubes
1 cup strongly brewed coffee, cooled
2 teaspoons Super Sweet Blend

1. Pour the almond milk into a quart jar. Add the whey protein and stir well. Add the ice cubes, followed by the coffee and sweetener. Stir well.

DF (IF USING COLLAGEN INSTEAD OF WHEY PROTEIN)

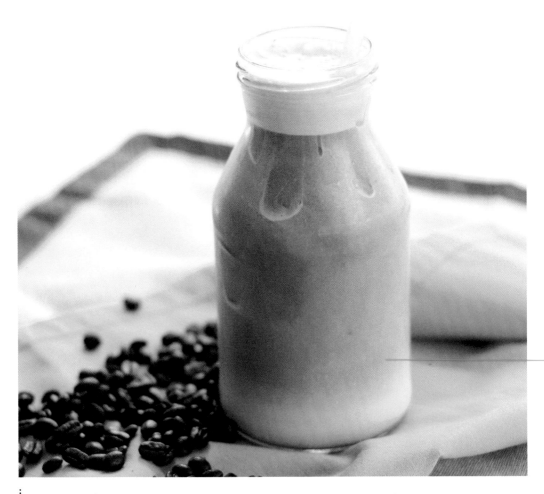

lemon-lime trim pop

Juice of ½ lemon (or 1 tablespoon
  lemon concentrate)

Juice of ½ lime (or 1 tablespoon lime
  concentrate)

2 doonks Pure Stevia Extract, or to
  taste

3 to 6 large ice cubes

12 ounces sparkling water

The THM plan offers you so many healthy hydrating drinks to choose from, but sometimes you just gotta have something bubbly! Get your pop fix with this revitalizing drink. Enjoy the bubbles dancing on your tongue and the zingy flavor of the citrus juice as it cleans and alkalizes your body!

1. Pour the juices into a large glass or jar, add the sweetener, and stir well. Add the ice cubes and then fill with the sparkling water.

NSI (IF YOU USE YOUR FAVORITE ON-PLAN SWEETENER) DF

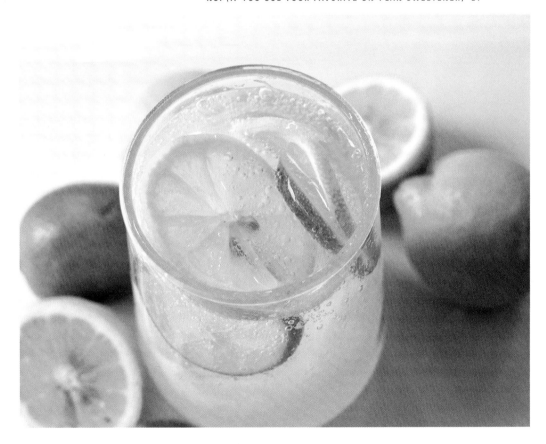

root beer float

SINGLE SERVE

1½ teaspoons root beer extract

1 teaspoon vanilla extract

¼ cup unsweetened almond or cashew milk

2 doonks Pure Stevia Extract, or to taste

1 tablespoon Pristine Whey Protein

4 to 6 large ice cubes

12 ounces sparkling water

So while there is no floating ice cream here, the creaminess and flavors of this drink make you feel like there is. How perfect on a hot day! You can find natural brands of root beer extract online or sometimes in health food stores and regular grocery stores.

1. Put the extracts in a large glass. Add the milk, sweetener, and protein powder, and whisk well. Add the ice cubes, then fill with the sparkling water.

NOTE: If preferred, just purchase stevia-sweetened root beer, pour a little into a glass, stir in the milk and protein powder, then fill the glass with the root beer.

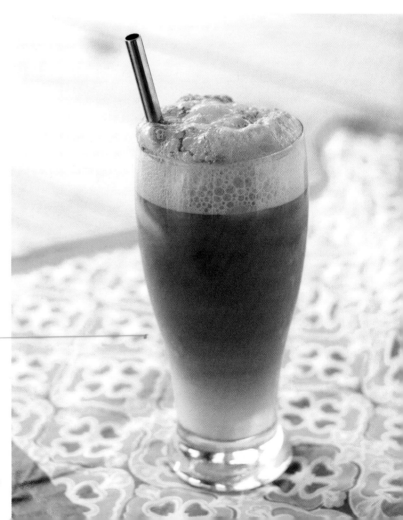

double fermented kefir

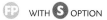
SINGLE SERVE — MAKES 2 CUPS

2 cups fermented kefir

1 to 2 tablespoons kefir grains

2 cups skim milk (or whole milk for **S** version)

SERENE CHATS: *Double fermenting multiplies the health benefits of kefir, which is a superfood cultured milk like a drinkable yogurt. The double fermentation eats up more of the lactose (milk sugars), so if you use skim milk to make your kefir, you can achieve a Fuel Pull cup of kefir. You would think that the double fermentation would create a more sour-tasting kefir, but it actually mellows the taste. I sometimes use whole milk for S purposes, but I only do this if I can get raw milk from grass-fed cows or goats (toxins are stored in the fats of animals). If I don't have such a source, I simply use skim (fat-free) milk from the grocery store.*

This recipe starts with 2 cups of 24-hour fermented kefir and kicks up from there. If you are completely new to kefir making, check out the instructions online—there are so many recipes for it. You'll need to get grains from a kefir-making friend or buy them online, but there are plenty to be found. This recipe makes a very manageable 2 cups per day. You can add a doonk or two of stevia and berries to stay in FP mode, or add other fruit like peaches for E. (Check out my video for making double fermented kefir in the video archives on our website.)

1. Drain the fermented kefir in a plastic colander with small holes. Use a plastic or wooden spoon (not metal) to stir vigorously so all the liquid is pushed through the holes into a sterilized pint jar.

2. Put the kefir grains back into the original pint jar and fill with the milk to continue the fermentation process. Cover the fermenting jar with a light cloth and place in a dark cupboard for one day to keep up your supply of fermented kefir.

3. Screw a tight lid onto the jar that now contains your kefir liquid and place in a dark cupboard to ferment for 24 hours, or up to 48 hours. (This second fermentation helps create the superfood-enzymes effect and you can now drink this with any meal or any snack.)

NOTE: You can make what we call a superfood-loaded kefir smoothie by blending the kefir with frozen berries, sweetener, a raw pastured egg yolk, superfood oil, and any other goodies you think will do your body good—like turmeric.

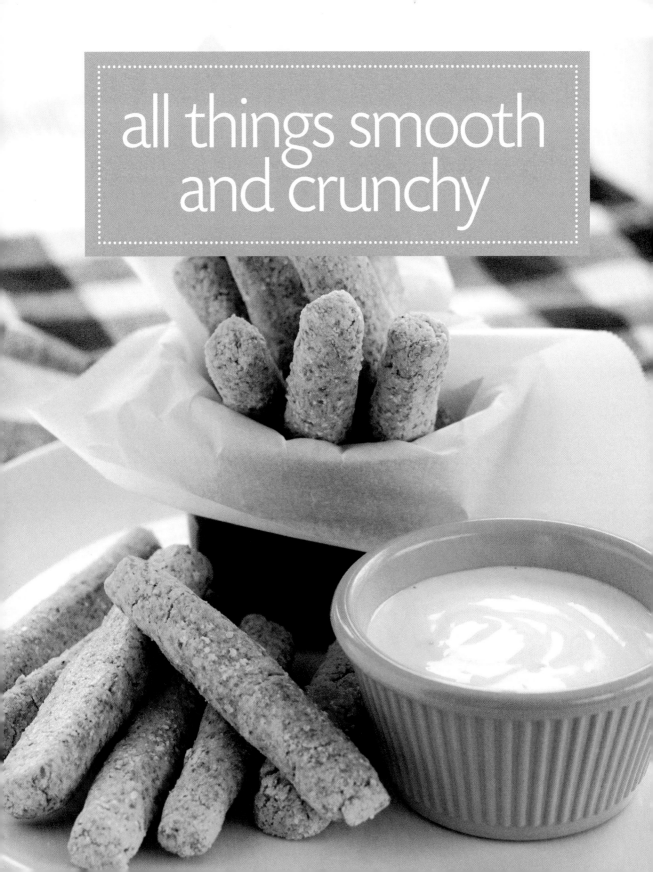

all things smooth
and crunchy

● = S   ● = E   ● = FP   MORE THAN ONE DOT INDICATES OPTIONS

CRACKERS, CHIPS, AND DIPS

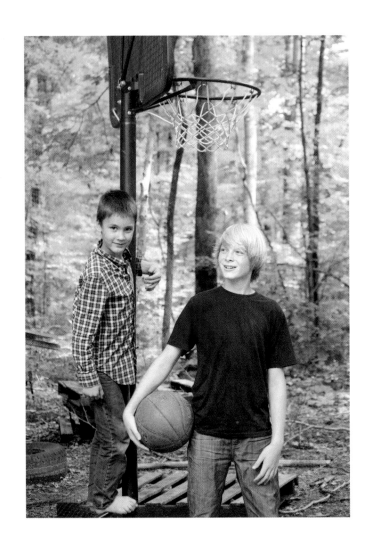

drive thru sue cheesy crackers

(S)

¼ cup plus 2 tablespoons finely grated Parmesan cheese (green can is fine)

¼ cup plus 1 tablespoon Trim Healthy Mama Baking Blend

4 tablespoons (½ stick) butter

2½ tablespoons water

3 ounces sharp cheddar cheese (does not have to be grated)

Scant ⅛ teaspoon Mineral Salt

⅛ teaspoon cayenne pepper

½ teaspoon paprika

Garlic powder to taste

PEARL CHATS: Easy, crunchy, and crisp. Don't dive into a box of Cheezits or fall for a bag of Doritos when you can make these in a jiffy! My husband and children love them. They're so much healthier for your growing children than those orange, fish-shaped crackers.

1. Preheat the oven to 350°F. Line two 9 × 13-inch baking sheets with parchment.

2. Put all the ingredients in a food processor and process well for 2 to 3 minutes. Don't worry if the mix is still a little crumbly.

3. Transfer the cheese mixture to a large bowl and press the crumbles together into a very loose dough. Grab teaspoon-size pieces and press into balls with your fingers (a fun job for children). Place the balls on the prepared baking sheets.

4. Press each little ball flat with 2 fingers or squish with the bottom of a jar. They should end up about the size of a small, thin zucchini slice, or about as big as a typical store-bought cheese cracker. Bake for 12 to 15 minutes, or until golden.

5. Allow the crackers to fully cool so they can crisp up. If crackers lose their crispness after a day or so, reheat in a 300°F oven for 5 to 10 minutes.

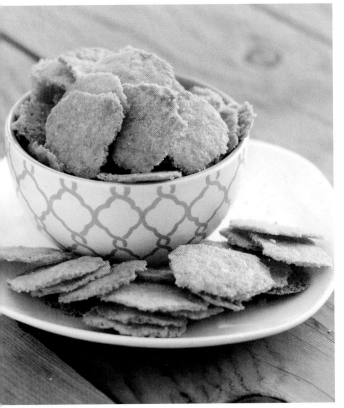

purist cheesy crackers

MULTIPLE SERVE — MAKES 1 EXTRA LARGE 11 × 15-INCH BAKING SHEET FULL OF CRACKERS

⅓ cup extra-virgin coconut oil

1 cup finely grated Parmesan cheese (green can is fine)

½ cup Trim Healthy Mama Baking Blend

½ teaspoon aluminum-free baking powder

3 tablespoons nutritional yeast

½ teaspoon onion powder

2 tablespoons Integral Collagen

5½ tablespoons unsweetened almond or cashew milk (or Foundation Milk, page 439)

OPTIONAL ADDITIONS

Toasted sesame oil (use just 3 tablespoons coconut oil and add 1 tablespoon sesame oil to the mix)

⅛ teaspoon black pepper

⅛ teaspoon cayenne pepper

1 teaspoon Liquid Smoke

¼ cup toasted sesame seeds (stir these in after processing)

SERENE CHATS: *I'm happy Pearl got herself a Drive Thru Sue cheese cracker replacement. My purist mindset doesn't allow me to eat pasteurized cheese very often, but I didn't like missing out! You may be wondering what makes my own crackers purist friendly? I may not be as fastidious as other purists, but I don't mind doing a little Parmesan cheese from time to time. I like to get most of my fat calories from superfood oils, avocados, or pastured raw dairy products, so I don't personally eat regular store-bought fatty cheeses unless they are raw (and then I gobble them up like a monster). My reasoning is that I simply don't like to waste calories, and I know that store-bought pasteurized cheese has a bunch of calories without much superfood return.*

Parmesan cheese is very light and is aged with only 1.5 grams of fat per tablespoon. Using a bit of "Parmy" for flavor and getting most of the calories from virgin coconut oil in these crisps makes their fat fuel more purist, and that gets placebo points from my brain. They also have a couple of nutritional powerhouses thrown in for good measure, like collagen and nutritional yeast. I mean, it's not like I'm so wound up that I won't eat some of Pearl's Drive Thru Sue Cheesy Crackers (page 449; which are very yummy) or have a piece of regular cheddar now and then, but if I'm going to make the effort to prepare something, it has to fit my purist reasoning.

1. Preheat the oven to 350°F. Line a large 11 × 15-inch baking sheet with parchment.

2. Put all the ingredients, including your chosen additions, except sesame seeds (if using), in a food processor and process until the mixture forms a ball of dough. Tear off pieces of dough and roll into little balls.

3. Place the balls on the prepared sheet and flatten with the back of a spoon (dip the spoon into a little cup of water to keep from getting sticky) or use your fingers. Or, you can roll out the dough and score little squares. Bake for 20 minutes. Alternatively, bake on the lowest setting your oven has just before you go to bed and let them crisp gently all night.

NOTE: The dough can be prepared ahead and stored in a zippy bag in the refrigerator for up to 2 weeks, or even frozen. Just allow it to soften at room temperature and then bake.

cheese chips

MULTIPLE SERVE

S

¾ cup egg whites (from carton
or 6 large eggs)

¼ teaspoon xanthan gum

2 teaspoons Rohnda's Ranch
Seasoning (page 492) or "Macho"
Nacho Seasoning (page 492), or Trim
Bouillon Mix (page 491)

¾ cup grated sharp cheddar cheese

Finely grated Parmesan cheese, for
sprinkling (optional)

These crunchy chips are a lighter S and just another way to get your crunch satisfaction. The Thinnies (page 455) are great easy chips/crackers, but there is only so much cheese you can eat, ya' know? Cheese is calorie dense, and sometimes you have to stop eating it before you feel quite ready. This chip recipe gives more bang for your cheesy-snacking buck. The calories are not nearly as dense, meaning you get to eat more—yippee!

1. Preheat the oven to 300°F. Line a large baking sheet with parchment.

2. In a medium mixing bowl, beat the egg whites and xanthan gum on medium speed until soft peaks form, approximately 3 minutes. Sprinkle the seasoning of choice onto the egg whites and beat on medium speed until the seasoning is well incorporated. Sprinkle the grated cheddar over the egg whites and gently fold in the cheese using a rubber spatula.

3. Using a tablespoon, put spoonfuls of the mixture onto the prepared baking sheet and, with the back of a spoon, gently flatten each mound into disks about 2 inches in diameter. Sprinkle each circle with grated Parmesan, if desired.

4. Bake for 20 minutes, or until the chips are a light golden brown. Turn off the oven and leave the chips in to cool for 20 to 30 minutes, or until firm and crisp.

5. Store in an airtight container for up to 2 days. To re-crisp, place on a baking sheet and put in a 300°F oven for 10 minutes.

NSI DF

crunkers

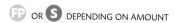

MULTIPLE SERVE – MAKES 2 LARGE 9 × 13-INCH BAKING SHEETS FULL OF CRACKERS (KEEP TO ⅛ RECIPE FOR **FP**)

1 cup Trim Healthy Mama Baking Blend

2 tablespoons ghee (clarified butter) or coconut oil

1 cup egg whites (carton or fresh) or same amount of water (for an egg-free version)

⅓ teaspoon Mineral Salt

½ teaspoon aluminum-free baking powder

SERENE CHATS: *At last, a cracker that is friendly to many of our allergen-free Mamas! If you have to avoid gluten, dairy, or even eggs, no worries; now you can have a neutral-tasting, crunchy cracker that is perfect topped with avocado or cheese and tomato (there is a little bit of almond flour in these crackers, though). We call these Crunkers because they're a cross between a sturdy cracker and a dunker for soups or dips. If you are both egg and dairy intolerant, a slice of Hello Cheese (page 487) sits perfectly on this cracker. Or smear it with Laughin' Mama Cheese (page 484), then top with sliced cucumber and a sprinkle of salt and pepper—yum! No more missing out for you!*

If you're not gluten intolerant—HEY, DON'T SKIP THIS RECIPE! Sorry, I had to raise my voice there, but this is not an exclusive allergen-free recipe, and I don't want anyone missing out! I tolerate gluten just fine, but I make these because I love them and so does my family. They are super easy to make, and you can munch on them and not fret about a fading waistline. Reclaim your girlish trim with crackers? Unheard of! But we're forging new trails as THMs, so get on board the pioneer wagon!

Use this as a basic recipe to beef up using your imagination. These crackers don't have a lot of flavor because you're going to put your flavorings on top of them. But you can make onion or herb and chive varieties. Create dried tomato and Italian herb crunchy crackers, too. Sprinkle in cheesy flavors like nutritional yeast, sesame oil, smoke flavoring, and a touch of lemon. You can even throw in some jalapeño heat, if you like. Have fun!

1. Line two 9 × 13-inch baking sheets with parchment or lightly grease a large baking stone.

2. Place all the ingredients in a food processor and process until smooth and well blended.

3. Divide the dough in half. Using a water-moistened rolling pin, roll out each ball of dough on the prepared baking sheet or on the greased baking stone. Moisten the rolling pin with a damp hand every time you roll in a different direction so it doesn't stick. Roll the dough out thinly, about the thickness of a saltine cracker, then score into desired shapes.

4. Place the baking sheets in the oven and set the oven to its lowest setting (preferably 150°F), but if your oven goes

down to only 175°F, that should be okay. Bake the sheets overnight or for 6 to 8 hours.

NOTE: Baking long and slow is key to making a non-bitter cracker that crunches well. You can roll out the dough earlier in the day when you have more energy (nobody wants to be cooking at 10 p.m.), then cover the baking sheets and store in the refrigerator. Put the sheets in the oven as the last thing you do before you go to bed.

DF

joseph's crackers ⓕⓟ

SINGLE SERVE

½ to 1 Joseph's pita (store bought), cut into triangles

PEARL CHATS: We Drive Thru Sue's humbly ask for grace from our fellow Purist Sistahs for this one. We can't help but love easy recipes, and this delivers. Turn your heads away from the microwave rays and avert your eyes from the not-quite-so-whole-foodsy ingredients in these crackers, dear pure ones. Don't worry, we're going to make some of the other crackers and chips too, but this recipe is just too simple for us to abandon. The commercial Joseph's bread products may not be perfect, but they can work on plan for some of us, and mercy, do they ever make a quick, practical cracker that you can put yummies on!

1. Put the pita triangles on a paper plate and microwave for 60 to 90 seconds, depending on whether you use ½ pita or a full pita. They should become golden in places. (Alternatively, place on a cookie sheet and bake for a few minutes at 375°F. Watch that they don't burn, as they brown quickly.)

NOTE: You can spray the pita triangles with coconut oil and sprinkle them with seasonings of choice before microwaving, but I never bother because I like to top them with cheddar cheese or butter and a little all-fruit jelly for an **S** or some light Laughing Cow cheese with tomato for **FP**.

NSI DF

mad melbas

Coconut oil cooking spray

1 cup Trim Healthy Mama Baking Blend

1 cup plus 2 tablespoons egg whites (carton or fresh)

8 small pinches Super Sweet Blend

4 pinches Mineral Salt

2 teaspoons aluminum-free baking powder

4 tablespoons water

OPTIONAL TOPPINGS

Coconut oil cooking spray

Mineral Salt

Garlic and onion powder

Black pepper

Finely grated Parmesan cheese

Ever see the classic movie *Alice in Wonderland,* in which the Mad Hatter and the crazy Cheshire Cat speak a bunch of senseless gibberish? We weren't acting any more sane when, at the end of many long months of cooking experiments for this book, we decided to come up with another FP cracker.

We loved our Crunkers (page 452), but knew that we couldn't really pig out on them and stay in FP range (did we mention we like to pig out?). We kept tweaking and tweaking one simple cracker, formulating changes and adjusting fat to protein to net carb ratios. Ugh! . . . with little scribbles on pieces of paper for various batch results taped and completely covering our fridges and parts of our walls. The cracker started tasting more and more like cardboard. Our husbands had to rescue us from our crazy-bin kitchens and take us out to dinner with a cooking ban for the night! We gave ourselves some "We really *do* love cooking" positive speech therapy and refreshed our noggins with a glass of Good Girl Moonshine (page 397) (that we halfway promise did not contain any hard liquor). Then the very simple solution jumped into our heads. How about we just turn our perfectly FP Swiss Bread recipe (page 196) into crackers—and by jingo, it worked!

These Mad Melbas and the following Swiss Crackers (page 457) were conceived from the ruins of our brains and we believe (though no one else will vouch for us) we have been almost sane ever since. Mad Melbas are crunchy, crispy, and perfect for loading goodies on. Woo-hoo! Off with our straitjackets!

1. Preheat the oven to 350°F. Lightly coat an 8-inch or 7 × 9-inch rectangular baking dish with coconut oil spray.

2. Combine all the ingredients in a medium bowl, blending with a whisk. Spread out into the prepared dish. (Alternatively, you could bake in a 12-cup muffin tin but the tops of the crackers may not look so perfectly "melba-ish.")

3. Bake for 20 to 25 minutes.

4. Allow to cool briefly in the dish and then invert to remove from the dish to cool completely.

5. Slice in half lengthwise. Now you will have two Melba loaves to slice into perfect Mad Melbas. Don't slice too crazy thin, slice nice thin pieces that will crisp up delightfully.

6. Lay the slices cut size down on a large baking sheet or baking stone, and if using, spray slices with coconut oil spray, then sprinkle on the toppings of choice. Bake at 350°F for an additional 10 or so minutes (keep a watch so they don't burn).

7. Turn the oven off and leave the crackers to cool slowly, the longer the better for them to crisp up. (Alternatively, you can bake them overnight on the lowest setting your oven allows; this is a foolproof way of never burning your Melbas.)

8. Remove from the oven, allow to cool, and store in zippered bags.

DF

thinnies ⓢ

MULTIPLE SERVE

Desired amount Sargento Ultra-Thin cheese slices

Here's another "cracker," and this one is so ridiculously easy. You need to use ultra-thin cheese slices to make this work, though. Sargento brand has natural cheese slices called Ultra-Thin. They work perfectly here.

1. Preheat the oven to 250°F. Line a baking sheet with parchment.

2. Cut each cheese slice into quarters. Lay the pieces on the prepared baking sheet and bake for 35 minutes, or until crispy looking.

NSI

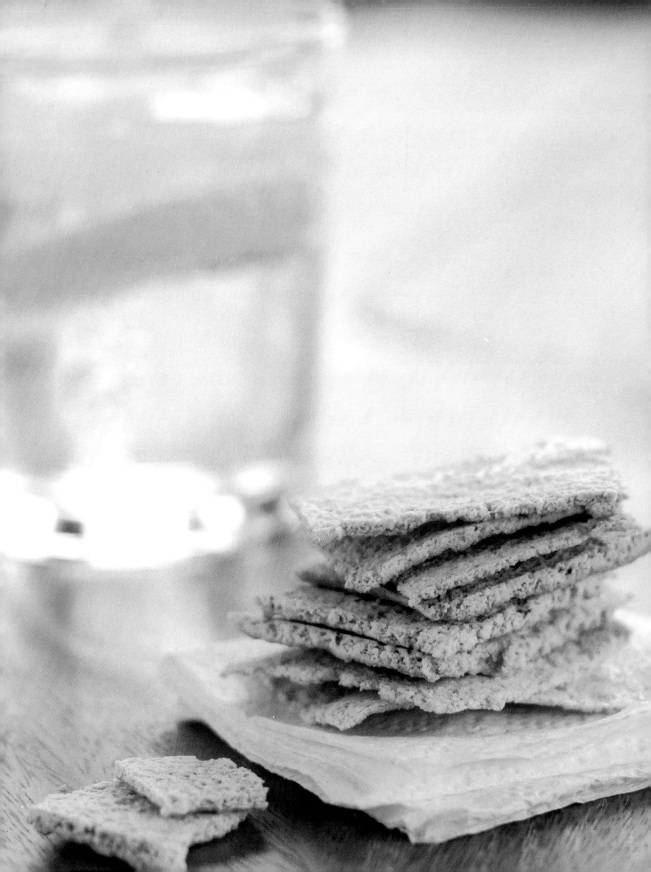

FP

Coconut oil cooking spray (optional)

1 cup Trim Healthy Mama Baking Blend (see Note)

1 cup plus 2 tablespoons egg whites (from carton or 9 large eggs)

8 small pinches Super Sweet Blend

4 pinches Mineral Salt

2 teaspoons aluminum-free baking powder

4 tablespoons water

These are more like regular crackers than the Mad Melbas on page 454. They can really shine if you are pregnant and nauseated, or recovering from a stomach virus and have no idea what to eat. During these times it can be tempting to eat empty carb crackers just to survive; maybe that is okay for a day or two—you gotta do what you gotta do sometimes—but getting too friendly with saltine crackers is not the best of relationships. They may look harmless, but those crackers are basically void of nutrition and are weight promoting to boot. They don't help baby, and they certainly don't help you.

Swiss Crackers offer the same neutral "dry cracker" fix without any of the negative effects. Instead of being blood-sugar spiking and carb laden, Swiss Crackers are high in protein. And with their glycine-rich collagen, they carry an incredibly balanced amino acid profile. Nauseated Mamas can graze on Swiss Crackers and sip on Good Girl Moonshine (page 397) made with sparkling water.

1. Lightly spray a large baking sheet with coconut oil spray or grease a baking stone.

2. Place all the ingredients in a medium bowl and whisk. Gather into a ball of dough, which will be very wet.

3. Spread the dough on the prepared baking sheet with your fingers until very thin, about the thickness of saltine crackers. Score with a knife into desired cracker shapes, marking where you will later break or cut the crackers after baking.

4. Set your oven to the lowest setting and bake until the crackers completely dry out and become crisp, about 4 hours. (Alternatively, bake for 10 minutes at 350°F, then turn off to crisp in the warm oven.)

NOTE: We find that any dough containing flax that is spread very thin and gets even slightly overbaked can lend a fishy taste (it's the omega-3 oils you are tasting). Our Baking Blend has a little bit of flax in it, and since this recipe is spread thin (and not baked as a bread first), we recommend the long and slow crisping method.

DF

crispy addictions

SERENE CHATS: *These babies are blazin'!!! Even coconut haters can't help but love them. I take them to parties and non-THMers devour them. Here are two manageable recipes for you to start with, but I make ginormous trays of both flavors, multiplying each recipe about 6 times. I put them in airtight zippered bags to take camping for the whole fam to munch on! We eat them around the campfire, in the car, in the kayak, at the beach, when we are starving at a restaurant because the food hasn't come yet, for breakfast, or as a late-night munchy. We are total junkies. They come with a warning from somebody on the other side of the addiction: Don't start if you want to keep any dignity or self-control. But, hey, if you're going to have an addiction, I couldn't think of a healthier one.*

CINNAMON CRISPY ADDICTIONS

MULTIPLE SERVE

4 cups largest flaked coconut you can find

1 teaspoon extra-virgin coconut oil

2½ teaspoons Super Sweet Blend, ground in a coffee grinder, or to taste

2 teaspoons ground cinnamon

1 teaspoon vanilla extract

3 to 4 pinches Mineral Salt, or to taste

These sweet, crispy coconut flakes are perfect for munching as a snack or for topping your Greek yogurt, NoGurt (see page 343), or Jigglegurt (page 345)—but they also make a great superfood breakfast full of middle-chain fatty acids when poured into a bowl and topped with unsweetened almond milk (or Foundation Milk, page 439) and a little extra Super Sweet Blend or Gentle Sweet sprinkled on top. Large-flake coconut is available at health food stores or online.

1. Place all the ingredients in a large mixing bowl and rub together between the palms of your hands to distribute the flavorings and mix the coconut. Spread on a large baking sheet and place in the oven at its lowest setting overnight.

2. In the morning, let the sheet cool. Once you taste them you will start the addiction and say goodbye to any other breakfast plans . . . 'cause once you start, you'll find it hard to stop.

3. Store leftovers in a gallon zippered bag from which you expel the air as much as possible, then place in the freezer. (This helps keep the crunch.)

NOTE: While the overnight baking gives the best results with ultimate crunch and less chance of burning, these can also bake at 350°F for 20 minutes, as long as you stir often and watch that they don't burn, then turn the oven down to 200°F, and crisp for 15 minutes to 1 hour, stirring from time to time.

DF

SAVORY CRISPY ADDICTIONS

⅛ to ¼ teaspoon garlic powder

1 teaspoon onion powder

1 teaspoon ground cumin

⅛ to ¼ teaspoon cayenne pepper (optional)

⅛ teaspoon black pepper

3 tablespoons hot sauce of choice

2 tablespoons nutritional yeast

2 tablespoons finely grated Parmesan cheese (green can is fine)

¼ teaspoon Mineral Salt

This version is not only great to munch on by itself but also fabulous on salads and to top fried eggs. These do not taste very coconutty; more like a savory potato chip that you just can't get enough of. Make the same way as in the master recipe, except omit the cinnamon and add the listed spices.

DF (IF YOU LEAVE OUT THE PARMESAN CHEESE BUT ADD ¼ TEASPOON MORE SALT AND 1 TABLESPOON MORE NUTRITIONAL YEAST)

crunch puffs

¾ cup egg whites (carton or fresh)

½ teaspoon xanthan gum (you need this; you cannot sub with Gluccie here)

Pinch of Mineral Salt

2 teaspoons Trim Healthy Mama Baking Blend

2 teaspoons Whole-Husk Psyllium Flakes

1 to 2 teaspoons "Macho" Nacho Seasoning (page 492), or Rohnda's Ranch Seasoning (page 492), or Trim Bouillon Mix (page 491) for savory puffs (omit for sweet versions; see bottom Note on page 462)

Coconut oil cooking spray

PEARL CHATS: If you are a late-night snacker who desires that savory or sweet crunch, let this **FP** snack come to your rescue. My husband is in this boat. Thankfully, he doesn't mind that I tell on him. "Honey, I just wrote about you in the book!" He just rolls his eyes and grins a little. Charlie can eat thousands of calories of nuts and cheese in the evening. No kidding! Even if he already had a hearty dinner! He sits there and keeps eating and eating. Hand to mouth, hand to mouth! It is the salty crunch he is after. It's amazing to me that he was able to lose his excess weight (45 pounds) on THM owing to the huge amounts of food he eats, but he's a guy and guys can sometimes do what we women cannot when it comes to weight loss. All that to say, while he still eats plenty of nuts and cheese, he also enjoys these puffs now, and since they are Fuel Pull, he can sit there and do his hand-to-mouth thing and I don't have to nag him—not that I would, of course (wink). If you like a crunchy side to your sandwich, the Macho Nacho version can help fill that void. Craving salty cheesiness? No problem. Cinnamonyness? Sure. Cocoa Peanuttyness? Yep, we got ya' covered.

1. Preheat the oven to 275°F. Line two 9 x 13-inch baking sheets with parchment.

2. In a medium bowl, beat the egg whites and xanthan gum on high speed until stiff peaks form, approximately 3 minutes. The egg whites should be stiff enough that if you tilt the bowl, the whites should not slide around.

3. Reduce the mixer speed to medium and slowly add the salt, Baking Blend, psyllium, and seasoning of choice. Increase the speed to high and beat for 1 more minute.

4. Place the mixture in a quart zippered freezer bag, seal the bag, and cut a ½-inch hole in one corner of the bag. Pipe the batter onto the prepared sheets in ½-inch balls (or 2-inch doodles). You will fill the trays completely full with balls.

5. Bake for 35 minutes. Turn the oven off and allow the puffs to sit in the closed oven another 25 minutes or so. Remove the puffs from the oven and allow to cool for about a minute. Pull any puffs apart that are stuck together.

6. Put the puffs in a bowl. Spray some coconut oil onto all the puffs.

7. Mix together the seasonings/flavorings for the desired recipe variation listed on the following page. Toss the puffs with half the seasoning/flavoring of choice (for savory puffs, be sure to match the seasoning you put into the batter). Spray again with coconut oil and sprinkle on the remaining seasoning/flavoring, tossing well for a double coat. (Remember that you can have up to a teaspoon of fat with an **FP**, so you don't need to be too stingy with the coconut oil spray. If you want to go full-on **S** with these, you can get real spray happy.)

8. Store any puffs you don't eat immediately in an airtight container for up to a couple of days. To re-crisp, place on a baking sheet and put in a 300°F oven for 10 minutes.

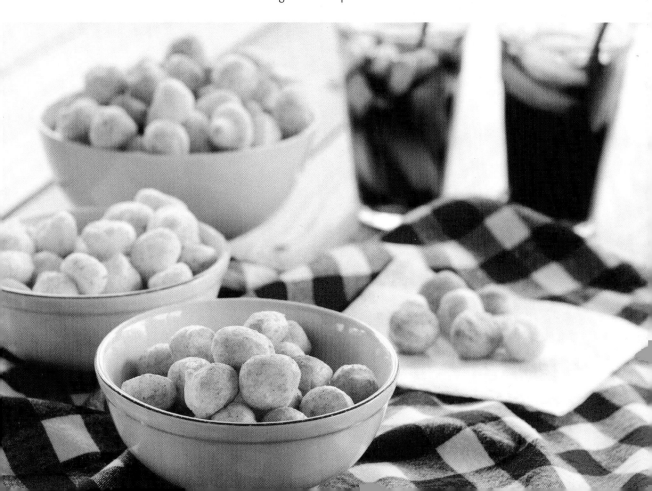

"MACHO" NACHO CRUNCH PUFFS

. . . .

1 tablespoon natural nacho cheese
   seasoning (see Note)
1 to 2 teaspoons "Macho" Nacho
   Seasoning (page 492)
1 tablespoon nutritional yeast

NOTE: You can find completely purist versions of nacho cheese seasoning online. Frontier Natural has a nice option, but if you're a Drive Thru Sue and don't care much about purism, use a simple MSG-free cheesy popcorn seasoning found at most grocery stores.

RANCH CRUNCH PUFFS

. . . .

2 teaspoons Rohnda's Ranch
   Seasoning (page 492)
1 tablespoon finely grated Parmesan
   cheese
1 tablespoon nutritional yeast

PEANUT COCOA CRUNCH PUFFS

. . . .

4 teaspoons Gentle Sweet
1 tablespoon Pressed Peanut flour
1 to 2 teaspoons unsweetened cocoa
   powder

CINNAMON CRUNCH PUFFS

. . . .

4 teaspoons Gentle Sweet
¾ teaspoon ground cinnamon

NOTE: The sweet versions do not work out so well if you put the sweetener into the actual puff mixture before cooking. Somehow it takes away the crunch factor.

DF (IF NOT USING THE VERSION THAT CALLS FOR NACHO CHEESE SEASONING)

pretzel sticks

MULTIPLE SERVE — MAKES 16 TO 20 STICKS

1 cup Trim Healthy Mama Baking
  Blend

½ teaspoon baking soda

2 teaspoons nutritional yeast

½ teaspoon Mineral Salt

½ cup egg whites (carton or fresh),
  lightly beaten, plus 1 to 2
  tablespoons egg whites, for coating

2 tablespoons unsweetened almond or
  cashew milk

½ teaspoon butter extract (optional)

Coarse salt, for sprinkling

These are reminiscent of those large soft pretzels you can buy at the mall. They are delicious with Honey Mustard Dip (page 468) or just eaten as is.

1. Preheat the oven to 350°F. Line a large baking sheet with parchment.

2. In a medium bowl, combine the Baking Blend, baking soda, nutritional yeast, and salt, whisking by hand. Add the beaten egg whites, almond milk, and butter flavoring (if using). Stir until the mixture becomes a dough.

3. Using 2 to 3 teaspoons' worth of dough, form little balls and roll them between your hands to shape into sticks 3 to 4 inches long. Lay the sticks on the prepared baking sheet. Brush each stick with a bit of egg white and sprinkle on a little coarse salt.

4. Bake the pretzels for 10 minutes, then flip over, brush on more egg white, and sprinkle on a bit more coarse salt. Bake for another 10 minutes.

5. For a crunchier pretzel, turn off the oven and let the pretzels remain in the oven to cool slowly.

D F

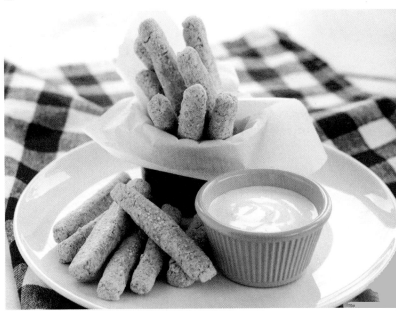

kale chips

 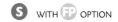
SINGLE SERVE — MAKES 1 LARGE 9 X 13-INCH BAKING SHEET FULL OF CHIPS

4 to 5 ounces kale leaves (about ⅓ of a
1-pound bag)

1 tablespoon coconut oil or melted
butter

2 to 3 generous pinches Mineral Salt

2 tablespoons nutritional yeast

These are addictive. And please don't be intimidated, as they are so simple to make. Most grocery stores have bags of prewashed kale leaves, perfect for chip making. You can get creative with the seasonings, too. Our favorite is the simple salt and nutritional yeast used here, but you can also sprinkle on Rohnda's Ranch Seasoning (page 492), or taco seasoning, or Trim Bouillon Mix (page 491)—or even some white vinegar. You can make several batches at a time if you want to share these with others.

1. Preheat the oven to 375°F. Line a large baking sheet or pan with parchment.

2. Lay the kale on the prepared baking sheet, pour on the coconut oil, and sprinkle with the salt and nutritional yeast. Toss all together with your hands, then spread out the kale evenly on the baking sheet.

3. Bake for 8 to 10 minutes, keeping a good eye out so that the kale doesn't burn (though we like ours a little browned and crisped).

NOTE: For an **FP** version, omit the oil or butter and spray the leaves with coconut oil spray before seasoning.

NSI (IF OMITTING THE NUTRITIONAL YEAST) DF

salmon mousse

SINGLE SERVE

½ (7-ounce) can salmon (see Note),
  including bones and skin (drained)
2 tablespoons ⅓ less fat cream cheese
2 rounded tablespoons cottage cheese
½ teaspoon Liquid Smoke
Juice of ½ lemon
Red pepper flakes (optional)

Power-packed with protein, healing glycine, and anti-inflammatory omega-3s, this mousse is a fabulous snack or part of a meal. It's perfect to pack in a cooler bag for a day out or if you work outside the home. Take along some cucumber or jicama slices to dip, or any of the crackers in this chapter, or if you're like us, grab a spoon and dig in—yum!

If you do work outside the home, it's a great idea to include this ultra-easy recipe as part of your prep day. Double or triple the recipe, then divide it into two or three individual containers with lids. The lemon disguises any fishy smell, so it should not offend your coworkers; they'll probably just be jealous of your good food! Don't be scared by the salmon taste, either; the smoke seasoning and lemon really turn it into something remarkably palatable, even for salmon skeptics.

One last thought before we stop gabbing and let you get on to the recipe. This uses canned salmon, and if possible buy the type with fish and bones included. You won't be grossed out because this recipe is processed and it becomes completely smooth. The fish and bones are the healthiest part for you!

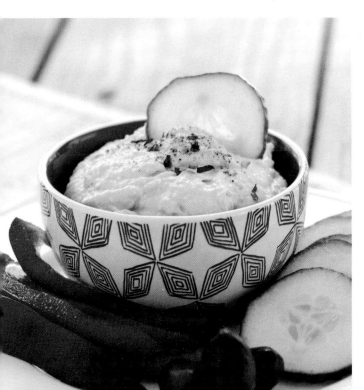

1. Put all the ingredients in a food processor and process until smooth.

NOTE: You can refrigerate the leftover half-can of salmon and use for any of the Quick Single Skillet Meals or Family Meals that call for salmon (see pages 79, 118, 122, and 124), or to top a single-serve salad.

NSI

2½ tablespoons Peanut Junkie Butter (page 481)

2½ tablespoons plain 0% Greek yogurt, or 2 tablespoons **FP** version of NoGurt (see page 343)

1 doonk Pure Stevia Extract, or to taste

This makes a great E afternoon snack with an apple!

1. Whisk together all the ingredients in a bowl.

DF (IF USING NOGURT)

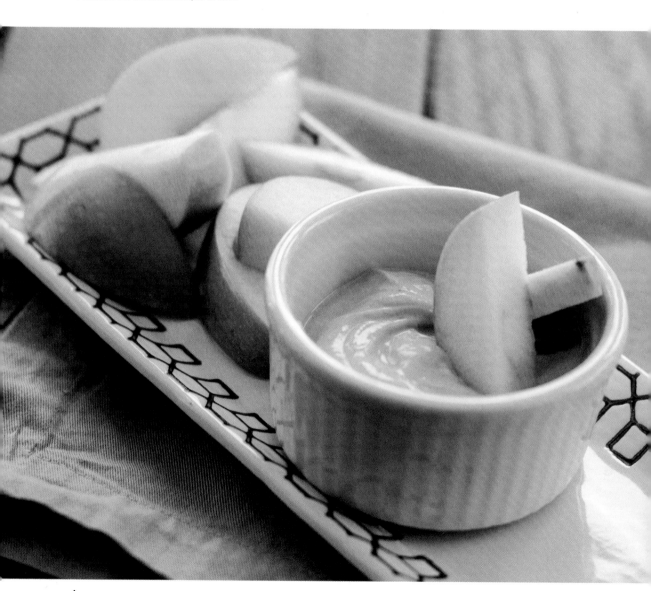

cheesy kale dip

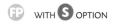 WITH **S** OPTION

MULTIPLE SERVE PARTY SIZE (YOU CAN HALVE INGREDIENTS FOR SMALLER GATHERING)

3 tablespoons chia seeds (see Note)

3 tablespoons nutritional yeast

3 tablespoons finely grated Parmesan
cheese (green can kind is fine)

1 teaspoon Mineral Salt

½ teaspoon garlic powder

½ teaspoon onion powder

½ teaspoon cayenne pepper

½ red bell pepper

Juice of 1 lemon

2 squirts Bragg liquid aminos, or
2 teaspoons tamari or soy sauce

12 ounces 1% or 2% cottage cheese

1 tablespoon MCT oil or extra-virgin
olive oil

8 ounces baby kale (half of a
prewashed 1-pound bag)

¼ to ½ cup water

½ cup chopped black or green olives
(for **S** option)

Sensationally green and surprisingly yummy! Not only is this great as a dip with crackers or crudités but you can serve it as a spread over Serene's Rustic Pizza Crust (page 212) topped with feta cheese, sun-dried tomatoes, and capers, and you have a Wow Factor pizza! You can also use this dip as the basis for a creamy kale soup; just add boiling water to 2 to 3 tablespoons of this dip and stir well. Garnish with pecorino romano and add a scoop of collagen. That's truly a healthy fast-food lunch idea when mealtime hits and you have no time to stop, think, or prepare.

1. Combine all the ingredients except the kale, water, and **S** option olives in a blender and process until very smooth.

2. Place the kale in a large saucepan with the water. Bring to a boil and then cover and turn down the heat to simmer until cooked; the vivid greens become darker when cooked, about 5 minutes. Drain the kale in a colander, then add the kale to a blender a bit at a time and blend until creamy smooth. Stir in the olives (if using).

3. Taste and adjust the seasonings to "own it." Chill and enjoy as a nutritional powerhouse protein dip.

NOTE: You could grind the chia seeds to a powder in a coffee grinder first to make the blending of the seeds more effective.

NSI (IF NOT INCLUDING NUTRITIONAL YEAST)

mrs. criddle's french onion dip (S)

½ cup mayonnaise

½ cup plain 0% Greek yogurt

2 tablespoons finely grated Parmesan cheese (green can kind is fine)

1 teaspoon onion powder

½ teaspoon garlic powder

1 teaspoon dried parsley, or
1 tablespoon finely diced fresh parsley

1 teaspoon dried chives, or
1 tablespoon finely diced fresh chives

Mineral Salt and pepper to taste

Sarah Criddle makes incredible THM recipes that are extremely popular in the THM community. This dip proves that. Check out more of her recipes at www.mrscriddles kitchen.com.

1. Mix together all the ingredients in a bowl. Place into a serving bowl and accompany with sliced crunchy veggies or crackers.

NSI

honey mustard dip (S)

2 tablespoons mayonnaise

2 tablespoon Greek yogurt

½ teaspoon apple cider vinegar

¾ teaspoon prepared yellow mustard

2 teaspoons Gentle Sweet, or to taste

This is great for dipping cooked chicken pieces or with Pretzel Sticks (page 463).

1. Combine all the ingredients in a bowl.

NSI (IF YOU USE YOUR FAVORITE ON-PLAN SWEETENER)

CONDIMENTS AND EXTRAS

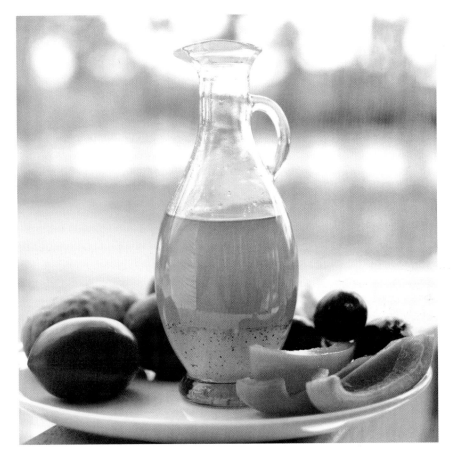

Tangy and Sweet Vinaigrette (page 472)

body-burn mayonnaise ⓢ

MULTIPLE SERVE — MAKES ABOUT 1 CUP

2 large egg yolks

1 tablespoon lemon juice or apple
cider vinegar

½ teaspoon Mineral Salt

1 teaspoon Dijon mustard, or
½ teaspoon dry mustard

1 doonk Pure Stevia Extract

½ cup MCT oil

½ cup mild-tasting cold-pressed oil,
like grapeseed oil

The MCT oil in this dressing is a metabolism reviver and helps protect your brain from the ravages of diseases like Alzheimer's. This mayo is a lovely golden color from the egg yolks and mustard. If you are a Drive Thru Sue, know that you can purchase regular mayonnaise from the store and it will still be on plan. But if you want to get adventurous and try your hand at homemade sometime, don't be skeered! It's easy and healthier.

1. Put all the ingredients except the oils in a blender, then run the blender on its slowest setting. Slowly add the oils a little at a time while the blender is running. (You can also try this in a bowl with a whisk; it will be a workout for your arm but you should get a similar result.) Chill in the fridge.

NOTE TO PURISTS: You can extend the refrigerator life of this by adding a couple tablespoons of whey water from your cheese making, then leaving the mayo to sit on the counter for a few hours before refrigerating.

NSI (IF YOU USE YOUR FAVORITE ON-PLAN SWEETENER) DF

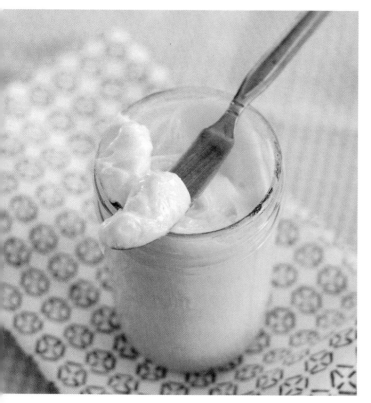

zesty avo cream dressing

S

MULTIPLE SERVE — MAKES ABOUT 1½ CUPS

1 medium avocado
1 cup plain 0% Greek yogurt
¼ cup extra-virgin olive oil
2 tablespoons fresh lemon or lime juice
½ cup fresh cilantro leaves
2 teaspoons hot sauce of choice
2 garlic cloves
1 teaspoon Mineral Salt

This beautiful green dressing harmonizes fabulously with the Zesty Southwestern Chop Up (page 182), but you can use it on any S salad. If you want to make this dairy-free, omit the yogurt and replace with another avocado—thin with a little water, if desired.

1. Place all the ingredients in a blender and blend well. Store in an airtight jar in the refrigerator until ready to use.

NSI DF (IF REPLACING YOGURT WITH EXTRA AVOCADO)

rohnda's ranch dressing

S

MULTIPLE SERVE — MAKES ABOUT 1¼ CUPS

¾ cup Body-Burn Mayonnaise
   (opposite; or use store-bought)
½ cup plain 0% Greek yogurt
1 to 2 garlic cloves, minced,
   or ½ to ¾ teaspoon powdered garlic
1 teaspoon dried parsley
½ teaspoon dried minced onion
½ teaspoon Mineral Salt
Dash of black pepper

1. Place all the ingredients in a medium bowl and mix well. Refrigerate at least 1 hour before serving.

NOTE: Check out Rohnda's Ranch Seasoning (page 492). You can use 1 tablespoon of that in place of the seasonings listed here.

NSI

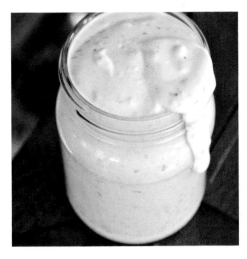

thousand island dressing ⓢ

¾ cup Body-Burn Mayonnaise (page 470; or use store-bought)

½ cup plain 0% Greek yogurt

5 tablespoons Trim Healthy Ketchup (page 482; or use store-bought sugar-free ketchup)

Several dashes of hot sauce of choice

½ cup dill relish

1½ teaspoons Super Sweet Blend, or 3 teaspoons Gentle Sweet, or to taste

If you enjoy the dressing from Reuben in a Bowl (page 73), make this larger amount and keep it handy in the fridge. It's been tweaked just a little from the original, but still has the same great flavors. And it works great on Trim Mac Salad (page 181) as well.

1. Combine all the ingredients in a blender and blend until smooth. Refrigerate until ready to serve.

NSI (IF YOU USE YOUR FAVORITE ON-PLAN SWEETENER)

tangy and sweet vinaigrette ⓢ

⅓ cup apple cider vinegar

2 doonks Pure Stevia Extract, or 1 teaspoon Super Sweet Blend, or to taste

1½ teaspoons minced garlic

½ teaspoon Mineral Salt

½ teaspoon freshly ground black pepper

¾ cup olive oil

Thanks to Jennifer Griffin for sharing another wonderful recipe with us.

1. Add all the ingredients to a blender and blend until smooth. Store in an airtight glass jar in the refrigerator until ready to use.

NSI (IF YOU USE YOUR FAVORITE ON-PLAN SWEETENER) DF

honey mustard dressing

½ cup Body-Burn Mayonnaise (page 470; or use store-bought)

½ cup plain 0% Greek yogurt

2 teaspoons apple cider vinegar

2 teaspoons prepared yellow mustard

1½ to 2 tablespoons Gentle Sweet, or to taste

1. Combine all the ingredients well and transfer to a squeeze bottle or jar with a lid. Refrigerate until ready to use.

NOTE: Be sure to check out the single-serve dip version of this recipe that accompanies Pretzel Sticks (page 468).

NSI (IF YOU USE YOUR FAVORITE ON-PLAN SWEETENER)

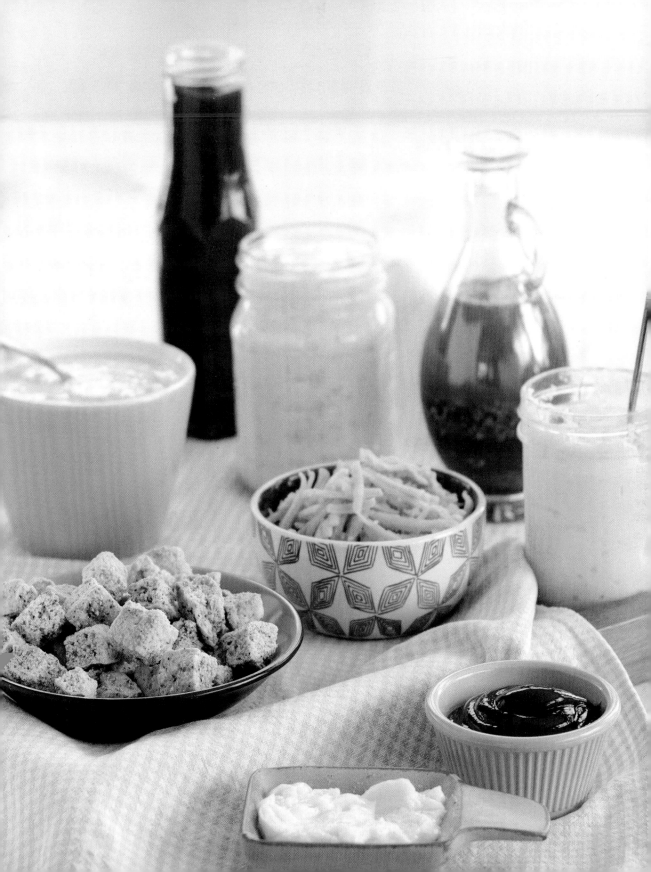

slim belly vinaigrette

SINGLE SERVE

2 tablespoons Slim Belly Jelly
  (page 478)
1 teaspoon apple cider vinegar
1 teaspoon white vinegar
1 teaspoon water, or as needed
Mineral Salt and pepper to taste

MULTIPLE SERVE — MAKES
ABOUT 2 CUPS
1 cup Slim Belly Jelly (page 478)
3 tablespoons apple cider vinegar
3 tablespoons white vinegar
3 tablespoons water, or as needed
Mineral Salt and pepper to taste

Sometimes the simplest things in life are the best. This recipe uses Slim Belly Jelly (page 478) and simply mixes some vinegar and water with it. It is sweet, wonderfully berryish, and a Fuel Pull.

1. Mix all the ingredients well in a blender or bowl. Use the single-serve batch right away. Store the multiple-serve batch in an airtight jar in the refrigerator until ready to use.

DF

tahini dressing

MULTIPLE SERVE — MAKES ABOUT 1½ CUPS

½ cup tahini (sesame paste)
½ cup water
¼ cup apple cider vinegar
2 tablespoons soy sauce or tamari,
  or 1 to 2 squirts Bragg or Coconut
  liquid aminos
1 doonk Pure Stevia Extract
⅛ teaspoon cayenne pepper
Black pepper to taste

Tahini is a paste made from sesame seeds. It can usually be found in the international aisle of your grocery store. Its very rich and flavorful taste makes for a wonderful change from typical dressings on green salads. It is also fantastic over sliced raw cabbage.

1. Put all the ingredients into a glass jar and whisk very well until you've got a smooth dressing texture. Refrigerate until ready to use.

NSI (IF YOU USE YOUR FAVORITE ON-PLAN SWEETENER) DF

grand greek dressing

MULTIPLE SERVE – MAKES ABOUT 1 CUP

¾ cup extra-virgin olive oil

Juice of 2 lemons

6 tablespoons red wine vinegar

4 garlic cloves, minced, or 1 teaspoon
  garlic powder

3 teaspoons dried oregano

1 teaspoon Mineral Salt

1 teaspoon black pepper

1 teaspoon onion powder

This dressing is the perfect accompaniment to the Grand Greek Salad (page 183), but it can go on any S salad to keep you happy and Greekified.

1. Whisk all the ingredients together in a bowl and transfer to a glass jar with an airtight lid. Refrigerate until ready to use.

NSI DF

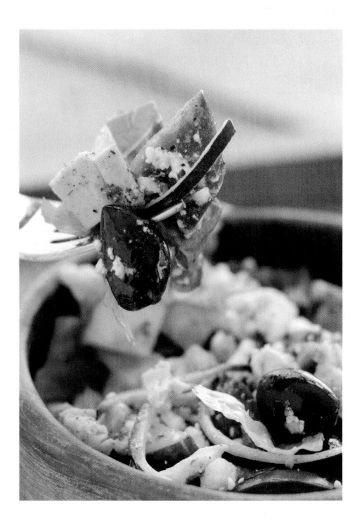

Coconut oil cooking spray

1 cup Trim Healthy Mama Baking Blend

4 to 6 small pinches Super Sweet Blend

4 pinches Mineral Salt

2 teaspoons aluminum-free baking powder

4 tablespoons water

1 cup plus 2 tablespoons egg whites (carton or fresh), lightly beaten

FOR SPRINKLING (SEE NOTE)

Coconut oil cooking spray

6 pinches Mineral Salt

6 pinches black pepper

Generous ¼ teaspoon garlic powder

1 teaspoon Italian seasoning mix

2 teaspoons finely grated Parmesan cheese (green can kind is fine)

These crunchy little squares of flavor don't taste like a substitute for croutons. We think they taste as good or better than the real thing! They satisfy a mouthful of salad crunch while working with your waistline, not against it. "Just leave off the croutons"—we've given that warning because croutons are usually the downfall of a healthy salad. They turn a slimming meal into a waist widener. Well, now Blendtons are here for your rescue. We don't have to nag about croutons any more—phew! Put that yummy bread crunch back in your salad, Mama! Keep some in a zippy in your purse, so you can throw them on a restaurant salad or, better yet, just eat them as a savory snack (our children love them like that). These also add the perfect crunch factor to a bowl of chili or soup.

This recipe uses the single-serve Swiss Bread recipe (page 196) times four. For your ease, we have quadrupled it here, but the flavors—oh, the flavors—are the magic here.

1. Preheat the oven to 350°F. Lightly coat a 12-cup muffin tin with coconut oil spray.

2. Whisk the Baking Blend, sweetener, salt, baking powder, water, and egg whites in a medium bowl until smooth.

3. Distribute the batter in 8 of the muffin holes, filling the remaining holes with water (for a steaming effect). Bake for 15 minutes. Remove the breads from the pan and let cool completely.

4. Chop the breads into croutons. Spread them on a baking sheet lightly coated with coconut oil spray, then spray the croutons lightly with coconut oil as well. Evenly sprinkle on the seasonings and toss. Add a final spray of coconut oil to set the spices on the croutons.

5. Bake the croutons in the oven overnight or for several hours during the day on the lowest setting possible. (Alternatively, bake at 350°F for 15 minutes, then turn off the oven and leave the Blendtons in the oven until they are cool and crispy.)

6. Store the Blendtons in an airtight container until ready to use so the air does not moisten them.

NOTE: Of course, this list of seasonings is just our suggestion and creates mild-tasting Blendtons. If you prefer more wham in each bite, simply increase amounts of seasonings or let your imagination run wild. For instance, try sprinkling with Rohnda's Ranch Seasoning (page 492) or the "Macho" Nacho Seasoning (page 492), or even the Trim Bouillon Mix (page 491).

DF (IF YOU SUBSTITUTE NUTRITIONAL YEAST FOR THE PARMESAN CHEESE)

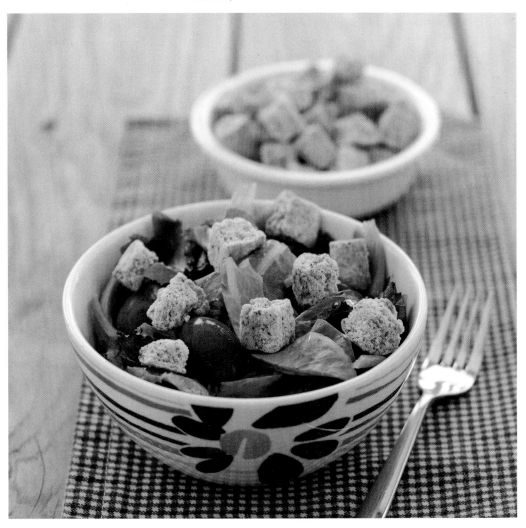

1½ cups water

2½ cups frozen berries

2 tablespoons lemon juice, or
   2 to 3 drops essential lemon oil

3 to 4 doonks Pure Stevia Extract,
   or 2½ to 3½ teaspoons Super
   Sweet Blend, or 5 to 7 teaspoons
   Gentle Sweet

¾ to 1½ teaspoons Gluccie

Put this on your pancakes, your donuts, in your yogurt—oh, the things you can do with SBJ!

1. Put the water, 1 cup of the berries, and all the other ingredients except the Gluccie in a blender and blend well.

2. Transfer the puree to a medium saucepan and add the rest of the berries. Bring the mixture to a boil, then turn down the heat to a simmer. Depending on whether you want a thicker or thinner jelly, start whisking in the Gluccie; use only ¾ teaspoon for a syrup-like consistency. Use the full amount for a set jelly. This jelly will thicken more as it sits in the fridge.

3. Taste and adjust the sweetness to "own it." Keep refrigerated until ready to use.

DF

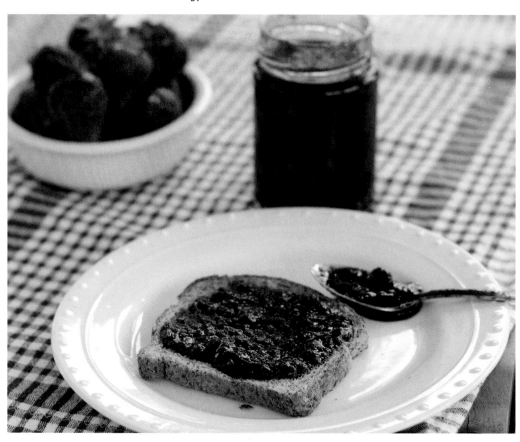

handy chocolate syrup ⓕⓟ

1 cup plus 2 tablespoons water
½ cup unsweetened cocoa powder
¾ cup Gentle Sweet
Scant ¼ teaspoon Mineral Salt
1 teaspoon vanilla extract

Drizzle this over anything you want to make chocolaty!

1. Put all the ingredients in a medium saucepan over medium-high heat, and whisk often while it comes to a boil. Take the saucepan off the heat, turn the heat to low, then return the saucepan to the heat and whisk well while the mixture simmers gently for a couple of minutes.

2. Allow the chocolate syrup to cool a little, then pour into a small jar with a lid. Store in the refrigerator until ready to use. The mixture will thicken more as it cools.

NSI (IF YOU USE YOUR FAVORITE ON-PLAN SWEETENER) DF

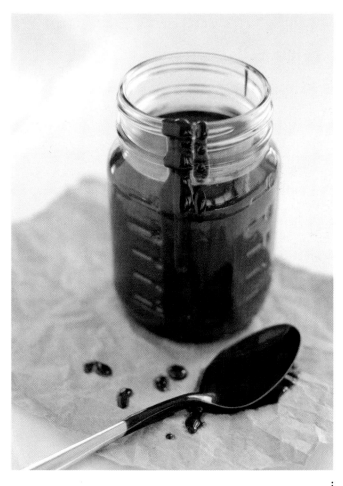

pancake syrup

MULTIPLE SERVE — MAKES ABOUT 1½ CUPS (TRY THIS AS WRITTEN THE FIRST TIME, BUT WE PREDICT IN THE FUTURE YOU'LL BE DOUBLING THE RECIPE)

1 cup water
2½ tablespoons Gentle Sweet
½ teaspoon maple extract
½ teaspoon butter extract
Pinch of Mineral Salt
¼ teaspoon blackstrap molasses (optional)
¼ teaspoon Gluccie

Why use the store-bought stuff with its fat-exploding sugar or health-destroying artificial sweeteners when this is a snap to make?

1. Put all the ingredients except the Gluccie in a small saucepan and bring to a simmer over medium heat. Reduce the heat to medium-low and slowly whisk in the Gluccie from a shaker. Simmer for a couple of minutes, whisking like crazy as it thickens.

2. Transfer the syrup to a jar and, when cool, cover and chill. As the syrup cools, it will continue to thicken.

NSI (IF YOU USE YOUR FAVORITE ON-PLAN SWEETENER AND SUBSTITUTE XANTHAN FOR GLUCCIE) DF

FP

6|17 7|25

¾ cup Pressed Peanut Flour

9 tablespoons water

¾ teaspoon MCT oil, or ½ teaspoon
  softened butter

⅓ teaspoon Mineral Salt, or to taste

½ teaspoon Gentle Sweet, or more
  to taste

While peanut butter is on plan, some of us tend to want to overdo it. You don't have to raise your hand, but Serene has hers waving high in the air! The awesome thing about this peanut butter is it can be used with E and FP meals, too! **Peanut Junkie Butter makes a mean PB and J sandwich on Soft Sprouted Bread (page 200) or Swiss Bread (page 196); hey, you can even put half a banana in your sandwich if you're so inclined! This is great for dipping sliced apples in or smeared on a small banana—and it offers some protein, too. It is also awesome smeared on any of the cracker recipes (see pages 449–457).**

1. Whisk all the ingredients in a small bowl, then transfer to a small jar with a lid. Cover and keep refrigerated until ready to use.

DF

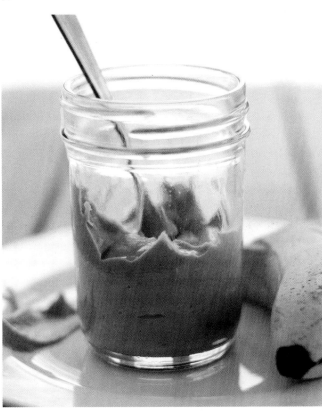

trim healthy ketchup

1 (6-ounce) can tomato paste

¾ cup water

2 tablespoons apple cider, red wine, or white vinegar

1 teaspoon Mineral Salt

⅓ teaspoon onion powder

2 teaspoons Super Sweet Blend, or 2 to 3 doonks Pure Stevia Extract

Most ketchups are laden with sugar. We don't get too worried if you order a low-carb burger with ketchup at a drive thru here and there, but it's a great idea to keep a healthier ketchup on hand at home so you can use it as liberally as you want. Whip this up in 2 minutes flat!

1. Whisk together all the ingredients in a small bowl, transfer to a glass jar, cover, and keep refrigerated.

NSI (IF YOU USE YOUR FAVORITE ON-PLAN SWEETENER) DF

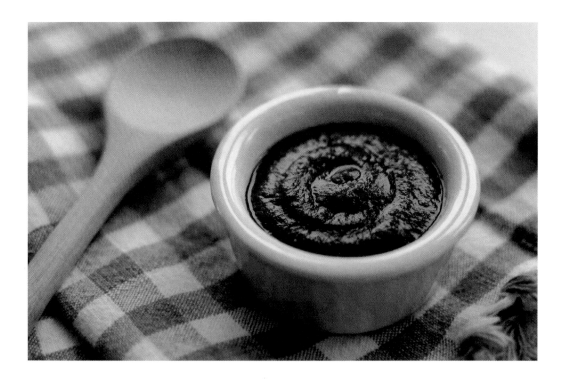

basic gravy

MULTIPLE SERVE – MAKES ABOUT 3 CUPS

3 cups water, broth, or bone stock
  (see pages 495–496)
1 teaspoon Mineral Salt
½ teaspoon onion powder
½ teaspoon garlic powder (optional)
Black and cayenne peppers to taste
2 tablespoons nutritional yeast
1 to 2 squirts Bragg liquid aminos
¾ to 1½ teaspoons Gluccie

While this gravy is excellent as a Fuel Pull, it really rocks out when it's made with some of the meat juices from a roasted, baked, or slow-cooked meat (then it's an S). Or add 3 tablespoons heavy cream for a decadent creamy S gravy.

1. Put all the ingredients except the Gluccie in a small saucepan over medium heat. Bring to a boil, then reduce the heat and simmer while you shake the Gluccie in slowly from a shaker, whisking like mad.

2. Stir for a few minutes while the gravy thickens a little more. Add a little Gluccie if needed, but don't overdo it, as the gravy will continue to thicken slowly.

3. Taste, adjust the seasonings, and "own it."

NSI (IF USING XANTHAN INSTEAD OF GLUCCIE AND OMITTING NUTRITIONAL YEAST) DF

laughin' mama cheese

1 cup water

1 teaspoon agar powder (not flakes; see Note)

1½ teaspoons Whole-Husk Psyllium Flakes

2 teaspoons Just Gelatin

1 tablespoon lemon juice

¼ cup nutritional yeast

1 scoop Integral Collagen

½ teaspoon Liquid Smoke

¾ teaspoon Mineral Salt

1 teaspoon onion powder

2 teaspoons toasted sesame oil

2 teaspoons tahini (sesame paste)

¼ teaspoon Sunflower Lecithin (optional; will give this cheese a little softer not-so-set texture)

SERENE CHATS: *Allergen-free and purist Mamas: Now you have something tasty and creamy to spread on your crackers or Crunkers (page 452), or to smear on your toast or your sand-wiches! A spreadable nondairy cheese—it's enough to make a Mama start laughing!*

It took us weeks and weeks of experimentation to come up with a soft "processed" type cheese spread that is dairy-free and that our purist Mamas could substitute for those little light cheese triangles. It had to be low in calories to fit in the FP cat-egory, as well as spreadable, a nutritious superfood, and free of most allergens. I'm one happy Mama now because, although I tolerate dairy very well, as a staunch purist I could never bring myself to use certain spreadable cheeses. I'm not looking down on Pearl and all her Drive Thru peeps for using that stuff, but my purist pals and I have never been able accept the fact that they have a preservative or two. Hey, I have to give Pearl credit, though. She was as determined as I was to create an alternative for those of us who care about this sort of thing.

While this doesn't taste exactly like those white processed triangles, I think it is way yummier and has a little more gour-met "foodie" flare. I now use Laughin' Mama anytime Pearl calls for the light Laughing Cow cheese wedges in her recipes. I'm finally able to enjoy her Loaded Potato Soup (page 117) and her Creamless Creamy Chicken (page 78)). Laughin' Mama has similar amounts of fat per serving, but feel free to halve the fat, if you want—take the 2 teaspoons of sesame oil and tahini down to 1 each. The cheese is still just as delicious; that is exactly what I do when I want to eat lots of this but still stay in FP mode. Stay within 1 to 3 tablespoons of this cheese as written for FP; other-wise, this will be a light S.

1. Bring the water to a near boil in a small saucepan over high heat. Add the agar and psyllium, and whisk well while bringing to a boil. Reduce the heat to low and whisk for 30 seconds.

2. Scrape the mixture into a blender using a spatula to make sure you get it all out of the pot. Add the remaining ingredi-ents and blend very well. Pour into a glass container, cover, and chill in the fridge until set.

NOTE: This recipe (and the other allergen-free cheese recipes) uses agar powder, which is a thickener made from a seaweed; it is easily available online and at some health food stores. It has been used as a thickener in Asian foods for centuries. Please do not confuse it with carrageenan; it has none of the same health concerns.

DF

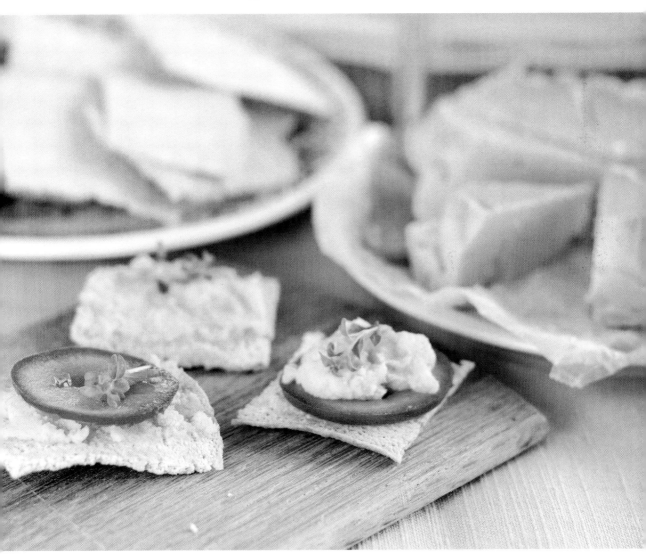

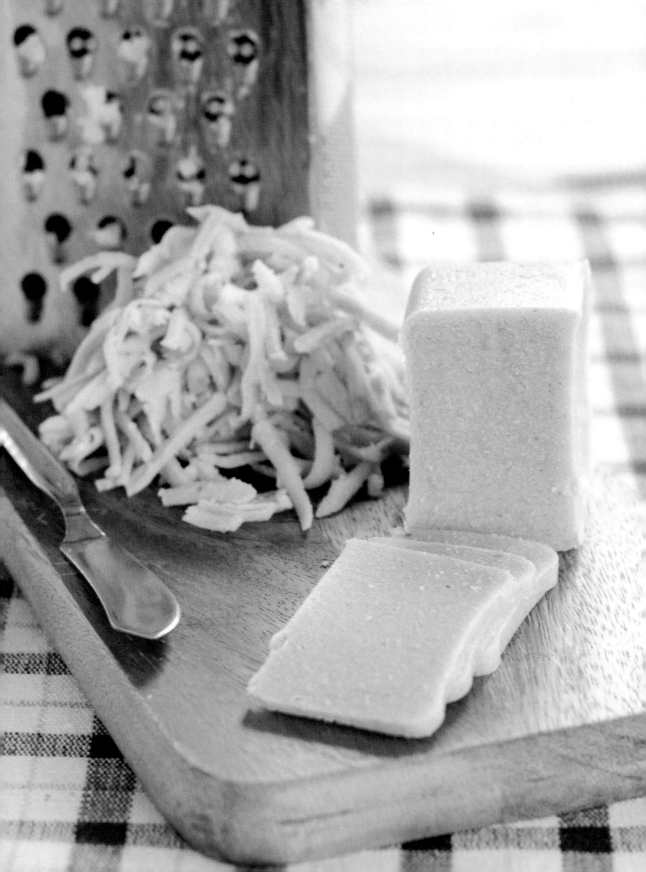

hello cheese ⓕ

1 cup water

2 teaspoons agar powder

2 tablespoons Trim Healthy Mama Baking Blend

¾ teaspoon Mineral Salt

1 teaspoon onion powder

¼ cup nutritional yeast

1 tablespoon lemon juice

1 scoop Integral Collagen

2 teaspoons toasted sesame oil (see Note)

2 teaspoons tahini (sesame paste; see Note)

1 teaspoon Liquid Smoke

Pinch of turmeric and paprika, for color (optional)

The taste for a good ol' slice of cheese is like a natural inborn instinct. It's one of nature's yummiest gifts, yet many have had to bid it farewell because of dairy sensitivities. Yes, there are vegan companies who make cheese substitutes, but those versions have their pitfalls. They are often laced with unstable vegetable oils and too often contain high-glycemic carbs like tapioca flour. Oh, and watch out for unsprouted or uncultured processed soy products in them as well. There are plenty of recipes for homemade dairy-free cheeses online, too, but most of them are excessively nut heavy, with oodles of dense calories in just a small piece of cheese.

We wanted our dairy-free Mamas to be able to say hello to an old friend. Now you can enjoy the cheese taste and satisfaction, but keep the door shut to inferior substitutes and processed junk. Here's a cheese that is suitable for most allergen-free diets (although it does contain a tiny bit of almond flour) and is high in satiating and cleansing fiber and rich in the amino acid glycine, which is frequently missing in modern diets.

You can slice it, shred it, grate it, and melt it—oh, and did we mention it is even Fuel Pull? Who has heard of a yummy cheese that is FP? Stay within 1 to 3 tablespoons for FP; otherwise, this will be a light S. Yeah, baby, eat some with your E meals as well! Heeeeeeelloooo, cheese!

1. Heat the water until almost boiling in a saucepan over high heat, then add the agar. Whisk well while bringing to a boil. Reduce the heat to low and whisk again for 30 seconds. Add the Baking Blend and bring back to a boil, and whisk well for another 30 seconds to 1 minute. Turn off the heat and add all the other ingredients, whisking well.

2. Use a spatula to transfer the mixture to a container with a lid and let cool. Place in the refrigerator to chill and set. Once set, cover the cheese so the edges do not harden.

NOTE: For an even lower-calorie option so that you can use more for **FPs** or **Es**, limit the tahini and sesame oil to 1 teaspoon each. It's still good this way.

DF

hello veggie cheese

½ cup roughly chopped celery

¼ medium onion

½ cup plus 2 tablespoons water

2 teaspoons agar powder

2 tablespoons Trim Healthy Baking Blend

1 tablespoon lemon juice

¾ teaspoon Mineral Salt

2 teaspoons toasted sesame oil (see Note)

2 teaspoons tahini (sesame paste; see Note)

1 scoop Integral Collagen

1 teaspoon Liquid Smoke

¼ cup nutritional yeast

Pinch of turmeric, for color (optional)

SERENE CHATS: *This is similar to the Hello Cheese (page 487), but the veggies give this a slightly more "aged" cheese taste. If you're a foodie and like to detect hints of flavors in every bite, try this version. This is actually my preference, even if Pearl doesn't like it as much. The natural saltiness of celery and the creamy savory taste of cooked onion lend the perfect gourmet touch to this cheese. Stay within 1 to 3 tablespoons for FP; otherwise, this will be a light S.*

1. Place the celery and onion in a small saucepan with 2 tablespoons water, cover, and bring to a boil over medium-high heat. Reduce the heat and simmer the veggies until they are tender.

2. Add the remaining ½ cup water to the saucepan; turn to high heat. When almost boiling, add the agar powder and whisk extremely well while bringing back to a boil. Reduce the heat slightly and whisk well for 30 seconds. Add the Baking Blend and keep whisking for another 30 seconds.

3. Turn off the heat. Add the remaining ingredients to the saucepan, then use a spatula to scrape the mixture into a blender. Blend until smooth.

4. Pour the cheesy mixture into a container and allow to cool. Put in the refrigerator to chill and set, then cover the container so the edges of the cheese do not harden.

NOTE: As with the other dairy-free cheese recipes, reduce tahini and oil by half so you can use even more for **FP** or **E**.

DF

nocream cheese berry spread

MULTIPLE SERVE — MAKES ABOUT 1¼ CUPS

2 teaspoons Just Gelatin

3 teaspoons cool water

1 cup hot (not quite boiling) water

1⅛ teaspoons agar powder

1½ teaspoons Whole-Husk Psyllium Flakes

¼ teaspoon Sunflower Lecithin

1 scoop Integral Collagen

1 tablespoon lemon juice

3 to 4 teaspoons MCT oil, or
  2 teaspoons ghee (clarified butter) or coconut oil

3 doonks Pure Stevia Extract

½ teaspoon Super Sweet Blend

4 pinches Mineral Salt

¼ teaspoon vanilla extract

¼ cup fresh or frozen tart raspberries or diced strawberries

1,000 mg ascorbic acid vitamin C (optional)

No dairy. No junk. No nuts. This delicious spread tastes like you are slathering a fattening slice of rich berry cheesecake on your toast. Try it spread on toasted Swiss Bread (page 196), Crunkers (page 452), Mad Melbas (pages 454), or Swiss Crackers (page 457), or on some sprouted or sourdough toast. Oh, and it is a delicious spread on the dairy-free version of Trim Healthy Pancakes or Waffles (page 259). Stay within 1 to 3 tablespoons for FP; otherwise, this will be a light S.

1. Put the gelatin in a little cup, add the cool water, and stir just a little to soften and dissolve.

2. Place the hot water, agar powder, psyllium, and dissolved gelatin in a small saucepan over medium-high heat and whisk well while bringing to a boil. Turn off the heat and stir well for 30 seconds.

3. Place the gelatin mixture in a blender and add all the remaining ingredients. Blend very well, then chill in the fridge until set.

DF

whipped nocream

MULTIPLE SERVE

1 teaspoon Just Gelatin

2 tablespoons cool water

2 tablespoons hot (not quite boiling) water

¼ cup unsweetened almond or cashew milk, or carton coconut milk

¼ cup extra-virgin coconut oil

1 scoop Pristine Whey Protein

2 pinches Mineral Salt

2 doonks Pure Stevia Extract

½ teaspoon vanilla extract

If you don't do well with dairy, this is a delightful whipped topping that can take its place. Or perhaps you are a purist who prefers not to use the store-bought pasteurized version of cream but can't get your hands on a source of the raw, pastured kind. No worries, Mate. We've got you covered here, too. While this is an S, it uses easier burn fats than heavy cream, so it is a nice change from time to time, for stubborn weight purposes. It sets up light and fluffy, and is a perfect topping for cakes, muffins, or fresh berries. This is not completely dairy-free, but it is lactose-free if you use the whey protein, which is a pure isolate and is tolerated well by many with dairy sensitivities. What a delight to indulge in something so delicious when it is whipped into wonderfulness with middle-chain triglyceride-rich virgin coconut oil.

Once this is spreadable, use it to ice cakes and muffins or to top donuts or fill cookie sandwiches. It is also absolutely divine just licked off the finger or in a parfait glass with sliced berries.

1. In a little cup, soften the gelatin in the cool water and then add the hot water to dissolve. Stir well to remove any lumps, then place in the fridge to set for a few minutes.

2. Place the gelatin in a blender with the milk, coconut oil, whey protein, salt, stevia, and vanilla. Blend until smooth, then transfer to a mixing bowl and beat until fluffy and high.

3. Place the whipped mixture in the refrigerator to firm up.

trim bouillon mix

MULTIPLE SERVE — MAKES ABOUT 1½ CUPS

1 cup nutritional yeast

3 tablespoons onion powder

2 tablespoons Mineral Salt

⅓ to ½ teaspoon Super Sweet Blend

1 tablespoon garlic powder

1½ teaspoons dried thyme

1 teaspoon dried sage

1 teaspoon paprika

½ teaspoon turmeric

2 teaspoon dried parsley

1 teaspoon Just Gelatin

DF

This is a delicious, concentrated base for many soups, or you can use it as the flavoring for a breading (when combined with Trim Healthy Baking Blend) for meats or veggies, or for sprouted tofu like our Chicken-Fried Tofu (page 173).

1. Place all the ingredients in a blender and blend to a dry even mix, making sure all the ingredients are powdered. Store in a zippered bag or glass container until ready to use. To make broth, add 1 tablespoon powder to 1 cup of boiling water.

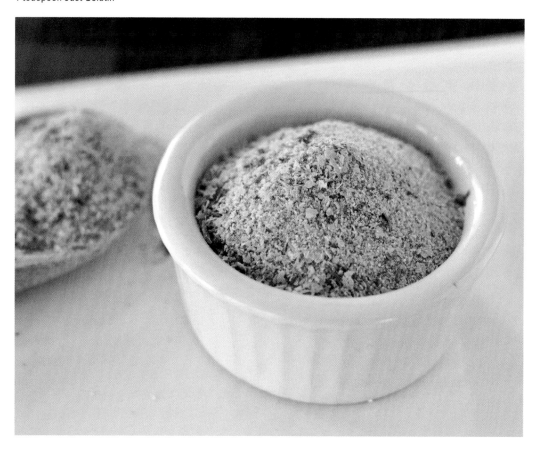

"macho" nacho seasoning

½ cup nutritional yeast
2 tablespoons dried minced onion
2 tablespoons garlic powder
2 tablespoons paprika
½ to 1 teaspoon red pepper flakes
4 teaspoons Mineral Salt
½ teaspoon black pepper
½ teaspoon turmeric (optional)
½ to 1 teaspoon Super Sweet Blend

This makes a great seasoning for Crunch Puffs (page 460), but it is also fabulous sprinkled on about anything else. It is super on E style popcorn and, of course, even better on Crossover popcorn with melted butter—hee, hee. Check out our guidelines for wise popcorn eating in "The Energizing Meal" chapter of *Trim Healthy Mama Plan*. For an E style popcorn, coat the popcorn with a little coconut oil spray, then sprinkle this over for great flavor.

1. Grind all the ingredients in a blender or food processor until a fine powder.

DF

rohnda's ranch seasoning

3 tablespoons garlic powder
6 tablespoons dried parsley
3 tablespoons dried minced onion
3 tablespoons Mineral Salt
¾ teaspoon black pepper

This is the bulk dry seasoning that goes into Rohnda's Ranch Dressing (page 471). You can store this mix in a jar and use it for sprinkling on crackers and chips, such as Cheese Chips (page 451) or use it in marinades. Use 1 flat tablespoon of this bulk version when making Rohnda's Ranch dressing.

1. Combine all the ingredients in a blender or food processor until well mixed, then store in an airtight jar until ready to use.

NSI DF

superfood salad sprinkles

S

MULTIPLE SERVE — MAKES 3 CUPS

1 cup finely grated Parmesan cheese
  (green can kind is fine) or ground
  white sesame seeds (for dairy-free;
  see Note)
1 cup golden flax meal
1 cup nutritional yeast
½ teaspoon Mineral Salt (plus
  ¼ teaspoon if using sesame seeds)
½ teaspoon black pepper
2 teaspoons Italian seasoning mix
1 teaspoon onion powder
½ teaspoon garlic powder
4 drops essential lemon oil, or
  ½ teaspoon lemon extract

We love this stuff! Use 2 tablespoons of it on any Salad, or mix with oil and vinegar as for the Superfood-Loaded Salad (page 192).

1. Place all the ingredients except the lemon oil in a bowl and whisk until there are no lumps. If using the lemon oil, put it on your hands and rub through the sprinkles. Place the sprinkles in a glass jar with a tight-fitting lid and store in the fridge for lots of yummy superfood salad meals.

NOTE: A variation on this recipe is to combine the regular mix with the dairy-free version. To do so, use ½ cup ground sesame and ½ cup grated Parmesan. Salads are delicious with the deep, delightful flavor of sesame.

DF (IF USING SESAME SEEDS IN PLACE OF PARMESAN CHEESE)

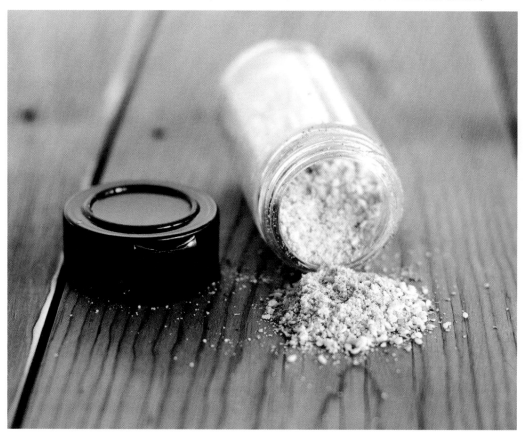

trimquik

½ cup Gentle Sweet

½ cup unsweetened cocoa powder

½ cup Pristine Whey Protein, or ¼ cup whey protein and ¼ cup Integral Collagen

¼ teaspoon Mineral Salt

Why buy NesQuik when you can enjoy TrimQuik? Now you can whip up protein-rich chocolate milk anytime you want in a flash. It's fabulous mixed with unsweetened almond or cashew milk. If you have growing children without weight issues, they can enjoy this with regular milk (raw whole milk being the most optimum for them).

1. Place all the ingredients in a blender and blend until smooth. Store in an airtight container in your cupboard.

SERVING IDEA: For easy chocolate milk, combine 2½ to 3 tablespoons TrimQuik with 1 large glass of milk in a blender, and spin until smooth and frothy. If you don't want to blend, put the TrimQuik in a glass with 2 tablespoons milk, stir well until blended to a paste, then add the rest of the milk, stirring again until smooth.

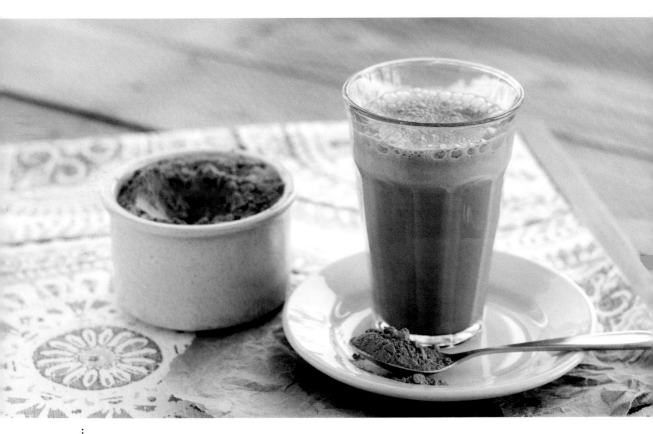

Carcasses and mixed bones from 3 Super Prepared Roasted Chickens (page 168), or approximately 2 pounds bones

2 tablespoons apple cider vinegar

2½ quarts cold water

OPTIONAL VEGGIES

1 medium onion, chopped in half (with skin)

1 garlic bulb, cut in half (with peel)

2 celery stalks, roughly chopped (with leaves)

1 large carrot, roughly chopped (with ends, unpeeled)

OPTIONAL HERBS

1 bay leaf

½ bunch fresh parsley

1 or 2 sprigs fresh thyme, or 3 to 4 fresh sage leaves

SERENE CHATS: *Hardly any work . . . cheap as dirt . . . better than any expensive health food supplement! All you need is leftover bones, water, and an old crockpot from a garage sale. Let the stock start a flowin'!*

It takes two big roasting chickens or three fryers to get roughly 2 pounds of bones, which is what you'll need to make this stock. This is without any meat attached. I know there are many recipes out there for stocks using bones with some meat on them, but I never have that option because there's never a morsel of meat left on the bone in my house. If you are using turkey, venison, or beef marrow bones, just use the same poundage recommendation. Don't stress about exact ounces—just get it somewhere in the ballpark. Another thing not to stress about are the veggies and herbs—just use what you have.

1. Place the bones in a large crockpot along with the vinegar and water. Add the veggies and herbs, and let sit for 30 minutes so the vinegar can begin pulling the goodness from the bones. (This is not a huge deal; if you start your stock at night before you go to bed and don't want to wait, just omit this step.)

2. Set the cooker on low and cook for 12 to 24 hours.

3. The next day, strain the stock in a colander. Put the stock in the refrigerator to allow the fat to rise and solidify on the top (see Note). Skim the fat (save it in zippered bags in the fridge or freezer for gravies and for flavoring **S** meals). Separate the stock into cup-size portions and freeze in zippies for future use.

NOTE: There is a gadget called a grease separator. This cup device catches and separates the grease from the stock immediately, so you don't have to deal with the cooling step.

NSI DF

drive thru sue bone stock

3 rotisserie chicken carcasses

2½ quarts cold water

2 tablespoons apple cider vinegar

1 medium carrot, broken in half

1 celery stalk, broken in half

1 medium onion, sliced in half
  (with skin)

PEARL CHATS: I mentioned to Serene that I'd never make stock because the process seems so complicated and laborious, and I just don't have time for all that. She looked at me in horror, "What Pearl???!!!! You mean you can't put your rotisserie chicken bones in your crockpot with a carrot and celery stick snapped in half???!!! What's wrong with you???!!!" I guess I needed a bit of my sister's tough love. It really is almost that simple. My fears were unfounded.

So my fellow Drive Thru Sue's, what are you waiting for? Shock yourself, your friends, and your family, and bring gourmet and homespun nutrition to your kitchen with this stripped-down to stupid-simple stock recipe! If you are single or have a small family, buy 1 chicken at a time and save the carcasses in bags in the freezer until you have enough, or save the bones from chicken legs and drums until you get 2 pounds.

1. Put all the ingredients in a crockpot and set it to low. Do it before bed and go to sleep, or do it in the morning and enjoy your day. Forget about it for 12 to 24 hours.

2. Strain your stock through a colander. Chill the stock in the fridge so the fat rises to the top.

3. Scrape off the fat and throw it away (although Serene would rather you freeze it in ice cube trays and use it for yummy meaty flavorings in **S** recipes, like gravies or frying up onions, and so on, but if that sounds like a lot of work, ignore Serene).

4. Separate the stock into cup-size portions and freeze in zippies for future use. Of course you will want to leave some in the fridge for this week.

NSI DF

appendix
THE MEAL RECAP

THE SATISFYING (S) MEAL

1. More fat, less carbs (anchored with protein)
2. Keep grains, sweet potatoes, and most fruits away from **S** meals

Build an S Meal
- Choose your protein (lean or fatty meat or fish, whole eggs, and egg whites).
- Add fats as desired.
- Add optional Fuel Pull foods like non-starchy veggies, berries, and cultured dairy.

TIPS
- Good fats can also include egg yolks, butter, red meat, coconut oil, and red palm oil, in addition to extra-virgin olive oil, nuts, and avocados.
- Non-starchy veggies can be any vegetable that is not a root vegetable (such as potato, sweet potato, or carrot) or corn.
- Nuts are also allowed in moderation.

S-Friendly Meats: All meats and fish, both fatty or lean (grass-fed is best but not mandatory)
S-Friendly Eggs: Whole eggs and egg whites

S-Friendly Dairy: Heavy cream; half-and-half; butter; all cheeses; sour cream; double-fermented kefir; both full-fat and reduced-fat forms of cottage cheese, ricotta cheese, feta cheese, and paneer; plain Greek yogurt, both 0% (stick to half cup as dessert or full cup for main protein) and full-fat; Laughing Cow Creamy Light Swiss cheese wedges (for non-purists)

S-Friendly Veggies: All non-starchy veggies. Don't go overboard with tomatoes, onions, peas, butternut squash, and acorn squash. Small amounts of carrots can squeeze in here and there.

S-Friendly Fruit: Up to 1 cup of all kinds of berries (except blueberries—keep those to ½ cup); lemons and limes

S-Friendly Nuts and Seeds: Raw or roasted seeds or nuts in moderation, nut butters without sugar in moderation, nut and seed flours in moderation

S-Friendly Condiments: Most cold-pressed oils; mayo; mustard; horseradish sauce; vinegar; salad dressings with 2 grams of carbs or less; olives; nutritional yeast; all broth and stock prepared without sugar, spices, and seasonings; unsweetened cocoa powders; sugar-free ketchup; sugar-free hot sauce

S-Friendly Grains and Beans: Keep these foods away from your **S** meals, with the exception of very small garnish amounts to be used occasionally.

S-Friendly Healthy Specialty Items: Pristine Whey Protein Powder (www.trimhealthy mama.com); Integral Collagen (www.trimhealthymama.com); Just Gelatin (www.trim healthymama.com); Trim Healthy Mama Baking Blend (www.trimhealthymama .com); Pressed Peanut Flour (www.trimhealthymama.com); Gluccie (www.trim healthymama.com); plan-approved sweeteners (www.trimhealthymama.com); Not Naughty Noodles or Not Naughty Rice (www.trimhealthymama.com); stevia-sweetened chocolate or a square or two of 85% dark chocolate, 100% cacao baker's chocolate; unsweetened nut milks such as almond, cashew, coconut, or flaxseed

S-Friendly "Personal Choice" Items: Joseph's low-carb pita or lavash bread, low-carb tortillas, fat-free Reddi-wip, Laughing Cow Creamy Light Swiss cheese wedges, Dreamfields pasta (limit to once a week)

THE ENERGIZING (E) MEAL

1. More healthy carbs, less fat (anchored with protein)

2. Your carbs include fruit, sweet potatoes, beans/legumes, and gentle whole grains like oatmeal or quinoa.

Build an E Meal

• Choose your lean protein.

• Add your carb (fruit, gentle whole grains, beans/legumes, or sweet potatoes).

- Add minimal fat (roughly 1 teaspoon); nuts and seeds are only used in garnish amounts.
- Add optional Fuel Pull foods like non-starchy veggies and berries and optional lean dairy.

TIPS
- Keep carbs to palm-size portions.
- MCT oil has the lowest amount of calories, so occasionally you can use 2 teaspoons with your **E** meal.
- Don't make corn your go-to grain.

E-Friendly Meat: All lean meats, chicken breast, tuna packed in water, salmon (look for less than 5 grams of fat), all other fish (not fried), venison, turkey breast, lean ground turkey or chicken (96% to 99% lean), lean deli meats (natural brands are best), ground meats with higher fat levels can be browned, drained, then rinsed well with hot water and used in **E** meals in up to 4-ounce portions

E-Friendly Egg Sources: Egg whites

E-Friendly Dairy: 0% plain Greek yogurt, low-fat or nonfat regular plain yogurt, plain low-fat or nonfat kefir, 1% cottage cheese (2% should be fine for purists who cannot find a suitable 1%), low-fat ricotta cheese (up to ¼ cup), skim mozzarella cheese (in small amounts), reduced-fat or 2% hard cheeses (small sprinkles only)

E-Friendly Grains: Brown rice (up to ¾ cup cooked serving); quinoa (up to ¾ cup cooked serving); whole barley (up to ¾ cup cooked serving); farro (up to ¾ cup cooked serving); oatmeal (up to 1¼ cups cooked serving); whole-grain bread in sprouted artisan sourdough, or dark rye form (2-piece servings); sprouted tortilla (1 large tortilla); sprouted whole-grain flours; sprouted whole-grain pasta; 4 Light Rye, Fiber, or Flax Seed Wasa crackers or 2 to 3 Multi-Grain, Hearty, Sourdough, or Whole Grain Wasa crackers (most Ryvita crackers are **E**-friendly, too); popcorn (4 to 5 cups of popped kernels spritzed with 1 teaspoon fat); baked blue corn chips

E-Friendly Fruit: All fruits in moderate quantities, e.g., 1 apple, 1 orange, 1 peach, 1 generous slice of cantaloupe; all berries in liberal quantities; use dried fruits very sparingly

E-Friendly Beans and Legumes: All beans and legumes including lentils and split peas—stick to 1 cup densely packed cooked, but more can be eaten when liquid is involved, i.e., chili or lentil soup

E-Friendly Veggies: All veggies except potatoes; enjoy sweet potatoes (1 medium) and carrots, both raw and cooked

E-Friendly Oils: 1 teaspoon oil (exception of occasional 2 teaspoons MCT oil)

E-Friendly Nuts: Limit nuts to garnish amounts or 1 teaspoon nut butters

E-Friendly Condiments: Mustard, horseradish sauce, hot sauce, low-fat dressings, mayo (up to 1 teaspoon), soy sauce/tamari/Bragg liquid aminos/Coconut aminos, all vinegars, all spices without sugar, unsweetened cocoa powder, nutritional yeast, all skimmed stock and broth (prepared without sugar)

E-Friendly Healthy Specialty Items: Pristine Whey Protein Powder (www.trimhealthy mama.com), Integral Collagen (www.trimhealthymama.com), Just Gelatin (www.trimhealthymama.com), Pressed Peanut Flour (www.trimhealthymama.com), Gluccie (www.trimhealthymama.com), plan-approved sweeteners (www.trim healthymama.com), Trim Healthy Mama Baking Blend (www.trimhealthy mama.com), Not Naughty Noodles and Not Naughty Rice (www.trimhealthy mama.com), unsweetened nut milks (avoid coconut milk for **E** meals)

E-Friendly "Personal Choice" Items: Joseph's low-carb pita or lavash bread (fruit, beans, or sweet potatoes will be needed for a proper **E** meal), low-carb tortillas (fruit, beans, or sweet potatoes will be needed for a proper **E** meal), fat-free Reddi-wip, Laughing Cow Creamy Light Swiss cheese wedges, Dreamfields pasta (limit to once a week; another carb source will be needed), light Progresso soups (another carb source will be needed)

FUEL PULLS

These are lighter foods that round out your plates and make your **S** and **E** meals complete (although they can be occasional full meals). They have low amounts of both fats and carbs.

Build a Fuel Pull Meal

• Choose your lean protein; limit meat to 3 to 4 ounces.
• Add minimal fat (roughly 1 teaspoon).
• Add other Fuel Pulls to your plate: generous non-starchy veggies, moderate berries, and optional lean dairy.

TIPS

• Limit nuts to garnish amounts or 1 teaspoon nut butters.
• Examples of non-starchy veggies: asparagus, broccoli, cabbage, cauliflower, cucumber, eggplant, mushrooms, jicama, tomatoes, yellow squash, zucchini, sugar snap peas, okra, onions, green onions, leeks, parsley, all leafy greens, radishes, spaghetti squash, pumpkin, chestnuts, baby Chinese corn
• Fuel Pulls shine as slimming snacks and desserts and help you avoid accidental Crossovers.

Fuel Pull–Friendly Meat: All lean meats in 3- to 4-ounce portions, chicken breast, tuna packed in water, salmon (look for less than 5 grams of fat), all other fish (not fried), venison, turkey breast, lean ground turkey or chicken (96% to 99% lean), lean deli meats (natural brands are best), ground meats with higher fat levels can be browned, drained, then rinsed well with hot water and used in FP meals in 3- to 4-ounce portions

Fuel Pull–Friendly Egg Sources: Egg whites

Fuel Pull–Friendly Dairy: 0% plain Greek yogurt, double-fermented nonfat kefir, 1% cottage cheese, low-fat ricotta cheese (up to ¼ cup), skim mozzarella cheese (in small amounts), reduced-fat 2% hard cheeses (small sprinkles only)

Fuel Pull–Friendly Veggies: All non-starchy veggies. Avoid potatoes, corn, sweet potatoes, and turnips.

Fuel Pull–Friendly Fruit: Up to 1 cup of all kinds of berries, lemons, and limes can be used, but keep blueberries to ½ cup.

Fuel Pull–Friendly Grains and Beans: 2 Light Rye, Fiber, or Flax Seed Wasa crackers or 2 Sesame Ryvita crackers; up to ¼ cup beans or oats occasionally (not in every Fuel Pull meal)

Fuel Pull–Friendly Oils: 1 teaspoon oil (exception of occasional 2 teaspoons MCT oil)

Fuel Pull–Friendly Condiments: Mustard; horseradish sauce; hot sauce; low-fat dressings; mayo (up to 1 teaspoon); soy sauce/tamari/Bragg liquid aminos/ Coconut aminos; all vinegars; all sugar-free spices; unsweetened cocoa powder; skimmed broth or stock prepared without sugar.

Fuel Pull–Friendly Healthy Specialty Items: Pristine Whey Protein Powder (www. trimhealthymama.com), Integral Collagen (www.trimhealthymama.com), Just Gelatin (www.trimhealthymama.com), Gluccie (www.trimhealthymama.com), plan-approved sweeteners (www.trimhealthymama.com), Trim Healthy Mama Baking Blend (www.trimhealthymama.com), Pressed Peanut Flour (www.trimhealthymama. com), Not Naughty Noodles and Not Naughty Rice (www.trimhealthymama.com), unsweetened nut milks (avoid coconut milk for FP)

Fuel Pull–Friendly "Personal Choice" Items: Joseph's low-carb pita or lavash bread, low-carb tortillas, fat-free Reddi-wip, Laughing Cow Creamy Light Swiss cheese wedges, light Progresso soups (avoid chowder versions)

CROSSOVERS (XO)

Crossovers merge the two fuels of fats and carbs for healthy tandem fueling. They keep to the **E** guidelines of carbs and add as many fats as desired.

Build a Crossover Meal
- Choose your protein (lean or fatty meat or fish, whole eggs and egg whites, or cultured dairy products).
- Add fats as desired (even if your protein source contains fat, other fats can be added).
- Add your carb in **E**-meal-safe amounts (fruit, gentle whole grains, beans/legumes, or sweet potatoes).

• Add optional Fuel Pull foods to your plate (non-starchy veggies, berries, and cultured dairy).

TIPS

1. People with extremely high metabolisms and healthy growing children will do well with mostly Crossover meals.

2. Pregnant and nursing women, as well as Maintenance Mamas, will benefit from including some Crossover meals.

S HELPERS (SH)

Add a little carb to your **S** meal for pleasure's sake, but not enough that it becomes a Crossover.

TIP

People who may not be used to eating meals with lower amounts of carbs, or people who suffer with hypoglycemia, may at first need **S** Helpers to help their bodies gently adapt to the pure **S** meal.

Same Foods List as S Meals (with these additional options):
⅓ to ½ cup quinoa
¼ cup brown rice
⅓ to ½ cup oatmeal
⅓ to ½ cup beans or lentils
½ piece of fruit like an apple or orange
½ medium sweet potato
1 piece of whole-grain sprouted, dark rye, or artisan sourdough bread toast
½ sprouted wrap or tortilla

index

THE ALLISON AND BARRETT FAMILIES

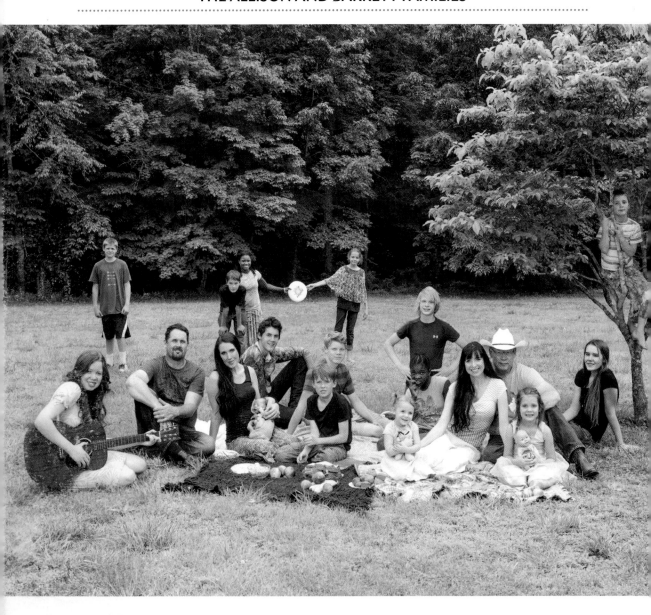

THE ALLISONS *(from oldest to youngest): Samuel Allison, Serene Allison, Arden Allison, Cherish Allison, Chalice Allison, Cedar Allison, Engedi Allison, Vision Allison, Shepherd Allison, Breeze Allison, Haven Allison, and Remnant Allison. (Serene and Sam also have three older children, two of whom are married, and three grandchildren.)*

THE BARRETTS *(from oldest to youngest): Charlie Barrett, Pearl Barrett, Meadow Barrett, Bowen Barrett, Rocky Barrett, Noble Barrett, and Autumn Barrett.*